Epidemiological Studies
A Practical Guide

Epidemiological Studies
A Practical Guide

THIRD EDITION

Alan J. Silman

Professor of Musculoskeletal Health, Botnar Research Institute,
Nuffield Department of Orthopaedics, Rheumatology and
Musculoskeletal Sciences, University of Oxford, UK

Gary J. Macfarlane

Professor of Epidemiology and Dean of Research (Life Sciences and
Medicine), University of Aberdeen, UK

Tatiana Macfarlane

Epidemiologist, Medicines Monitoring Unit, University of Dundee, UK;
Honorary Reader, Epidemiology Group, School of Medicine, Medical
Sciences and Nutrition, University of Aberdeen, UK

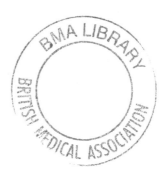

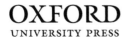

OXFORD
UNIVERSITY PRESS

Great Clarendon Street, Oxford, OX2 6DP,
United Kingdom

Oxford University Press is a department of the University of Oxford.
It furthers the University's objective of excellence in research, scholarship,
and education by publishing worldwide. Oxford is a registered trade mark of
Oxford University Press in the UK and in certain other countries

First Edition published in 1995
Second Edition published in 2002
Third Edition published in 2019

Impression: 1

Published in the United States of America by Oxford University Press
198 Madison Avenue, New York, NY 10016, United States of America

British Library Cataloguing in Publication Data
Data available

Library of Congress Control Number: 2018945620

ISBN 978-0-19-881472-6

Printed and bound by
CPI Group (UK) Ltd, Croydon, CR0 4YY

To our families, with love and gratitude for their support.

Preface

Epidemiological Studies: A Practical Guide was conceived as a practical handbook for those who wanted to conduct an epidemiological study and to provide the necessary toolkit from design to conduct and analysis of the results that emerged. The aim is that students and researchers could use this volume as a source of guidance for the necessary steps that would need to be undertaken to complete a study from 'start to finish'.

There are many excellent texts on the basis of epidemiology, the concepts behind the approach to studying diseases and their risk factors in populations, and the challenges and limitations of the results that emerge. From an academic perspective, such insights are important to understand and question the nature of what emerges from epidemiological investigations.

This volume is different. It focuses on the challenges of epidemiological data collection and allows the reader to conduct a study in confidence. This includes practical but highly relevant topics such as how to choose the right population to study, how to maximize participation and retention, and how to frame questions so subjects will provide the information required from the bedrock of the material presented. Whereas there are many software packages available for epidemiological data analysis, success in analysis is predicated on ensuring that the data are checked for quality and presented in appropriate formats.

Since the second edition published in 2002, much has changed in terms of the epidemiological thinking that underpins study design and conduct, the nature of information technology, and the growing 'digital world' that has transformed the possibilities for population data gathering. Equally important are the changes in Western societies that, on the one hand, expect that data from individuals and populations are maximally exploited, while on the other hand, have increased concerns about personal confidentiality and the potential misuse of large data sets.

In light of these changes, much of the material in this edition is either completely new or has been subject to considerable revision. We have now included consideration of modern study designs, such as case-crossover and case–cohort studies. Although migrant and ecological studies are now less commonly encountered in practice, it remains important to understand them and these are still covered. In addition, although it is open to debate whether intervention studies are part of epidemiology, randomized controlled trials are undoubtedly one way to study aetiology and we have thus included consideration of intervention trials in this edition.

Analysis of secondary data, with a specific focus on exploiting routine health and other data sources, mining disease registers, and linking with health records as well as material from biobanks, has become a much more important approach for epidemiological research. The different challenges they present, in comparison to primary data collection, are considered. These latter topics have their own methodologies and concerns which are in many ways different from the traditional epidemiological data collection which underpins much of this book.

With the increasing numbers of studies being conducted, there is increasing understanding that it is not the results of an individual study (conducted in one setting with a particular design and possible biases) which matters, but the coherence of evidence across all studies. Two new chapters, one on systematic reviews (which *summarize* the totality of evidence), and the other on meta-analysis (which *quantifies* the combined effect) have thus been added. There is also an increasing focus on the implications of results (i.e. what do they mean in terms of how we intervene to either prevent the onset or improve the outcome of a condition). Key to this is an understanding of whether an observed association is causal or not, and this is newly considered in this edition.

This edition also reflects the new digital world covering such aspects as the use of electronic and mobile technology to collect data, together with the changing legal constraints and ethical issues in collecting and storing personal data. The book still retains the simple approaches to calculation of the main measures of epidemiological concern. However, we take account of the greater availability and range of software to undertake statistical analysis, allowing more sophisticated analysis.

In most chapters we have now added a 'Further reading' section to allow readers, if desired, to explore specific topics in further detail and which often provides examples of the issues discussed.

Acknowledgements

The authors acknowledge the help of Jacqui Oliver in preparing the manuscript for submission and of Ruth Silman for detailed proof reading.

Contents

List of Abbreviations *xiii*

Biography *xv*

Part A **Introduction**

1 Scope of epidemiological enquiry and overview of main problem areas *3*

Part B **Measuring the occurrence of disease**

2 Which measure of disease occurrence? *13*

3 Comparing rates between and within populations *19*

4 Studies of disease occurrence: The population *28*

5 Studies of disease occurrence: Assessing disease status in study populations *34*

Part C **Studying associations between exposures and disease**

6 Which type of epidemiological study? *47*

7 Quantifying the association between exposures and diseases: Which measure? *63*

Part D **Selection of populations and samples to study in studies of disease aetiology**

8 Studies of disease causation *71*

9 Use of secondary data *90*

Part E **Information from epidemiological studies**

10 Collecting information *101*

11 Obtaining valid information *108*

12 Repeatability *114*

13 Participation in epidemiology studies *121*

14 Feasibility and pilot studies *136*

Part F **Analysis and interpretation of epidemiological data**

15 Preparation of collected primary data for statistical analysis *145*

16 Introductory data analysis: Descriptive epidemiology *155*

17 Introductory data analysis: Analytical epidemiology *168*

18 Confounding *192*

19 Bias *202*

20 Association or causation *211*

Part G Coherence of evidence across studies

21 Reviews of evidence *221*

22 Meta-analysis *233*

Part H Other practical issues

23 Ethical issues in epidemiology *249*

24 The costs of an epidemiological study *260*

Index *271*

List of Abbreviations

BMI	body mass index
CEBM	Centre for Evidence-Based Medicine
CPRD	Clinical Practice Research Datalink
CRD	Centre for Reviews and Dissemination
DARE	Database of Abstracts of Reviews of Effects
DASR	directly age-standardized rate
EMA	European Medicines Agency
EQUATOR	Enhancing the QUAlity and Transparency of health Research
EVIPNet	Evidence-Informed Policy Network
FDA	Food and Drug Administration
GLOBOCAN	Global Cancer Incidence, Mortality and Prevalence
GPRD	General Practice Research Database
HBPM	home blood pressure monitoring
HMO	health maintenance organization
IARC	International Agency for Research on Cancer
ICTRP	International Clinical Trials Registry Platform
IPD	individual patient data
IQR	Interquartile Range
IR	Incidence Rate
MeSH	medical subject headings
MI	myocardial infarction
NHANES	National Health and Nutritional Examination Surveys
NICE	National Institute for Health and Care Excellence
NHS	National Health Service
NOS	Newcastle-Ottawa Scale
OA	osteoarthritis
OCEBM	Oxford Centre for Evidence-Based Medicine
OCP	oral contraceptive pill
OHR	occupational hygiene review
PRISMA	Preferred Reporting Items for Systematic Review and Meta Analysis
RA	rheumatoid arthritis
ROC	receiver operating characteristic
SE	standard error
SIGN	Scottish Intercollegiate Guidelines Network
SIR	standardized incidence ratio
SMR	standardized mortality ratio
SNP	single nucleotide polymorphism
SPR	standardized prevalence ratio
SRDR	Systematic Review Data Repository
STROBE	Strengthening the Reporting of Observational Studies in Epidemiology
URTI	upper respiratory tract infection
UTI	urinary tract infection

Biography

Alan J. Silman is an epidemiologist and rheumatologist. He was Director of Arthritis Research UK's Epidemiology Unit at the University of Manchester from 1988 to 2006, before moving on to become Arthritis Research UK's first Medical Director from 2007 to 2014. Since 2015 he has been Professor of Musculoskeletal Health at the University of Oxford, working in the fields of comorbidity and big data.

Gary J. Macfarlane trained in statistics and then medicine at the University of Glasgow before undertaking a PhD in epidemiology at the University of Bristol. He was a cancer epidemiologist at the European Institute of Oncology, Milan, held the Chair in Epidemiology at the University of Manchester, and currently holds the same position at the University of Aberdeen (as well as being a Consultant in the Department of Public Health at NHS Grampian) with a research focus on musculoskeletal conditions.

Tatiana Macfarlane trained in mathematics at the Lomonosov Moscow State University. She was a cancer epidemiologist at the Blokhin Cancer Research Centre in Moscow, the International Agency for Research on Cancer in Lyons, and the European Institute of Oncology in Milan. She undertook a PhD in epidemiology at the University of Manchester where she was Lecturer, then Senior Lecturer. She was a Reader in Epidemiology at the University of Aberdeen and is currently an epidemiologist at the University of Dundee.

Part A

Introduction

Chapter 1

Scope of epidemiological enquiry and overview of main problem areas

1.1 Introduction

Epidemiology is classically defined as the study of the distribution of disease and its determinants in human populations. In other words, it provides the answers to questions on how many people have a disease, how this varies by time and place, and what specific factors put individuals at risk. The 'epidemiology' section in a medical textbook chapter on a particular disease will provide data on these aspects. There is an alternative and broader view of epidemiology, which is that it is a tool for studying diseases as they occur in human populations. The focus can also be on diagnosis, outcome, and the results of interventions, as well as on causes. This broader definition allows a substantially greater scope for the kinds of question that can be addressed both by those studying the health of populations and by those whose main focus is the study of disease in patient groups.

1.2 Scope of epidemiological research

The list in Table 1.1 represents the vast array of topics that epidemiologists would consider as relevant to their discipline.

In practice, epidemiological methods are appropriate for applying outside disease to other human traits and behaviours, for example, in the fields of education, social care, and criminology. There are also subspecialties within epidemiology typically based on specific expertise related to particular exposures (Table 1.2).[1]

1.3 Applications of epidemiology

1.3.1 Disease definition

Most diseases lack a clear diagnostic test that totally discriminates between disease and normality, although infectious disease and trauma are two obvious exceptions. Most often the diagnosis is based on clinical opinion, with the latter based on experience, prejudice, or arbitrary rules. In the absence of a standardized definition of disease, results from aetiological, prognostic, or therapeutic studies cannot be directly compared. The development of disease criteria is a separate topic in itself which requires a careful epidemiological study of the occurrence of specific features in cases determined by a notional gold standard, such as the expert clinician's diagnosis. These features are then compared with those from an appropriate group of non-cases and the level of agreement evaluated. Similar approaches apply to grading severity of a disease. Clinical trials in particular need to ensure like is compared with like, and 'clinician diagnostic opinion' is rarely sufficient.

Table 1.1 Questions relevant for epidemiological enquiry

Disease definition	What characteristics or combination of characteristics best discriminate an affected (including grade of severity) from an unaffected individual?
Disease occurrence	What is the rate of development of new cases in a population?
	What is the proportion of current disease within a population?
	What are the influences of age, sex, time, and geography on the points above?
Disease causation	What are the risk factors for disease development and what are their relative strengths with respect to an individual and a population?
Disease outcome	What is the outcome following disease onset and what are the risk factors, including their relative strengths, for a poor outcome?
Disease management	What is the relative effectiveness of proposed therapeutic interventions? (Included within this are health service research questions related to the relative effectiveness of proposed health service delivery options.)
Disease prevention	What is the relative effectiveness of proposed preventive strategies including screening?

Example 1.i

Clinical trials in the field of mental health rely on the use of an agreed list of categories and criteria: The American Psychiatric Association's Diagnostic and Statistical Manual (DSM-5) of mental disorders that in the latest version, for example, discriminate between Asperger's syndrome and more severe forms of autism spectrum disorder and suggest how severity should be classified.

Table 1.2 Subspecialty areas in chronic disease epidemiology

Subspecialty	Specific areas of expertise
Genetic epidemiology	Understanding how inheritance within families influences risk
	How populations change in their genetic structure
	Handling data sets with up to one million variables
Pharmaco-epidemiology	Availability and limitations of data on exposure to drugs, dosage, and adherence
	Complexities of separating out the effects of a drug from the indications it was given for (methods also apply to other interventions such as surgical procedures, etc.)
Nutritional epidemiology	Methods of diet enquiry and patterns of diet intake in free-living populations
	Separating out effects of dietary components when they are strongly related to other components of diet
	Exposure assessment techniques
Occupational epidemiology	Methods of assessing occupational (and in a related field environmental toxins) exposure based on understanding of job demands and activities

1.3.2 **Disease occurrence**

This is the classical focus of epidemiological study and the available approaches to measure occurrence are discussed in Chapter 2. Data on occurrence are of interest in their own right, but are also relevant both to the clinician, in weighing up different diagnostic likelihoods in the face of the same evidence, and to those providing health services. A more detailed study will uncover differences in occurrence between sexes and across age groups, over time and between different geographical populations. Indeed, the age and sex effects on disease occurrence are normally so strong that it is absolutely fundamental to gather such data in order to compare disease occurrence both between populations and within the same population over time. These issues are discussed in Chapter 3. In addition, marked differences between occurrence in different population groups may provide aetiological clues for further enquiry. The approach used to assess disease occurrence may be extrapolated to assessing specific outcomes in a disease population.

Example 1.ii

A group of diabetologists wanted to undertake an epidemiological study to identify the number of persons with diabetic eye disease in a population of patients with diabetes.

1.3.3 **Disease causation**

Similarly, the use of epidemiology to unravel possible causative pathways is one of its most frequent roles. It is, however, too simplistic for most chronic diseases to restrict consideration of their influence on disease risk just as present or absent. It is the strength of any disease association with possible risk factor variables that is of more interest.

Example 1.iii

In planning a study on whether workers exposed to organic dusts were at increased risk of various lung diseases, the investigators aimed to discover: (i) whether or not there was an increased risk; (ii) the level of any increase for the major lung disorders considered; and (iii) how these risks compared with those from smoking in the same population.

1.3.4 **Risk and association**

It is appropriate, at this stage, to clarify the meaning of the terms 'risk' and 'association'. In common use, association indicates a relationship with no indication as to the underlying path. As an example, there is an association between an individual's height and his/her weight, although there are several possible paths: (i) the taller an individual the greater will be the weight; (ii) (unlikely) the heavier an individual the greater will be the height; or (iii) there are common factors (e.g. genetic) that influence both height and weight. By contrast, risk implies that the pathway is known (or worthy of investigation). Thus, in the previous example, the question can be addressed whether height is a risk factor for being overweight. In practice, epidemiological investigations aim to uncover associations that, using other information, may then be considered as risks.

1.3.5 **Disease outcome**

Investigations concerning the frequency and prediction of specific disease outcomes in patient populations may be considered as the clinical epidemiological parallels of studies of disease occurrence and causation in normal populations. Thus, the *population* epidemiologist may wish to ascertain the incidence of, and risk factors for, angina in a stated population; whereas the *clinical* epidemiologist may wish to ascertain the incidence of, and risk factors for, subsequent myocardial infarction and sudden death in patients with angina. The methodological concepts, however, are identical.

1.3.6 Disease management and disease prevention

Investigating the relationship between a predictor and disease onset has its parallel with that of a predictor and disease outcome as mentioned earlier. Where the predictor is an external presumed beneficial intervention then epidemiological method can be used to determine the value (and/or harms) of such interventions. Such studies can be 'observational' insofar as they examine the outcomes of treatments as they are used and prescribed with all the biases that will be discussed. Indeed, the use of such natural experiments can provide key insights into the benefits of a proposed prevention strategy.

Example 1.iv

The effectiveness of adding fluoride to drinking water to prevent dental caries was supported by comparing the prevalence of dental decay in children living in areas with and without fluoridation. It would have been difficult to have undertaken a randomized trial on this topic.

Alternatively, a clinical trial can be established as a particular type of epidemiological study to compare the effectiveness of two or more particular therapeutic interventions. Epidemiologically, the clinical trial can be considered as an experimental study where the investigator has intervened to alter the 'exposure' (e.g. management), in order to measure the effect on disease occurrence or outcome. The term 'intervention study' describes this broad activity. The intervention trial concepts can be applied to health service delivery to answer questions such as whether policy A is likely to be more effective than policy B in reducing waiting lists. Health service research questions such as this require the same rigorous epidemiological approach. In most developed countries with increasing economic pressure to contain health service costs, there is considerable demand (and funding) for epidemiologists to apply their expertise in this area. An extension of this is the use of the intervention trial to assess the effectiveness of a population-wide preventive strategy. Population-based primary prevention trials can indeed be considered as clinical trials on a massive scale. Screening for preclinical disease is a widely practised preventive strategy and the evaluation of screening as a tool for reducing morbidity/mortality can be considered under the same heading.

1.3.7 Pooling results from several studies

Given all the difficulties in undertaking studies in human populations it is not surprising that all kinds of epidemiological studies, addressing the same question, might emerge with quite different results. This could be due to chance, differences in study populations, or differences in measures of exposure and disease. Pooling information across all studies which have examined an exposure-disease relationship allows you to assess the overall evidence and its consistency. There is an epidemiological skill in assessing information that seems to be producing conflicting results as well as statistical approaches to pool the data using meta-analysis techniques. Results which are consistent across studies conducted in different geographical areas, different study populations, study designs and using alternative ways of measuring exposure and disease, provide more compelling evidence that an association exists. These are discussed at length in Chapters 21 and 22.

1.4 **What are the major issues in conducting epidemiological research?**

The greatest challenge in epidemiology is the large number of methodological issues that could affect the results and their interpretation. The concerns stem in large from the basic tenet that epidemiology deals with 'free living', and frequently healthy, human populations. The consequences of this are: (i) methods of study have to be simple and non-invasive; (ii) subjects, as compared with laboratory animals, may choose to participate or not, or even withdraw from participation during a study; and (iii) obtaining accurate information is often a balance between the ideal and the practical. In addition, since many important diseases are relatively rare, studies often need to be large in scope, long in duration, or both, with consequences both for the resources required and for the patience and longevity of the investigator.

There are a substantial number of problems to be considered in undertaking any epidemiological study. These are listed in Table 1.3, which provides the framework for the rest of the volume, and are discussed in outline next.

1.4.1 **Study design**

The first demand is to clearly frame and thereafter focus on the specific questions posed. In Chapters 4 and 5, the various options for studies of disease occurrence and causation are outlined. A decision must be made about the choice of study design that can best answer the question posed, taking into account the often-conflicting demands of scientific validity and practicality.

1.4.2 **Population selection**

The subjects to be studied must be defined both in terms of the group(s) from which they are to be selected and, in selecting individuals, the inclusion and exclusion rules. Specific problems arise in comparative studies when it is necessary to recruit two or more groups based on their disease or on their risk factor status. Problems in population selection are one of the major reasons for a study's

Table 1.3 Major problem areas for epidemiological research

Study design	What is the question posed—what type of study can best answer the question and is most practicable?
Population selection	Who should be studied? How many should be studied?
Information gathering	How should the information be obtained? Is the information obtained correct? Is the method used to obtain the information consistent?
Analysis	How should the data gathered be prepared for analysis? What are the appropriate analytical methods?
Interpretation of results	Can any associations observed be explained by confounding? Are the results explained by bias? Are the results generalizable?
Logistics	Is the research ethical? Is the research affordable?

conclusions being invalid. A specific difficulty is that of sample size. Cost, time, or other practical considerations may limit the availability of subjects for study. A scientific approach to sample size estimation is given for the different study design options later on in the book (Chapter 8). Non-response or loss to follow-up can reduce the number of subjects available for analysis and an adequately large study at the onset may prove too small by the end.

1.4.3 Information quality

This major issue relates to the quality of the data obtained (Chapters 11 and 12). There is a particular problem when the approach requires a subject to recall past symptoms or exposures. The most appropriate method for obtaining information must be selected. This might, for example, be a choice between interview and self-administered questionnaire. Other sources of information such as data collected prior to the study, often for another purpose such as the medical record, may be available. The classical approach is to consider the quality of information obtained under the headings of: (i) *validity* (i.e. does the measurement give the true answer), and (ii) *repeatability* (i.e. is the same answer obtained from the same person when repeated measures are made?).

1.4.4 Data handling and analysis

The time spent on this activity is frequently longer than that spent on the data collection itself. In particular, there is a need to ensure that the data set used for analysis is complete with minimal missing data and free of errors. Once the quality of the data set is assured then it is necessary to choose the appropriate method(s) of analysis. These aspects are discussed in detail in Chapters 15–17.

1.4.5 Interpreting the results

The first issue is that of confounding (see Chapter 18). Put simply, it is often difficult in human populations to distinguish between attributes that frequently occur together. Thus, in studies to determine the effect of cigarette smoking on the risk for a particular disease, a positive association may be observed that does not relate to the direct impact of smoking on risk, but reflects the joint association between a *confounder*, such as alcohol consumption, which is linked to both cigarette smoking and the disease under study. One of the major advances in the practice of epidemiology in the past decade has been the simultaneous development of user-friendly software and accessible hardware that permit the analysis of the impact of one or more potential confounders in a way that manual methods of statistical analysis could not achieve.

The second issue is whether the results obtained could be explained by bias (see Chapter 19), either in the selection of subjects, in the subjects who chose to participate, or in the gathering of information.

In general, one issue is how far an epidemiological study, however robust the findings from its own methods, can be taken to imply a causative relationship. This is a topic of increasing interest and discussed in greater length in Chapter 20.

The third issue is whether the results are generalizable.

Example 1.v

A study has been conducted among university students examining the relationship between coffee consumption and migraine headaches. Students with migraine were more than twice as likely to consume, on average, more than two cups of coffee per day. Though this might be true for migraine in students, the more relevant scientific question is whether this association is generalizable to a wider population?

1.4.6 **Logistical issues**

Two important areas to be addressed are those of ethics and cost (Chapters 23 and 24). Studying free-living individuals imposes ethical constraints on the investigators, and the need for cost containment is self-evident. Indeed, these issues must be considered early on, as they are likely to influence the final study design.

Note

1. There is a specific set of expertise required in identifying causes of an outbreak (e.g. of an infectious disease) but these are not considered specifically in this book.

Part B

Measuring the occurrence of disease

Chapter 2

Which measure of disease occurrence?

2.1 Introduction

Measuring disease occurrence is the basic activity of epidemiology, and the following section provides the background to choosing the most appropriate measure(s) of disease occurrence for the aims of the study. The term 'disease' can also be taken in this context to describe any personal attribute. Thus, the concepts described apply equally well to assessing the occurrence of a symptom (such as fatigue), the development of a particular disability, or the frequency of a medical intervention such as hip replacement in a population. The first step is to distinguish between incidence and prevalence. These two terms are frequently confused and a simple distinction is to consider incidence as measuring disease *onsets* and prevalence as measuring disease *states*.

2.2 Incidence

The *incidence* of a disease is the number of new onsets in a defined population within a specified period of time. It will be noted that this measure does not make any reference to the size of population studied and therefore to compare the incidence between a large city and a small village does not make sense. To overcome this problem, a denominator is required and two measures— the *incidence proportion* (also called *risk* or *cumulative incidence*) and the *incidence rate* can be calculated.

Incidence proportion is the proportion of a population (free of the disease of interest at the start of study) that develop the disease under study during follow-up.

$$\text{Incidence proportion} = \frac{\text{Number of new study disease onsets during follow-up}}{\text{Total population free of study disease at start of study}}$$

This proportion is often multiplied by 100 and expressed as a percentage.

The incidence rate uses the same numerator (number of new disease onsets) but the denominator is the sum of the time at risk of developing the disease under study across each individual subject giving a measure of person–time at risk, most commonly express as person-years at risk. At its simplest, if two disease-free individuals are observed, one for three years and the other for five years, and both remain disease-free then they have contributed eight person-years at risk of developing the disease under study.

$$\text{Incidence rate} = \frac{\text{Number of new study disease onsets during follow-up}}{\text{Total person-years at risk of developing study disease}}$$

For ease of interpretation, this is usually multiplied by a constant (e.g. 1,000 or 10,000).

It should be noted that mortality is a special case of incidence where death is the 'disease onset' being studied. Thus (in an analogous fashion to incidence rate) mortality rate is defined as:

$$\text{Mortality rate} = \frac{\text{Number of deaths during follow-up}}{\text{Total person-years of observation}\left(\text{at risk of dying}\right)}$$

Example 2.i

A study recruited 1,000 adults aged 60–69 years in good musculoskeletal health. When recontacted five years later, 43 had undergone a hip replacement operation.
    Incidence = 32 relevant 'events' in the follow-up period

$$\text{Incidence proportion} = \frac{43}{1,000} = \frac{\text{Events in follow-up period}}{\text{Number in population}}$$

$$= 0.043$$
$$= 4.3\%$$

Therefore, the incidence proportion was 0.043 (i.e. 4.3% of the study population had a hip replacement during the follow-up period).

Example 2.ii

In a study of the incidence of upper respiratory tract infection (URTI) at a local school during the course of a year, there were 743 children registered at some point during the school year. However, since some children joined/left during the school year, the total person-years of follow-up was only 695 person-years. There were 32 children who had a new URTI during the school year.
    Incidence = 32 'relevant' events in follow-up period

$$\text{Incidence rate} = \frac{32}{695} = \frac{\text{Events in follow-up period}}{\text{Person-years at risk}}$$

$$= 0.046$$
$$= 46 \text{ per } 1,000 \text{ person-years at risk}$$

Since the measure is theoretically a measure of density of events, it is sometimes also referred to as incidence density.

2.2.1 Approaches to measuring incidence

There are several different approaches to measuring incidence. *First-ever incidence* is restricted to the inclusion of only those subjects who present with their first disease episode from a particular pathology during a particular time period. It might, however, be of greater concern to record all episodes, '*the episode incidence*', irrespective of whether it is the first occurrence or a recurrence.

In Example 2.ii, if one is interested in *first-ever incidence* during the study, then when a study subject is confirmed as having a URTI then they will afterwards contribute no further time to the denominator since they are no longer at risk of a first URTI. Thus, if a study subject develops a URTI after 0.5 years of follow-up, this will be the total time period 'at risk' they contribute to the denominator, since they are no longer 'at risk' of having a first URTI. In contrast if one is interested in *episode incidence*, then persons who had a URTI during follow-up would still contribute person-years of follow-up to the denominator, since they would remain at risk of developing further episodes.

Example 2.iii

To gain an idea of the age distribution of onset of coronary artery disease, the cardiovascular epidemiologist might wish to study the incidence of first myocardial infarction. By contrast, the public health physician might wish to know the episode incidence in order to provide an appropriate level of acute care facilities.

There is the assumption that it is always possible to distinguish between a recurrent episode of an existing pathological process and a new episode from a separate pathological process. This is frequently not the case.

Example 2.iv

An investigator considered the options for estimating the incidence of low back pain. The problem was that low back pain is associated with multiple episodes in a single individual during a lifetime, which might result from single or multiple causes. The decision was made to consider the proportion of adult males who experienced an episode of low back pain over a one-year period. This is the incidence proportion (or cumulative incidence). This is a risk rather than a rate and is expressed as a proportion.

A risk is the combined effect of rates operating over a specific time period. This approach is often used in follow-up studies to compare the subsequent development of a disease in groups determined by their exposure, particularly when outcome is only measured at defined time points and the timing of onset of the 'outcome' is difficult to accurately determine, such as for pain. It can be measured over a variety of periods (e.g. several years, an age range, or lifetime).

Cumulative incidence is also frequently used in communicating to a wider audience the population importance of a particular condition.

Example 2.v

Cumulative cancer incidence (risk) aged 0–84 years for males and females in Great Britain born in 1930 is 0.47 and 0.36, respectively. For persons born in 1980 we do not know the comparable figure, since this cohort has not yet reached 84 years of age.

The reader will appreciate from the definition given for cumulative incidence that it does not take account of all-cause mortality (i.e. the risk of dying from any cause). It is possible therefore for the cumulative incidence of a disease to increase, even though there has been no change to the underlying incidence rate. This will happen if there has been a decrease in all-cause mortality rates (i.e. more people remain alive for longer and therefore are at risk for getting the disease under study). More sophisticated techniques are therefore required to take account of such 'competing risks' (see 'Further reading').

Example 2.vi

In the investigation of an outbreak of gastroenteritis after a banquet, an investigator calculated the cumulative incidence, during the following one-week period, of developing infection in those who did and did not eat each of the particular foods available.

2.3 **Prevalence**

The prevalence of disease is the proportion of individuals in a population with a disease or other personal attribute. It is a *proportion* and not a *rate*, since there is no time element involved. It should therefore be referred to as *prevalence proportion*, although the erroneous term *prevalence rate* is frequently seen used. Prevalence is often expressed per multiple of the population (e.g. 1,000 or 10,000).

Example 2.vii

A questionnaire was distributed to the workforce of a large industrial company on a particular working day. Of the 1,534 workers, 178 reported headaches on the survey day.

$$\text{Prevalence} = \frac{178}{1,534}$$

$$= 0.12$$
$$= 12 \text{ per } 100 \text{ workers}$$

There are also several different approaches to measuring prevalence.

2.3.1 **Approaches to measuring prevalence**

Point prevalence records all those with a disease at a notional point in time. In reality the disease status of currently living individuals is assessed at varying points in time, but those who are positive are all assumed to be in the same disease state on 'prevalence day'. Thus, a point prevalence estimate should be in the form of: the proportion of the population with disease on, for example, 2 December 2016 is 35 per 1,000 of the population. Alternatively, a study may have posted out a questionnaire which asked respondents whether they had experienced 'flu-like' symptoms in the past 24 hours. It found that 9 per 100 population reported these symptoms. Note that in this case it is still an estimate of prevalence, even though not all individuals will have completed the questionnaire on the same day or time of day.

Period prevalence takes account of the common situation that diseases vary within an individual in their clinical manifestations and that an individual sufferer may not be *in state* at a single point in time. The most suitable approach is to describe the occurrence at any time within a defined *period*. Examples include migraine and sleep disturbance, reflecting the fact that within a nominated period an individual may experience these, but not necessarily at a single arbitrary point in time. What time period should be chosen when measuring period prevalence? There is no single answer to this, but the decision should be influenced by the period over which respondents can validly recall the condition of interest and also the pattern of natural history (e.g. does the condition of interest vary day to day or season to season?).

Example 2.viii

A population survey was used to measure the prevalence of mood disorder. Questionnaires were sent out by post and respondents were asked to answer mood questions with reference to the previous four weeks, and to provide details of the day when they completed the questionnaire. The sending out of questionnaires was staggered throughout the calendar year in order to determine whether the four-week prevalence of mood disorder varied throughout the year. The results were as follows:

Questionnaires completed:
October–March

$$\text{Four-week prevalence} = \frac{321}{2,765} = \frac{\text{cases}}{\text{population}}$$

$$= 0.12$$
$$= 12 \text{ per } 100 \text{ respondents}$$

April–September

$$\text{Four-week prevalence} = \frac{172}{2,934} = \frac{\text{cases}}{\text{population}}$$

$$= 0.06$$
$$= 6 \text{ per } 100 \text{ respondents}$$

The four-week prevalence (which could be called a one-month prevalence) in this study is double in the autumn/winter months compared to the spring/summer months.

2.4 **Choice of measure**

By implication, from the previous paragraphs, it is the nature of the disease itself that determines the appropriate choice of measure. A summary of the issues is given in Table 2.1. The choice of measure has important practical implications because the methodological approaches vary considerably (see Chapter 6). The table can only offer guidance and the decision is not always obvious. Knowledge of the natural history and variation of presentation of disease is important.

The key to the methods to be used is almost always the study aims and objectives. Unless these are clear, it will be difficult to know the appropriate study design to use.

Example 2.ix

For conditions such as severe mental disorder, the healthcare planner would need knowledge of point prevalence as a priority. By contrast, the perinatal epidemiologist would focus on the incidence during the first year of life.

Table 2.1 Appropriate measures of disease occurrence (*optimal measure shown first)

Disease characteristics	Examples	Appropriate measures*
A		
Clearly defined onset	Acute appendicitis	First-ever incidence
Single episode	Colon cancer	Incidence proportion
Terminated by death, spontaneous resolution, or therapy	Major trauma	
B		
Clearly defined onset	Myocardial infarction	Episode incidence
Possible multiple, but infrequent episodes	Influenza	Incidence proportion
Short duration	Fracture	
Episodes terminated by death, spontaneous resolution, or therapy		
C		
Clearly defined onset	Insulin-dependent diabetes	First-ever incidence
Chronic relatively stable disease state or requiring long-term therapy	Renal failure	Point prevalence
		Incidence proportion
D		
Clearly defined onset	Rheumatoid arthritis	First-ever incidence
Single or multiple episodes	Peptic ulcer	Incidence proportion
Variable duration		
E		
Ill-defined onset	Hypertension	Point prevalence
Chronic relatively stable disease state or requiring long-term therapy	Hip osteoarthritis	
	Deafness	
F		
Ill-defined onset	Asthma	Period prevalence
Multiple episodes with periods of disease absence	Migraine	Episode incidence

Further reading

Competing risks

Ahmad AS, Ormiston-Smith N, Sasieni PD (2015). Trends in the lifetime risk of developing cancer in Great Britain: comparison of risk for those born from 1930 to 1960. *Br J Cancer*, **112**(5), 943–47.

Andersen PK, Geskus RB, de Witte T, Putter H (2012). Competing risks in epidemiology: possibilities and pitfalls. *Int J Epidemiol*, **41**(3), 861–70.

Chapter 3

Comparing rates between and within populations

3.1 **Introduction**

The previous chapter has outlined types of rates and their measurement. For the public health specialist concerned with the provision of services, measurement of disease occurrence may be an end in itself. For the epidemiologist, however, measurement of rates will commonly be the beginning of a process whose aim is to understand the aetiology of a disease. In order to formulate hypotheses, the rate of a disease under study in a population may be compared with the rate in other populations, or in the same population at different time points. Those populations (or population groups) with particularly high or low rates can be identified and features of these populations determined in order to formulate hypotheses on the influence of disease to be tested in a formal epidemiological study. If the rates are increasing (or decreasing), the factors responsible for such a change need to be determined.

Whatever the comparison being made, either between populations, between subgroups of a larger population, or in one population over a period of time, it is important that comparisons are made on a like-for-like basis. As an example, increasing incidence rates of stroke within a single population may be a consequence of the population ageing or it may reflect a real increase in rates. If the rates of disease change within a population are found to be real, then further investigation of the pattern of change can also provide clues to the possible reasons.

Example 3.i

An epidemiologist compared the prevalence of a given disease in two districts of their health board. Both districts had the same population size (n = 6,100) but the prevalence was very different. There were 67 cases in District A (prevalence 11.0 per 1,000) and 145 cases in District B (prevalence 23.8 per 1,000).

They then investigated the difference further by documenting the disease prevalence by age group in the two districts.

Looking at Table 3.1 next, what is noticeable?

The first observation is that despite the fact that all-ages prevalence is double in District B, when one looks at age-specific prevalence, it is lower in District B in every age group. How can these apparently contradictory observations be explained?

There are two reasons for these observations. Firstly, age is strongly related to the disease under study. In both districts, prevalence increases with older age. Secondly, there is a large difference in age distribution between the two districts. District B has a much greater proportion of people in older age groups. Therefore, although District B has lower prevalence at each age group, there are more older people among whom the disease is more common and thus they have a higher number of persons with the disease overall.

This is an example of *confounding*, an important concept in epidemiology which is discussed in more detail in Chapter 18. A relationship between an 'exposure' (here it is area of residence) and a disease under study is confounded if the potential confounder is a risk factor for the disease and its distribution varies accordingly to levels of the exposure under study. Here age is a risk factor

Table 3.1 A comparison between the prevalence of a given disease in two districts

Age group (years)	District A			District B		
	Population	Persons with disease (n)	Prevalence per 1,000	Population	Persons with disease (n)	Prevalence per 1,000
All ages	6,100	67	11.0	6,100	145	23.8
0–14	500	2	4	400	1	2.5
15–29	2,000	8	4	300	1	3.3
30–44	2,000	12	6	1,000	5	5
45–60	1,000	10	10	2,000	18	9
61–74	500	20	40	2,000	70	35
75+	100	15	150	400	50	125

for the disease and age does vary between the two districts and thus it does satisfy the criteria to be a confounder in this relationship.

Therefore, disease occurrence (incidence or prevalence) should be compared between populations taking account of such confounding variables; standardization is one way to do this.

3.2 Standardization

Standardization is one procedure for the control of variables that may confound an observed relationship, and is discussed in Chapter 18 with information provided on the specific calculations involved. In this section, the general approach will be covered considering age, the most common such factor on which to standardize when comparing rates between populations (since such data is usually readily available). The principles outlined can apply to other factors such as gender and social class, and also when comparing rates within the same population over time.

There are two methods of standardization: direct and indirect. They are equally applicable to incidence rates and prevalence proportions. See Section 16.4 for information on calculations.

3.2.1 Direct standardization

Using Example 3.i, disease prevalence has been measured in two districts A and B, but as just noted disease prevalence is strongly related to age and the age structure is markedly different in the two districts. The rates in the two districts need to be compared taking account of the different age structure. (Note: this example relates to age but could equally apply to any other factors on which data is available and which potentially confounds a relationship. Other examples are gender and socioeconomic status.)

Direct standardization (for age) calculates what the overall disease rate would have been in a population if it had a specified structure with respect to the potentially confounding variable (i.e. in this case, age structure). This specified age structure is referred to as the 'standard population'. The standard population could be one of the populations considered within a study (e.g. District A); it could be a third population (e.g. the age structure of the region in which Districts A and B are located), or it could be a real or imaginary third population.

Does it matter which population is chosen as the standard? The role of the 'standard population' is to provide weightings for age-specific rates in study populations based on the proportion of the standard population which is in each age group. Therefore if a standard population with a young age structure is chosen then greater weight will be given in the process of 'standardization' of each study population to rates at young ages. In terms of interpretation it makes sense to choose a standard population with an age structure that is close to the populations being compared. For example, if cancer incidence rates are being compared across several European countries, a suitable standard population could be the age structure of all European populations together. It is also desirable to use a population structure to which other investigators have access, thus further facilitating comparison of rates. One such standard, which has been proposed and widely used when comparing disease rates globally, is the World Health Organization (WHO) world standard population which is based on the estimated age structure across all countries. The standard has changed over time, to reflect changing population structure, particularly lower mortality rates in childhood and at older ages. The WHO World Standard Population for 2000–2025 is shown in Table 3.2. Directly standardized rates have the advantage that they can be compared with any other rate which has been directly standardized to the same population. A disadvantage, however,

Table 3.2 World Health Organization (WHO) world standard population 2000–2025

Age group (years)	WHO world standard (%)	WHO world standard population (n)
0–4	8.86	8,569
5–9	8.69	86,870
10–14	8.60	85,970
15–19	8.47	84,670
20–24	8.22	82,171
25–29	7.93	79,272
30–34	7.61	76,073
35–39	7.15	71,475
40–44	6.59	65,877
45–49	6.04	60,379
50–54	5.37	53,681
55–59	4.55	45,484
60–64	3.72	37,187
65–69	2.96	29,590
70–74	2.21	22,092
75–79	1.52	15,195
80–84	0.91	9,097
85–89	0.44	4,398
90–94	0.15	1,500
95–99	0.04	400
100+	0.005	50
Total	100	1,000,000

is that problems can arise when study populations do not have sufficient numbers of cases to calculate robust age-specific rates.

Example 3.ii

A small seaside town appeared to have a very high prevalence of blindness compared with the rest of the region in which it was situated. However, the town was a popular location for elderly people in retirement. After direct standardization to the region's population, the prevalence of blindness was still 25% higher suggesting that there was an influence that could not be explained by age.

3.2.2 **Indirect standardization**

In contrast to direct standardization, which involves the use of population weights, indirect standardization involves the use of a set of age-specific rates from a standard population. These age-specific rates are then applied to the age structure of the study population to obtain the 'expected' number of cases of disease if these rates had applied to the study population. This 'expected' number of cases is then compared to the actual number of cases 'observed' in the study population. The ratio of observed/expected numbers of cases, multiplied by the crude rate in the study population is an indirectly standardized rate and can be compared with the crude rate in the standard population. Most commonly, however, it is the observed/expected numbers of cases (multiplied by 100) which is reported. If the ratio is 100, this shows that the observed and expected number of cases are the same, greater than 100 implies that the number of cases observed is more than would be expected if the age-specific rates in the standard population had applied, and lower than 100 implies less cases than would have been expected. This ratio is called the standardized incidence ratio (SIR), standardized mortality ratio (SMR), or standardized prevalence ratio (SPR), depending on the specific measure being considered. Given that in each comparison the 'weight' applied in indirect standardization is the population structure of the study population, then technically the only valid comparison is between the study and standard populations used to derive the standardized ratios (i.e. two standardized ratios should not be compared).

Example 3.iii

There were 35 cases of cataracts in Oldtown and 23 in Youngtown. If Youngtown's age-specific rates of cataracts were applied to the age structure of Oldtown, 34.4 cases would have been expected in Oldtown. In this case Youngtown is being defined as the standard population. Thus, the SPR is 102 and the difference in the number of cases between the towns can be explained by differences in the age of the residents, rather than by different age-specific rates of cataracts.

Example 3.iv

Table 3.3 shows a comparison of incidence rates of squamous cell carcinoma of the oesophagus according to occupational status/groups in the Nordic Occupational Cancer Study, using indirect standardization. The age and gender structure of workers in these groups is likely to be different (and age/gender is related to cancer risk). How common occupations are may differ between individual countries (and cancer incidence varies between countries). Therefore, the standardization has used country, age group, and gender-specific incidence rates. It should be noted that each comparison is of incidence in a specific group defined by their occupation/occupational status against the whole study population. Comparisons cannot be made between working groups directly. Thus, one cannot deduce that the SIR in cooks and stewards compared to assistant nurses is 253/145.

Table 3.3 Standardized incidence ratio of squamous cell carcinoma of the oesophagus according to occupation

Occupational groups	Squamous cell cancer of the oesophagus	
	SIR	95% Confidence interval
Painters	119	101–139
Beverage workers	187	89–343
Artistic workers	150	117–191
Postal workers	105	84–129
Economically inactive	165	153–176
Welders	108	87–132
Launderers	86	43–154
Cooks and stewards	253	194–325
Journalists	129	85–187
Building caretakers	120	98–144
Assistant nurses	145	77–248
All categories	100	

Source: data from Jansson C, Oh JK, Martinsen JI, Lagergren J, *et al*. (2015). Occupation and risk of oesophageal adenocarcinoma and squamous-cell carcinoma: the Nordic Occupational Cancer Study. *International Journal of Cancer*. Volume 137, Issue 3, pp. 590–7.

3.3 **Comparison of rates over time**

The previous section has considered the comparison of rates between populations. A special case of such a comparison is monitoring rates in a single population over time. Changing all-ages (crude) rates within a population could be a reflection of changes in age-specific rates or it could be a reflection of a population getting older with time. Thus, it is important to make comparisons with respect to a defined 'standard population' either by direct or indirect age standardization.

Example 3.v

A region monitored the incidence of hip fractures over the period 1990–2015 and noticed a steady increase over this time. The region had experienced on outflow of younger people during this time and hip fracture is more common among older people. A further analysis used the 1990 population age structure as the 'standard population' and standardized the incidence rates in all subsequent years to the population in this year. This demonstrated that there was no important change in the incidence of hip fracture over this period using standardized rates, and the apparent increase in the all-ages rate could be explained by changes in population age structure.

A comparison of trends in mortality rates, among men, using indirect standardization is shown in Table 3.4. Information on cancer mortality trends in selected European populations is given for 1985, 1991, and 2000. For each country the mortality rates in 1991 have been defined the 'standard population'. Thus, the age-specific rates in 1991 have been applied to the age structure of the population in both 1985 and 2000 to calculate SMR. By definition the SMR in each country is 100 in 1991. It can be seen from the tables that, although the number of cancer deaths has increased

Table 3.4 Trends in cancer mortality, among males, in selected European countries 1985–2000

Countries/ Year	1985		1991[1] (Reference)	2000	
	SMR[2]	N	SMR	SMR	N
Belgium	107	15,687	100	95	17,422
France	103	80,074	100	90	96,890
Germany	100	97,710	100	88	117,543
Greece	99	11,007	100	99	13,823
Italy	101	73,385	100	86	97,342
Netherlands	104	19,343	100	90	23,114
Spain	93	40,189	100	103	50,630
Sweden	102	10,282	100	94	11,367
United Kingdom	104	82,222	100	85	93,457

[1] Comparisons are standardized for age group

[2] Standardized mortality ratio

Source: data from P. Boyle, A. d'Onofrio, P. Maisonneuve, G. Severi, C. Robertson, M. Tubiana, U. Veronesi; Measuring progress against cancer in Europe: has the 15% decline targeted for 2000 come about?, *Annals of Oncology*, Volume 14, Issue 8, 1 August 2003, Pages 1312–25, https://doi.org/10.1093/annonc/mdg353

in every country between 1985 and 2000 the SMR has decreased in all but two countries. In the United Kingdom it can be seen that the number of cancer deaths in men has increased by around 14% (from 82,222 to 93,457). However, once changes to the population have been taken into account (age structure and population size) the SMR has decreased substantially from 104 to 85.

An alternative approach to comparing rates would have been to directly standardize them. The standard population could be from one of the years under study in one of the countries, or in all the countries combined. An alternative would be to use an 'external' population, but it would not make sense to use the WHO world standard population in this case since this population has a quite different structure to all the countries in this study.

3.3.1 **Age-specific rates**

The evaluation of changes in rates of disease in a population, in addition to standardization for age, should include examination of changes in age-specific rates over time. The pattern of changes in age-specific rates can give some indication of possible aetiology and can also help in the prediction of future rates.

Example 3.vi

A decrease in mortality rates from bladder cancer was observed in a population. On examination of cancer mortality rates within five-year age groups the decrease was noted to have occurred at all ages at the same calendar period. Such effects are known as 'time-period effects' (i.e. those changes which affect all age groups at or from a given calendar time period). It was considered that they may have resulted from an artefactual cause such as a change in registration procedure or coding rules. When this was discounted it was believed that recent improvements in the treatment of the disease and patients presenting earlier had resulted in improved survival rates and thus decreased mortality.

Changes in rates may show a time-period effect (as in Example 3.vi). Alternatively, the change in rates may manifest as a 'cohort effect'. Such an effect is associated with different risks of disease between generations and are a consequence of changes in long-term habits such as diet.

Figure 3.1 shows increases in tongue cancer incidence in persons aged 35–64 years (particularly in males) in Scotland between 1960 and 1989. There was no increase observed at older ages (data not shown). Rates in younger and middle-aged males increased steadily over this period from around 1 per 100,000 person-years to around 3 per 100,000 person-years. Further investigation of this increase is shown in Figure 3.2. Here incidence rates for five-year age groups are plotted for persons aged 40–84 years, not according to the time that the cancer was diagnosed but according to the birth cohort to which they belong. For example, persons in the age group 45–49 years who were diagnosed with tongue cancer in 1960–1964 will have been born between 1911 and 1919 (and therefore are plotted against the midpoint of this range, 1915). Similarly, persons aged 50–54 years who were diagnosed between 1965 and 1969 will also be part of the same birth cohort and are also plotted against 1915. Reading vertically from 1915, one can see the tongue cancer incidence rates experienced by people born in the birth cohort centred on 1915. Moving to the left or right one can see the experience of persons born in early or later birth cohorts. If rates are changing according to birth cohort (rather than by time period), then patterns will be evident. Data are not available for every age group and every birth cohort since for the earliest born persons routine statistics may not have been available for them at younger ages while the latest born persons will not yet have reached old age. The data in Figure 3.2 demonstrate that among men in cohorts born up to around 1910 rates were falling in each group for which data is available. Thereafter, in subsequent birth cohorts, rates increased again at each group. Since data is not available at older ages

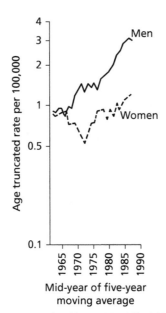

Figure 3.1 Tongue cancer incidence in Scotland (per 100,000) 1960–1989 among men and women age 35–64 years.

Reproduced with permission from Macfarlane GJ, Boyle P, Scully C (1992). Oral cancer in Scotland: changing incidence and mortality. *BMJ*. Volume 305, Issue 6862, pp. 1121–3. © 1992 BMJ Publishing Group Ltd.

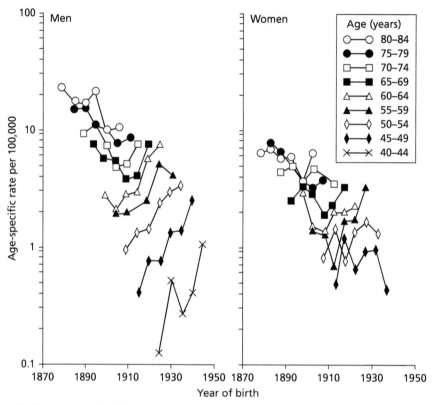

Figure 3.2 Tongue cancer incidence (per 100,000) in Scotland among men and women by year of birth.

Reproduced with permission from Macfarlane GJ, Boyle P, Scully C (1992). Oral cancer in Scotland: changing incidence and mortality. *BMJ*. Volume 305, Issue 6862, pp. 1121–3. © 1992 BMJ Publishing Group Ltd.

(at the time of this study) it is not known if such changes would continue into older ages. There is no clear pattern among women by birth cohort.

There are statistical methodologies available (age–period–cohort models) to more formally evaluate the role of age, period, and cohort effects on changing rates. The particular challenge in assigning changes in rates between these effects is that once two variables are known (such as a person's age and the time period of observation) this defines the birth cohort to which they belong, but these are beyond the scope of the current text (see 'Further reading').

Further reading

WHO world standard population

Ahmad OB, Boschi-Pinto C, Lopez AD, *et al.* (2001). Age-standardization of rates: a new WHO standard. GPE Discussion Paper Series: No 31 EIP/GPE/EBD. World Health Organization, Geneva, Switzerland. Available at: http://www.who.int/healthinfo/paper31.pdf

Direct standardization

Sorlie PD, Thom TJ, Manolio T, *et al.* (1999). Age-adjusted death rates: consequences of the Year 2000 standard. *Ann Epidemiol*, **9**(2), 93–100.

Indirect standardization

Boyle P, d'Onofrio A, Maisonneuve P, *et al.* (2003). Measuring progress against cancer in Europe: has the 15% decline targeted for 2000 come about? *Ann Oncol*, **14**(8), 1312–25.

Jansson C, Oh JK, Martinsen JI, *et al.* (2015). Occupation and risk of oesophageal adenocarcinoma and squamous-cell carcinoma: the Nordic Occupational Cancer Study. *Int J Cancer*, **137**(3), 590–97.

Evaluating changes in rates by birth cohort

Macfarlane GJ, Boyle P, Scully C (1992). Oral cancer in Scotland: changing incidence and mortality. *BMJ*, **305**(6862), 1121–23.

Age-period-cohort modelling

Bell A, Jones K (2013). The impossibility of separating age, period and cohort effects. *Soc Sci Med*, **93**, 163–65.

Chapter 4

Studies of disease occurrence
The population

4.1 Introduction

This chapter reviews the options for population selection in undertaking investigations aimed at estimating the occurrence of a disease in a target population. The same principles apply, however, if the object of the study is to investigate the occurrence of a risk factor, such as cigarette smoking, or other human attribute. The first requirement is to identify the target population to which the occurrence estimate will apply.

Example 4.i

In many countries, data are routinely collected on infectious diseases and on cancers based on national notification systems. Incidence rates are calculated using national population data derived from a census as the denominator. As censuses occur only at defined time intervals (e.g. 10 years apart), the population used in the denominator will be estimated, adjusted to take account of subsequent births, deaths, and estimated migrations. For the sake of convenience, disease events occurring in any single calendar year are usually related to the estimated mid-year population.

In practice, most epidemiological surveys use a variety of subnational populations. These may be defined by geopolitical boundaries such as an administrative area (e.g. persons resident within a local authority/metropolitan area for the purposes of receiving services and paying local taxes) or electoral district. Alternatively, a true geographical boundary may be used, derived either from a map or, where possible, based on postcodes. Another approach is to use populations registered for other purposes, such as those registered with a general practitioner or other health provider. Some epidemiological studies target particular age groups such as children or older people. In such groups possibilities may include school registers, or lists of persons receiving state pensions.

In each of these circumstances an evaluation will be required to determine to what extent these represent population sampling frames. These will be location-specific and will depend on local circumstances. For example, a true geographical sample (based on residence) will provide a population sampling frame for the defined population. Using lists of persons receiving state pensions may provide a suitable population sampling frame for older persons if everyone receives such a pension. If, however, a pension is only provided to persons with low incomes, then it will not.

Example 4.ii

In a study to determine the prevalence at birth of congenital dislocation of the hip, the investigators used a national birth register to identify their target population.

The choice of the appropriate target population for measuring disease prevalence is determined by five factors: representativeness, availability, access population, data accuracy, and size. These are discussed next and issues of sample size are considered in Section 4.5.

4.2 **Identifying a target population: Representativeness**

An epidemiological study of the prevalence of a specific disease conducted in a suburb of a large city will provide an estimate of prevalence only in that suburb. Although it is often relatively easy to allow for age and sex differences between the sample studied and a wider population (see Chapter 18), other differences such as socioeconomic and related factors might suggest that such estimates cannot be applied more widely, even to the neighbouring city itself. It would be even more problematic to apply such prevalence estimates to a suburb of a city in another country where there might be important differences in healthcare provision, lifestyle, and cultural factors.

In theory, most epidemiological investigations have as their unstated aim the derivation of 'national' estimates. Although governmental and related institutions often attempt national sample surveys for specific purposes, this approach is rarely practical or available to other investigators. In practice, therefore, for most diseases, published estimates of incidence and prevalence are based on local studies. This potential lack of representativeness is never an easy dilemma to solve. The most practical approach, if the aim is to present a 'national' view, is to choose a study population (populations) that is not extreme, for example, in its socioeconomic distribution, but includes persons across the distribution of relevant factors. This will either allow formal statistical adjustment of the results or at least provide relevant information about the sample to enable the 'reader' to interpret the results. National census data, for example, might provide information as to the study population's ranking in relation to some key variables, such as socioeconomic or ethnic mix, but may not have information on lifestyle variables such as physical activity and diet. Ultimately, however, estimates from studies can strictly be applied only to the population from whom the sample was selected. Alternatively, the same methodology can be used in several geographically and socially disparate populations.

The issue of representativeness can be a controversial topic—some believe that this is an essential feature of any sample, and earlier it has been discussed why it is generally important in measuring prevalence. However, in some circumstances a sample should not be representative; for example, if one wanted to estimate the prevalence of osteoporosis in a region and whether this varied by ethnic group. If there was a relatively low number of persons resident who were non-Caucasian, a sample which reflected the target population would likely not produce enough non-Caucasians to robustly estimate the prevalence in ethnic groups. In this case it would be necessary to oversample from ethnic groups (see Section 4.6). In Chapter 6, when study designs to examine disease aetiology are considered, we will see that representativeness is generally not required (see 'Further reading').

Example 4.iii

A major study was carried out in the United Kingdom (UK) to examine the prevalence of ischaemic heart disease in middle-aged males. The investigators used identical methods to study population samples in diverse geographical areas. These areas were chosen to include areas from each of the four countries within the UK to include urban, suburban, and rural areas, and to include areas, using available government statistics, across the spectrum of levels of average income per household.

4.3 **Identifying a target population: Availability**

As discussed next, there are two approaches to measuring disease occurrence. These are: (i) the 'catchment population' approach, which counts the number of ascertained cases (based on normal clinical referral and diagnosis) and relates that numerator to the denominator or population served by those clinical facilities; and (ii) the population survey approach, where each member of the study sample is individually investigated to accurately classify their disease status.

Example 4.iv

In order to determine the incidence of acute appendicitis in a small town, the investigators assumed that all cases that arose within that population would be admitted to one of two local acute hospitals. The population base was the estimated size of the geographical based population served by those hospitals. The researchers excluded cases that lived outside that area, but also had to allow for some residents being admitted to hospitals away from their home town.

The choice of the target population is determined by which of these approaches is to be used. Thus, in the catchment population approach it is only necessary to have available the actual numbers in the target population from which the cases were ascertained, and knowledge of their individual identities is not required. Conversely, for a population survey, it is necessary to have a list of individuals and contact details (usually their address), in order that contact can be made. This would require that a population register exists for the purposes, for example, for voting or obtaining an identity card. Where this is not available, then investigators will need to consider whether a suitable alternative exists.

For example, in the United Kingdom, one may consider general practitioner lists and persons on the electoral register. The former is particularly suitable since healthcare in the UK is free at the point of receipt and patients must register with a general practitioner to whom they should first consult for healthcare. Thus, it is estimated that the vast majority of the population are registered. These registers are held within the practice and at a national level. General practitioner lists also provide age, which can be useful for defining a target population and drawing a sample. In other countries, true geopolitical population listings are available providing age and other key variables. There is, however, a considerable advantage in using a register derived for health purposes, in that it provides the subject and the investigator with a strong motive for recruitment and participation. In some countries enrolment to receive healthcare services (e.g. in the United States) with the health maintenance organizations (HMO), is not universal and those registered are not representative of any geographical group and are likely to represent particularly socioeconomic groups.

4.4 **Identifying a target population: Access**

The existence of a population register does not imply that the investigator will be able to access it for research purposes. Indeed, over the past decades there have been greater controls with respect to access, in terms of who can access population registers and what they can access. Government-held registers are often unavailable to researchers, and identifiable data from the UK census is not available for 100 years! Previously, access to medical registers was discussed in terms of identifying a target population (sampling frame). However, researchers will not have individual consent for accessing such data. In order to access such information, routes of access which may be available are:

a) application to an 'access committee' making a case that the research question is so important that the public good from providing an answer outweighs the fact that people's information is being accessed without their consent;

b) that the data is initially accessed by persons who do have permission to access, who then approach persons about participation in the study (on behalf of the researcher).

The former approach will, by definition, only be considered to apply to a small number of subjects. The latter, while providing a route of access to the required data, does rely on the availability of approved persons to access the data and that the researcher will not have any information on persons approached, but who did not respond.

There are also commercial organizations which sell mailing lists or provide access to 'people panels' who have volunteered to take part (normally paid) in research studies. Apart from the cost, however, such lists are not derived from population samples, they are compiled from several sources and are likely to be highly selective (e.g. in terms of age, social class, economic factors).

4.5 **Identifying a target population: Data accuracy**

Errors in the denominator population can lead to important errors in the disease estimates obtained. In the catchment population approach, the denominator population is normally obtained from population census estimates, which might be inaccurate owing both to initial errors in their compilation and estimates of population change since the date of the survey due to births, deaths, and migration. Calculations are often undertaken to obtain projected population sizes between censuses (interpolation) or after the last census conducted (extrapolation). In reality, for rare disease, it may not matter if there is a 10% error in the denominator population, although it is important to remember that errors may be greater in certain population subgroups, for example, young adults and persons in cities (who have high mobility). In inner-city populations, if there was 30% mobility each year, for every notional 100 persons living at a stated address within that area at the start of a year, only 70 would still reside at that same address at the end of the year. A further problem is that those who are mobile are likely to have different health states from those who are more static. In the population survey approach, the denominator can normally be corrected by knowledge of errors. Deaths and migration frequently come to light during the course of the investigation. These factors can also affect health registers, whereby people have moved away and their registrations have not been cancelled. A register that is very inaccurate can lead both to an initial underestimate of the population size which it is necessary to survey as well as contributing significantly to costs.

4.6 **Identifying a target population: Study size**

Once the target population has been selected, it is necessary to calculate whether it is large enough to provide robust estimates of disease occurrence. Further, if the aim is also to derive robust estimates in each (say) 10-year age group by sex then the number in the target population in each stratum needs to be sufficiently large. If this is required, using a sampling frame which includes age would be advantageous. The determination of sample size is dependent on two, fairly obvious, aspects: (i) the approximate expected occurrence—the rarer the disease, the larger the population required; and (ii) the precision required for the estimate—the more precise the estimate, the larger the population required. Statistically, the calculation of sample size is based on the estimated prevalence (of course, if the actual prevalence was known there would be no need to undertake the study!), and the size of the confidence interval required around it (95% confidence intervals are most common). An example of sample sizes for some typical situations is shown in Table 4.1. There is a variety of software available to allow the reader to calculate the sample size of a survey for their own particular study situation and requirements (see 'Further reading').

Example 4. v

Using the data presented in Table 4.1, one can see that if the best estimate for prevalence of obesity in a town is 20% and it is required to estimate prevalence with a confidence interval of width 6% (i.e. +/- 3%) then one would require 682 participants in the population survey. If it estimated that in the sample drawn from the

Table 4.1 Approximate sample size requirements for population surveys

Expected frequency (%)	Precision required (within +/– %)	Sample size required ^
0.5	0.2	4,755
	0.1	18,763
1	0.5	1,519
	0.2	9,418
2	1	752
	0.5	3,003
5	2	456
	1	1,821
10	3	384
	2	864
	1	3,445
20	5	246
	3	682
	1	6,109

^ These figures assume the population sampling frame is very large and are based on a 95% confidence that the true frequency will lie within the limits given.

sampling frame that 5% of persons are no longer resident in the town when checked on the electoral register and among persons mailed, that only 30% agree to take part, then one requires to draw an initial sample of 2,392 (i.e. 682 × (100/30) × (100/95)).

4.7 **Sampling from a population**

In many surveys it will not be necessary or feasible to study everyone in the target population. In such instances it will only be necessary to study a sample. The basic unit in a study (e.g. a person) is referred to as the sampling unit; while the sampling frame consists of all the relevant sampling units (e.g. a list of all adults aged 18–65 years resident in a town). Those subjects selected for participation in the study are referred to as the study sample. In order that the sample is likely to be representative of the target population from which it is drawn, selection nearly always involves some element of randomness, that is, the chance of any subject included in the sampling frame (or within a subgroup, for example, defined by age group, of the sampling frame) being selected is equal.

The most common method employed is simple random sampling. In this method each of the sampling units in the sampling frame would have the same probability of being selected as part of the study sample. This could be achieved by allocating each unit a number and then selecting a sample of a predetermined size using random number tables or a computer program's random number generator. In such circumstances each person has the same probability of being selected for the sample. As discussed previously, in estimating the prevalence of a disease in a population one may wish to have a predetermined level of precision in each 10-year age group. This can be achieved by stratified random sampling. The sampling frame would be divided into strata defined by age groups, and thereafter subjects selected at random.

In some studies, it may be necessary to interview subjects or make a clinical diagnosis. It is unlikely to be feasible to interview or examine all subjects in the study sample.

Example 4.vi

A study wished to examine the prevalence of asthma (defined by clinical diagnosis) but it would have been extremely time-consuming and resource-intensive to examine all subjects in a large study sample. Most subjects would not have asthma. Instead, a multistage sampling procedure was employed. The study sample was selected using simple random sampling. Each of the study sample received a postal 'screening' questionnaire. Selection of subjects for the second (clinical) stage of the study then depended on responses to the first-stage questionnaire. This method allowed the prevalence of asthma in the target population to be estimated with efficient use of resources.

Finally, multistage (cluster) sampling is commonly used. The clusters may, for example, be towns, schools, or general practices. The first stage is to select a cluster sample and thereafter from each of the selected clusters to sample individual units (e.g. residents, schoolchildren, patients). This can be particularly efficient if, for example, the study procedures necessitate a visit by the participant and thus these are concentrated in certain geographical areas or health service facilities (Example 4.vii).

Example 4.vii

A study was designed to estimate the prevalence of dental decay among seven-year-old children in Rose County (USA). Firstly, a sample of schools was randomly selected from all those within the county. Thereafter, from the seven-year-old children attending these schools, a further simple random sample of individual children was selected.

Further reading

Representativeness

Rothman KJ, Gallacher JE, Hatch EE (2013). Why representativeness should be avoided. *Int J Epidemiol*, **42**(4), 1012–24.

Software for calculating survey sample requirements

Open Source Epidemiologic Statistics for Public Health. Available at: http://www.openepi.com/Menu/OE_Menu.htm—see Sample Size section and Proportion subsection) [Accessed April 2017].

Chapter 5

Studies of disease occurrence
Assessing disease status in study populations

5.1 **Introduction**

Chapter 4 has given definitions for measures of disease occurrence, but the practical challenge for an epidemiologist can be how these should be determined in practice. There may be, for example, national cancer registers which allow a date of diagnosis to be determined and in which case this is relatively straightforward. However, in terms of measuring incidence where there are no registers measuring disease onset and where it is practically difficult to measure this (or to have a proxy for such), then an alternative approach needs to be taken.

5.2 **Approaches to measuring incidence**

Four possible approaches to measuring disease incidence in a target population are (Fig. 5.1):

   i) a single population survey identifying those with disease onset during a defined time period;
  ii) two population surveys, separated by an interval of time to permit identification of those cases of disease that develop between the two surveys;
 iii) a retrospective review of diagnosed cases attending clinical facilities serving the defined target or 'catchment' population;
  iv) a prospective registration system (which could include routine health records) for recording either all new diagnosed cases or disease onsets within the defined target or 'catchment' population.

The choice of appropriate strategy is guided by several considerations as outlined in the flowchart (Fig. 5.2). The first question is whether all individuals with the disease in question are likely to seek medical attention and be diagnosed. If this is not so, for example, in self-limiting acute viral illnesses, minor trauma, or common symptoms, then a population survey approach is essential. Even if most individuals with the disease are likely to seek medical attention, it is necessary to determine firstly, where they consult such as family practice, hospital outpatient, and emergency services. Different people may present to different types of medical facilities. Secondly, one needs to determine whether the catchment population approach is appropriate. In cities, for instance, there is a wide choice of clinical facilities and it may be impossible to identify those facilities that will cover all the individuals, from the target population, who may develop the disease. This is particularly true in countries where there is a private healthcare system but even in public healthcare systems it can be challenging. It thus may be necessary to use a population survey strategy.

Example 5.i

A study aimed to investigate the incidence of myocardial infarction in a target population. Preliminary enquiries revealed that many such episodes resulted in admission to hospitals outside the immediate geographical area, including, for example, hospitals local to where the cases were employed. Surveying local hospitals was therefore abandoned as a strategy for assessing incidence. By contrast, in the ideal situation of a single central facility that provides the only healthcare to a population, the catchment population approach, using available records, is feasible.

(i) Single populaion survey

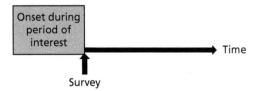

Survey

(ii) Duplicate populaion surveys

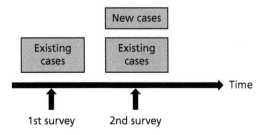

1st survey   2nd survey

(iii) Retrospecive review of diagnosed cases

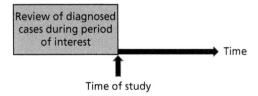

Time of study

(iv) Prospective review of diagnosed cases

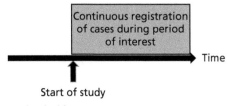

Start of study

Figure 5.1 Approaches to measuring incidence.

Example 5.ii

The Rochester Epidemiology Project is based on the necessity that all inhabitants from Olmsted County, Minnesota, United States, seek their medical care either from the Mayo Clinic or a linked medical practice. It is possible to identify Olmsted County residents from the Mayo's diagnostic database, which should include all the diagnosed cases that have arisen within that target population. As a consequence, there have been a large number of studies estimating incidence of a variety of diseases from that source (see 'Further reading' for an example studying Parkinson's disease).

In situations where there is not an existing database that will permit easy identification of patients previously diagnosed with disease, then it will be necessary to establish a prospective system. In this approach, the investigator specifically recruits all relevant physicians to notify any new case, with the specific disorder under investigation, to the study. A study using this method would need to assess the completeness of the notification system. If a population survey is required, a single survey will normally suffice if the disease onset can be easily recalled and defined

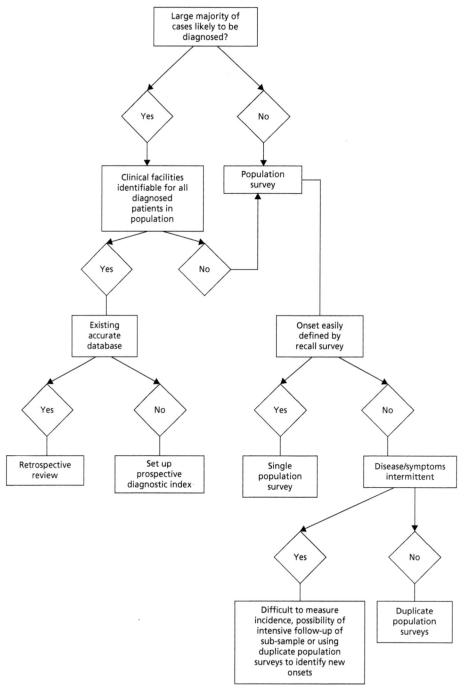

Figure 5.2 Choosing the appropriate strategy.

by the subjects surveyed. Alternatively, if onset is unlikely to be recalled, duplicate cross-sectional surveys must be undertaken. For diseases or symptoms of an episodic nature, even such duplicate surveys may not be able to measure incidence, since some episodes occurring entirely between surveys may be missed. Where the latter circumstances exist (e.g. headache), then a single population survey asking about episode onsets within a defined recent period (e.g. the past month or three months) is likely to be the best approach.

Example 5.iii

A study was conducted to identify the incidence of knee pain consultations. The decision was whether to identify incidence cases by population survey or by search of general practitioner records. Using the former approach, the concern was whether people would remember consultations for knee pain within a one-year time period, while in the latter approach the concern was whether practitioners had actually recorded knee pain as the reason for consultation (acknowledging that people consult with multiple symptoms). A feasibility study was thus conducted to determine whether persons remember knee pain consultation recorded in the notes and whether reports of knee pain consultations can be identified in general practitioner records (see 'Further reading').

5.2.1 Diagnosed cases: Retrospective review or prospective notification?

As indicated already, the presence of an existing diagnostic database (or disease register) will permit the use of the retrospective approach to ascertain cases diagnosed in the past. The problem is that only rarely are such databases accurate or cover all relevant departments. Thus, a gastroenterology department within a hospital may keep an index of all new cases of peptic ulcer, but such an index would exclude cases attending a geriatric or general medical unit, for example. In Scotland, Scandinavia, and some other countries, there are population-based databases of all hospital inpatient admissions. Thus, provided that the disorder leads to an inpatient stay, such as acute appendicitis or fracture of the neck of femur, these data sources can be useful in providing incidence estimates. They would not, however, be useful for measuring the incidence of myocardial infarction, since persons who had a myocardial infarction but who died before being admitted to hospital, would not be recorded by such a system. The diagnostic accuracy of these databases often needs to be determined because those recording the data do not have a vested interest in the data quality, at least as far as the specific question is concerned. The other problem is that it may not be possible to identify all the health facilities serving a catchment population. Specifically, private hospitals and similar institutions may not have a statutory requirement to provide data but in some areas, for some disorders, they may be a source of an important proportion of cases.

Clinical team compliance

Other factors to be taken into consideration are shown in Table 5.1. With an existing database it is not necessary to ensure compliance of the clinical team, though it will be necessary to gain appropriate permissions to access the data. The term *databases* can be used to cover many different sources of data including local department record, an entire hospital or organization's data system, or a national disease register. Whichever it is, it will be necessary to assess the completeness of the database both in terms of identifying cases of disease and in the extent and quality of the data collected on these patients (e.g. missing data). One of the problems with prospective notification is that this normally requires contacting all relevant clinical teams and asking for their help in identifying and notifying cases. If the disease is rare, or the notification procedure complex, it may be impossible to attain complete ascertainment. Constant reminders are required and the most

Table 5.1 Retrospective review or prospective notification to identify cases of disease

Attribute	Retrospective review	Prospective notification
Existing diagnostic database	required	not required
Physician compliance	not required	required
Diagnostic verification	may be difficult to ascertain	can be incorporated
Under-ascertainment	may be difficult to determine	may be high
Expense	low	medium

successful schemes, which are clerically time-consuming, involve circulating all relevant clinical teams at least monthly or even weekly for common diseases. It is preferable, if resources allow, to have study personnel (or to provide resources for local nurses) dedicated to the task of identifying eligible clinic patients.

More recently it has been possible to interrogate clinical record systems to count potential cases. However, due to data protection and ethics issues, normally special permission for access to such data is necessary (since the researcher may be gaining access to the information without the individual consent of the patients). Further, if the researcher needs access to case notes to verify diagnosis or collect further clinical details then explicit consent is likely to be required or the information extracted by members of the clinical care team who have permission to access the system. If it is necessary, for example, to interview study subjects or to undertake further investigations, initial contact with the potential study participant will usually need to come from the clinical care teams. Researchers will only be aware of those who have agreed to participate, although it can be possible to have permission to have access to group data on non-participants such as the number of males/females or age group.

Example 5.iv

In a study aimed at ascertaining all new cases of Crohn's disease in a target population, the investigators were aware that no diagnostic database existed. They wrote monthly to all local general physicians, gastroenterologists, paediatricians, and gastrointestinal surgeons asking for notification of new cases diagnosed in the previous month.

Compliance may be enhanced by offering a small financial inducement for every patient notified, although the value of this tactic is unclear!

Problems with rare diseases

If the disease under study is very rare, the retrospective approach, provided that the database goes back far enough, will permit an answer to be obtained in a much shorter time than the prospective approach, which might require several years of case ascertainment to derive sufficient numbers of cases for reasonably robust estimates of prevalence. Similarly, if time trends are of interest, only the retrospective approach can yield an answer in a reasonable time frame.

5.2.2 **Defining cases with the catchment population approach**

There are inevitably two issues in defining the numerator for the catchment population approach to incidence studies. These can be considered as case ascertainment and case verification (although the principles are also relevant to the population survey approach). There is a need to ensure that all cases have been ascertained and also that all cases ascertained are verified to have the disease.

Case ascertainment

Under-ascertainment is a distinct possibility in the catchment population approach, both retrospective and prospective. The major causes are, in the former, diagnostic misclassification and, in the latter, non-compliance by the participating physicians in addition to the already-mentioned issue of referral practices (i.e. non-referral or referral to another clinical facility). One approach to checking for under-ascertainment in the retrospective approach is to review a sample of medical records of individuals with a related diagnosis. In the prospective approach, if the disease is relatively common the population survey approach may be suitable, or using estimates from both specialist and primary care settings may be another option (see 'Further reading').

Example 5.v

A surgeon wished to determine the incidence of acute appendicitis in the local population. In addition to gathering all those listed as having that diagnosis from the target hospitals, he reviewed a random sample of records from those with acute abdominal pain to determine whether any additional cases of acute appendicitis had come to light.

In the prospective approach, one useful strategy—if there are enough cases—is to compare the rates of notification from different physicians or clinical departments. Obviously, depending on their practices and interests, there will be an inevitable variation in the number of cases reported, but very large variation may indicate that cases are being missed in some settings.

Example 5.vi

In response to a local survey of eight urologists for notifications of cases to determine the incidence of renal colic, five of the surgeons notified an average of ten cases and the remaining three only notified two cases each within the study period. Further investigation suggested that the last three surgeons had not identified all eligible cases.

Case verification

Diagnostic verification involves setting up a series of rules to ensure that the cases notified actually have the disease. This will inevitably involve, at the minimum, a review of medical records to establish the basis for the diagnostic assignment and might also require the investigator to interview, examine, or even investigate the subjects identified to confirm the diagnosis. The advantage of the prospective approach is that because the data collection is contemporaneous, the investigator can both provide the inclusion rules to the participating physicians and check, if necessary, with the patient. For patients registered some time ago, such diagnostic information is very difficult to obtain.

Example 5.vii

In a prospective study of the incidence of acute appendicitis, the registration form sought details of findings at surgery and from histology in addition to the clinical diagnosis.

Finally, it is apparent that any prospective system is more costly than a recall system that relies on trawling through existing databases, although even the costs of the former are substantially more modest than those involved in a population survey.

5.2.3 **Use of cross-sectional population surveys to assess incidence**

Single or duplicate surveys?

Incidence estimates may be derived either from a single or from duplicate population surveys. In situations (Table 5.2) where the disease has a clear onset and is easily recalled by the subject, a single cross-sectional survey will permit an estimate of the incidence. With disorders which have a major impact such as myocardial infarction, then retrospective recall of the event in a single cross-sectional survey might provide an accurate estimate of the occurrence, even over a fairly prolonged period. However, by definition, persons who have a myocardial infarction may not survive and thus 'incident episodes' resulting in death prior to the cross-sectional survey would be missed. With disorders such as gastroenteritis following a point source outbreak, an enquiry fairly close in time to the event is necessary to ascertain cumulative incidence.

Some disorders, though characterized by a clearly defined onset, present as multiple episodes of short duration, for example, epileptic fits and pain. The problem in studying such disorders is that in cross-sectional surveys, recall by the individual of the date of onset of each episode may be poor. It is thus necessary to undertake duplicate surveys, relatively close in time, to derive accurate estimates of the number of episodes that occurred in the interval.

Finally, for those disorders where the date of onset is difficult or impossible to define, such as hypertension, it may be possible to derive an estimate of incidence based on the number who change their disease status between two cross-sectional surveys. This is calculated as a risk, which is the number of new cases at the second survey divided by the number of persons studied. The interval between surveys could be long. However, people who develop hypertension after the initial survey which resolves before the second will be missed. For conditions which do not resolve, such as rheumatoid arthritis, this is not an issue.

Left censorship

One major problem with any cross-sectional (survey) approach to measure incidence is referred to as left censorship. This problem results from retrospective enquiries, which, by their nature, exclude those who were in the target population and had an incident event during the period of interest that was not ascertained, due to death, migration, or even full recovery. In circumstances where the length of an episode could be very short, for example, low back pain, unless the follow-up interval is also very short, follow-up surveys may miss new onsets. Conversely, intensive follow-up of subjects enquiring about specific symptoms may lead to subjects reporting even very minor symptoms.

Table 5.2 Single or duplicate population surveys for measuring incidence

Attribute	Example	Survey approach
Onset easy to recall and accurately date	Food poisoning outbreak	Single retrospective survey
Onset easy to recall but difficult to date	Acute low back pain	Duplicate retrospective surveys with short interval or intensive follow-up of population sample
Onset not recallable by subject	Rheumatoid arthritis	Duplicate surveys, interval not so important

Example 5.viii

A retrospective survey aimed to determine the incidence of myocardial infarction in the previous five years. This method would miss detection of those individuals who had developed an acute infarction and had died as a result. Such subjects clearly would not be able to be surveyed, seriously underestimating the true incidence.

Other more subtle examples of this bias might reflect those who have developed the disease and moved subsequently to a different location, perhaps because of loss of job or seeking a different climate, and similarly they would not be ascertained.

5.3 Approaches to measuring prevalence

As with studying incidence, there are several approaches to measuring prevalence:

 i) retrospective review of diagnosed cases;
 ii) prospective recording of current diagnosed cases;
 iii) population survey.

In a similar manner there are the alternatives of: (i) review of diagnosed cases from a catchment population, or (ii) a population survey. With prevalence, the more usual approach is to undertake a special survey, but there are circumstances where it can be acceptable to use the cheaper and quicker catchment population method.

5.3.1 Catchment population methods for measuring prevalence

There are several requirements before such an approach can be used for deriving prevalence data:

◆ diagnostic register available;

◆ substantial majority of cases likely to be diagnosed;

◆ registers available to cover all individuals in catchment population;

◆ vital status (dead/alive) known on prevalence day;

◆ residence known on prevalence day;

◆ disease status known on prevalence day.

There must be a database available covering the disorder in question; most cases that arise within a population would be expected to be diagnosed and therefore incorporated into the database, and the clinic facilities surveyed should cover the catchment population. In addition, because (the normally quoted) point prevalence requires knowledge that an individual is in 'disease state' on a specific day (prevalence day), there are other assumptions that need to be met. These are: (i) each of the cases on the register is still a resident of the catchment population on prevalence day (as opposed to the date of onset); (ii) as part of the aforementioned, each of the cases is known to be alive on prevalence day; (iii) each of the cases is still in 'disease state' on prevalence day. Thus, there are only a small number of conditions that would fit these requirements such as cystic fibrosis and insulin-dependent diabetes.

Example 5.ix

In the case of type I (insulin-dependent) diabetes in childhood, it is reasonable to assume that all cases that arise will be diagnosed in a recognized clinical facility, and the relevant institutions for a particular target population should be identifiable. As the condition is (to all intents and purposes) irreversible, disease presence at diagnosis is equivalent to disease presence on prevalence day in those still alive. Given that virtually all children will probably be followed up in a clinic, it should be possible to trace the current residence of all the cases. Thus, the point prevalence at an arbitrary date can be estimated.

Prospective measurement of prevalence

This approach is reasonable for assessing the period prevalence of conditions that are fairly common and occur in episodes that normally require clinical attendance at some time during an arbitrary period.

Example 5.x

It is unlikely that all cases of asthma will attend hospital. However, it may be reasonable to assume that, in a given year, if there is any significant morbidity from asthma, then the sufferer will need to make contact with primary care to seek attention, attend a routine assessment, or at least request medication, at the primary care level. Thus, to determine period prevalence, a system can be instituted to target primary care physicians and other practice staff to document, prospectively, all attendances (or more generally 'encounters') with persons who have diagnosed asthma during the period of (say) one year, to estimate the one-year period prevalence.

In some countries, general practice computerized records results in the automatic recording of all consultations, visits, and prescriptions.

5.3.2 **Population surveys**

Prevalence day does not need to be on the same day for each study subject. Population surveys may be conducted over a period of several months. On a postal questionnaire it will probably relate to when the questionnaire is filled in (and perhaps a prior period, such as the previous month). Nevertheless, in presenting results a notional 'prevalence day' is assumed in calculating point prevalence rates. The most frequently used approach to deriving prevalence is the population survey, where a target population is identified and an attempt is made to classify the disease state (present or absent) of every individual on 'prevalence day'.

Example 5.xi

A study attempted to estimate the prevalence of shoulder pain. During the preparatory phase for the study which would involve a home interview, it became apparent that symptoms were most commonly intermittent and that ascertaining disease status at a single time point (point prevalence) was not appropriate. Doing so would mean that many persons with shoulder pain would be classified as not having such symptoms since they did not have pain during the actual interview. It was therefore decided to ask whether persons had experience shoulder pain 'within the past seven days'—and thus the study would ascertain the one-week period prevalence.

Approaches to population surveys

The approach to be taken depends on the information required to classify disease accurately. A hierarchy of strategies for population prevalence surveys of increasing complexity and cost is as follows:

◆ postal or telephone survey;
◆ postal screening survey with telephone or postal follow-up;
◆ postal screening survey with interview or examination follow-up;
◆ interview survey;
◆ interview screening survey with examination;
◆ interview screening survey with investigation;
◆ investigation survey.

Thus, at the lowest level, a postal survey may provide all the necessary information and has been used, for example, in surveys of diseases whose diagnosis is essentially based on history alone, such as angina and chronic bronchitis. If the questions are prone to misinterpretation or error, an interview may be required either by telephone or in person either at the subject's home or on special premises. Detailed aspects of the relative advantages of a questionnaire over an interview for obtaining epidemiological information are given in Chapter 10. It may be necessary to undertake a restricted physical examination, for example, blood pressure measurement.

Obviously direct contact is required when investigations such as blood, urine, or radiological testing are required. A cost-effective approach is often to undertake a two-stage screening procedure if the nature of the disease makes it appropriate. The first stage is thus a postal or telephone interview to all, with follow-up of subjects depending on the results of the initial screen.

Example 5.xii

Investigators wished to determine the prevalence of periodontal disease among persons aged 18 years and over registered with general practitioners based in Hightown. They decided that a diagnosis could only be made by clinical examination, but it was not feasible to examine all adults in the town. A screening questionnaire about oral health was sent to all adults in the town. Only persons screening positive to the questionnaire were invited to attend for examination. It was assumed that persons screening negative, not reporting oral symptoms, were very unlikely to have periodontal disease. However, this was checked by also inviting a small number of screen negative persons to an examination.

Example 5.xiii

There are standard criteria for determining whether someone has dementia. However, conducting such assessments on a population sample (even restricted to older ages) to determine the prevalence of dementia is not feasible in terms of time and cost. Therefore, investigators firstly recruited a sample of persons aged 60 years and older in a specific geographical area and asked them to complete a screening questionnaire (the Mini-Mental State Examination) for cognitive impairment. Those screening positive were then invited for an assessment with a family member, friend, or carer. This allowed investigators to estimate the prevalence of dementia (see 'Further reading').

5.4 **Other (indirect) measures**

It will be appreciated that when measuring incidence, determining the date of disease 'onset' may only be an approximation. For example, the date of onset of cancer recorded will usually refer to a date of diagnosis, even though symptoms are likely to have been present some time previously. Indeed, the true onset of the cancer will predate even symptom onset. In some circumstances it may not be possible to measure incidence and some proxy measure may be used. If the disease under investigation has very poor survival rates, then mortality may be a good approximation to disease onset.

Example 5.xiv

In an international study of lung cancer, some countries involved did not routinely measure lung cancer incidence. However, since the survival rate from lung cancer is very poor (approximately 3% at five years) it was considered reasonable to use available mortality data.

In other circumstances it may be possible to use healthcare data to approximate disease state or onset. This may not capture all persons in the disease state or with the disease onset of interest, but it is likely to reflect those of a certain severity or perceived severity. Investigators will, however, have to consider the quality of the data recording and whether it is in a form suitable for the purposes of the study.

Example 5.xv

Investigators wished to determine the prevalence of hypothyroidism (an underactive thyroid) in a small town. They did not have the resources to investigate all the residents. Instead they obtained permission to scrutinize the medical records of the single general practice in the town. It was possible to determine from the computerized and paper medical records the number of residents who had been formally diagnosed during the previous year.

There will be occasions where the recorded data of the condition of interest may not be suitable for use for a variety of reasons (e.g. not closely enough related to incidence, poor quality of the data, and so on).

Example 5.xvi

A company had requested local investigators to determine how common back pain was among their workforce. Analysis of the company absenteeism records showed that back pain was by far the most common reason self-reported by workers for short-term absences. However, in many cases the records were incomplete and there was no cause given. The investigators thought that the quality of the records, the inconsistent way in which the information was recorded, and the fact that many people with back pain may not have taken time off work meant that they had to undertake a special enquiry for that purpose.

Overall, the decision would need to be made on the basis of specific needs relating to an individual project where actual incidence data were not available, to ascertain whether an alternative (proxy) measure may be suitable.

Further reading

Adelman S, Blanchard M, Rait G, Leavey G, Livingston G (2011). Prevalence of dementia in African-Caribbean compared with UK-born White older people: two-stage cross-sectional study. *Br J Psychiatry*, **199**(2), 119–25.

Dean LE, Macfarlane GJ, Jones GT (2016). Differences in the prevalence of ankylosing spondylitis in primary and secondary care: only one-third of patients are managed in rheumatology. *Rheumatology (Oxford)*, **55**(10), 1820–5.

Jordan K, Jinks C, Croft P (2006). Health care utilization: measurement using primary care records and patient recall both showed bias. *J Clin Epidemiol*, **59**(8), 791–7.

Savica R, Grossardt BR, Bower JH, Ahlskog JE, Rocca WA (2016). Time trends in the incidence of Parkinson disease. *JAMA Neurol*, **73**(8), 981–9.

Part C

Studying associations between exposures and disease

Chapter 6

Which type of epidemiological study?

6.1 Introduction

Assuming there is a scientific hypothesis which is suitably answered by an epidemiological approach, the subsequent decision is which type of study is appropriate. The decision will be based not only on methodological but also on practical considerations. For example, the most appropriate study may be too expensive or take too long to provide an answer. In such circumstances a compromise will need to be made—to undertake a study which can be conducted within the budget and time available and which delivers information which is suitable for answering the hypothesis.

6.2 Cross-sectional study

The key feature about a cross-sectional study is that it studies a whole population or a random sample of a population and collects information about current disease state (i.e. prevalent disease) and also measures exposures of interest. In some instances, the study may base determination of disease status on a period of time (e.g. past month).

Example 6.i

A questionnaire was sent to all individuals aged over 65 years resident in a town. They were asked about whether they had fallen in their home during the past month. In addition, information was collected on general health, current medication, and aspects about the layout of their home. The investigators wished to determine the one-month period prevalence of falls and whether the risk of falling was higher in the presence of any of the risk factors about which information was collected.

The principal advantages of the cross-sectional study are normally that it is relatively inexpensive and can be conducted within a short timescale. The principal disadvantage is the lack of information on temporality of disease state and exposures (Example 6.ii). In addition, a cross-sectional survey, in identifying prevalent cases, will preferentially identify chronic cases (and survivors). Those with only short-lived symptoms or disease, or who have died shortly after disease onset, are less likely to be 'in disease state' at the time of survey. In Figure 6.1, of the seven back pain subjects on which data is presented, four subjects (A, D, E, and F) reported back pain at the time of survey. All these subjects have more long-standing symptoms in comparison to the other subjects who experience back pain and who were back pain free at the time of survey (subjects C and G). This must be borne in mind when interpreting relationships with risk factors.

Example 6.ii

A cross-sectional survey was conducted among adult residents of a single town to determine whether mental disorder was more common among those from lower socioeconomic groups. The study found that mental disorder was twice as common in the lowest socioeconomic group in comparison to the highest group. In interpreting these results, the investigators considered that this observation was consistent with the hypothesis that some aspect of the circumstances and lifestyle of those of low social status predisposed them to the onset of a mental disorder. However, they also realized that the consequences of having a mental disorder may, through changing or loss of employment, result in their socioeconomic status falling. The study therefore, while demonstrating an association, has not established the temporal order of events.

In addition to measuring prevalence and determining the association of risk factors with disease, cross-sectional studies may be the method through which other study designs are conducted. For example, a cross-sectional study may be conducted to be used as a sampling frame for cases of a disease and controls for a case–control study (albeit one which used prevalent cases). A cohort study may consist of a series of cross-sectional studies which determine new disease onsets. A series of cross-sectional studies may also be used to determine time-trends in the prevalence of disease, and when investigating possible clustering of disease in time and geographical location. They may also be the method through which information is collected on participants in a migrant study.

6.3 **The case–control study**

In this type of study, persons with the disease of interest are identified (*cases*) together with a sample of those without the disease (*controls*). The cases and controls are then compared with respect to their exposure to potential risk factors. Exposure information may relate to current and/ or past exposures.

Example 6.iii

A study investigated the possible role of alcohol consumption in the aetiology of cancer of the stomach. Cases were persons, resident in Eastern county, diagnosed with stomach cancer during 2015–2016. Controls were selected at random from persons registered with the same family doctor, of the same gender, and born within two calendar years of the case. Information was then collected from all cases and controls on alcohol consumption. Cases and controls were asked about alcohol consumption 5, 10, and 20 years previously, reflecting the likely long time period between exposure and development of cancer.

Case–control studies are typically either population based (as in Example 6.iii) where the study identifies all cases which have arisen within a specific time period in a defined population, or hospital based (as in Example 6.iv) where the study identifies all cases which have been diagnosed

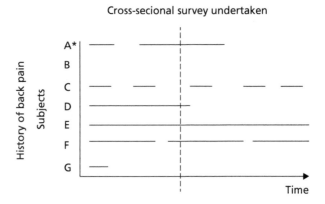

* Timelines indicate when individual subjects have experienced back pain

Figure 6.1 A cross-sectional study of back pain.

within a specific time period within one or more clinical facilities. The latter is often an easier study to conduct, but the case group may not be representative of persons with the disease. For example, the hospital unit(s) chosen may be a regional referral centre and specialized in more complex clinical cases. The aforementioned designs use incident cases. This is often preferable as it reduces the issue of measuring exposures which are consequences rather than antecedents of the disease. However, it is possible to conduct case–control studies using prevalent cases and, as just discussed, these may be identified, for example, through a cross-sectional study. Cases included in such studies are more likely to be chronic and the challenge is that the study of aetiological factors may be mixed up with the study of factors for persistence or survival.

Example 6.iv

All individuals admitted to a local coronary care unit with a diagnosis of myocardial infarction (MI) were enrolled as cases in a case–control study and information gathered on their diet during the previous year. Controls were randomly selected from persons admitted to the hospital on the same day (for reasons other than an MI) and who were of the same gender, born within two years, and of the same social class. Information on diet during the previous year was also collected from these controls.

The case–control approach is particularly suitable when the disease is rare, and when the aim is to investigate the effect of many exposures on one disease. Subjects will be required to report current or recall past 'exposures' and there will be an issue of firstly, whether they will be able to recall such exposures accurately and secondly, whether recall is similar in cases and controls. The issue of recall bias is discussed in Section 19.4. For some exposures, concerns about recall may be able to be overcome by the use of documentary records (Examples 6.v and 6.vi).

Example 6.v

A case–control study of chronic pain in adulthood, gathered information relating to adverse events prior to the age of 16. The study found that all events in childhood about which information was collected from participant interview, were associated with case status. The authors were concerned about recall of such events. In particular, the study investigators were worried that cases may be more likely to remember events which occurred, compared with controls. Therefore, two events were chosen which were most likely to have accessible documented evidence for their occurrence: hospitalizations and operations. When medical record information was used, the associations were much weaker or non-existent. Controls were much more likely not to report on interview, hospitalizations and operations which were documented in their medical records (see 'Further reading').

Example 6.vi

A case–control study of Parkinson's disease found that cases were more likely to self-report exposure to pesticides. However, because of concerns over differential recall of exposure between cases and controls, participants who reported exposure at levels greater than expected in the general population underwent an occupational hygiene review (OHR). Using the information from the OHR, the association between case status and pesticide exposure was reduced and case status was more strongly related to working in farming. This suggests that an exposure linked to farming, but not pesticides, may be linked to Parkinson's disease (see 'Further reading').

Using incident cases and asking about past exposures, reduces concern about temporality of events (i.e. interest is in exposures which precede onset of disease). In many situations it will be clear that the exposures reported predated disease onset (Example 6.vii). However, in some situations it will not be clear whether exposures measured in a case–control study could be a consequence of disease (Example 6.viii).

Example 6.vii

A case–control study was undertaken to test the hypothesis that the younger a child is in a school year, the greater risk of emotional and behavioural problems. Children aged 5–15 years of age were included and those with a psychiatric diagnosis (cases) were compared to those without (controls). Risk of being a case was increased among those with a lower 'relative age' in the school year. In this example, it is reasonable to assume that being young in a school year is not a consequence of having a psychiatric diagnosis (see 'Further reading').

Example 6.viii

A case–control study of pancreatic cancer investigated whether there were differences in telomere length between cases and controls. Telomeres are the end of chromosomes and are hypothesized to be involved in the pathogenesis of disease. Cases were more likely to have short telomeres compared to controls. However, in interpreting the results it is not clear that such differences precede the development of pancreatic cancer—they may be a consequence of having the disease (see 'Further reading').

The crucial aspects in any such study will be the criteria for cases and controls and the sampling frame(s) from which they are selected, and also whether cases and controls are matched. Matching is a technique which can be used to control for confounding factors (i.e. risk factors for the disease of interest and related to the exposure of interest) and may involve matching cases and controls at the individual or group level. This is discussed in detail in Chapter 8.

In order to ensure the comparability of information from cases and controls, study procedures should ensure that the collection of information is as similar as possible. This will include the information being collected by the same techniques (e.g. interviewer, questionnaire) in the same setting (e.g. hospital, home) and at the same calendar time. Ideally, if the study involves face-to-face interview, the interviewer should not be aware of the case or control status of the subject, although this is often not practical. However, it is possible, usually, to ensure that the interviewer is not aware of the specific hypotheses under investigation: this reduces the possibility of observer bias, which is discussed further in Section 19.4.

In most situations the case–control study will be able to be conducted in the short to medium term. The rate-limiting step in study conduct will usually be the identification of cases, and for particularly rare diseases it may be necessary to have recruitment on a national or international basis, in order to identify enough cases within a reasonable time period.

6.4 **The cohort study**

A cohort study involves one or more groups of subjects, defined by their exposure status and free of the disease of interest, being followed through time to identify disease onset. The purpose is to determine whether initial exposure status influences risk of subsequent disease. Two particular types of cohort study are the *prospective cohort study* and the *retrospective cohort study*. The only difference between these approaches is with respect to the timing of collecting exposure and disease information (Fig. 6.2).

In the prospective approach, cohort(s) are identified by their exposure status presently and are followed-up to determine any future disease onset (Example 6.ix). The retrospective approach identifies the exposure status of cohort(s) in the past and in a parallel sense they are 'followed-up' until the present time, when their disease status is determined (Example 6.x). The latter approach will undoubtedly be quicker and less expensive, but may not always be appropriate or possible.

A retrospective study will:

◆ rely on there being sufficient information available on past exposure status and on being able to determine current disease status;

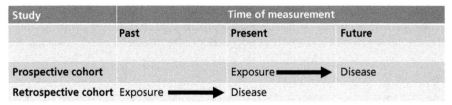

Figure 6.2 Design of prospective and retrospective cohort studies.

♦ involve identification of cohort subjects on national (disease) registers or individually tracing subjects;

and may need to consider whether information is available:

♦ on changes in exposure status;

♦ on other risk factors for the disease which are potentially associated with the exposure status of interest, that is, confounding factors (see Chapter 18).

The major advantages of a prospective study are that it can be determined which exposure is measured and how; if and when change in exposure status is measured; procedures to allow future identification and tracing can be implemented; the nature and timing of outcome measures can be determined. Consequently, however, the timescale of the study will be considerably longer and for some outcomes such as cancer and death, may be as long as 20–30 years.

Overall, the cohort approach is suitable when the disease outcome is common, and is particularly suited to determine the effects of exposure on a variety of disease outcomes. Given exposure status when measured will refer to 'current status' and this is measured prior to disease onset, the issues of temporality of disease/exposure, problems with recall, and particularly recall bias will not, in general, affect cohort studies. For this reason in particular, prospective studies can deliver high-quality epidemiological evidence in relation to effects of exposures.

Example 6.ix

A study enrolled persons 30–44 years of age who were non-smokers. It collected information on sociodemographic and lifestyle factors on participants and persons with whom they lived. It planned to follow-up participants and collect similar information annually. One of the principal objectives was to determine whether non-smokers who lived with smokers (i.e. who were likely to be exposed to passive smoke) had a higher risk of respiratory disease than non-smokers who lived with other non-smokers. The investigators determined that they would need to follow-up the cohort for 25 years in order for enough disease outcomes to have developed.

Example 6.x

Investigators wished to determine whether low birth weight was associated with an increased risk of cardiovascular death. They identified a register set up in the 1960s which recorded all births in a region and which included information on aspects of pregnancy and birth. This allowed the investigators to identify low birth weight (and other) babies. They then identified from national registers those persons who were now alive/ dead and if they had died, whether it was related to cardiovascular disease.

In some instances, it is beneficial to combine the case–control and cohort approaches: namely a case–control study nested within a cohort study (known as a *nested case–control study*). Assessment of exposure, or one aspect of exposure, may be very time-consuming and costly, and instead of undertaking measurement on everyone in a cohort, it may be more prudent to wait to determine which subjects in a cohort develop the disease under study (i.e. the cases for the nested case–control study). When a case occurs, a control is selected from persons in the cohort who are in follow-up at that time and who have not developed the disease of interest (Example 6.xi).

Example 6.xi

Investigators undertook a prospective cohort study to investigate the aetiology of colorectal cancer. One area of interest was the role of medications (specifically non-steroidal anti-inflammatory drugs). Medication history was determined by medical record review which was time-consuming (and therefore expensive) to collect. Therefore, medication review was only undertaken for cases (when they were identified) and persons selected as controls.

6.5 **Other observational studies**

6.5.1 **Case-crossover study**

It has been noted that MI (heart attacks) occur in a diurnal pattern with a peak in the late morning, troughs in the late evening and during the night. Investigating the aetiology is most obviously answered by a case–control study with cases defined as persons diagnosed with a MI and controls persons without such a diagnosis. All subjects could be asked about activities in the three-hour period before the MI (cases), while controls could be asked about activities in a reference three-hour period. If the case–control study was individually matched, the reference period for controls could be the same as their matched cases.

An alternative approach is the case-crossover study (Example 6.xii). In this design, cases are persons who had been diagnosed with a MI and exposures recorded in, say, the three-hour period prior to the myocardial infarction. Exposures would be compared with those in the same persons during a reference three-hour period to answer the question 'What was unusual about the period before the myocardial infarction?'. The reference period could be, for example, the same three-hour period: 24 hours prior, the previous working or non-working day, or the previous week (Fig. 6.3).

This design is potentially useful if:

◆ The onset of the outcome of interest is measurable (e.g. the precise time of onset of a motor vehicle accident is usually possible, but it is more difficult to pinpoint the onset of an episode of fatigue);

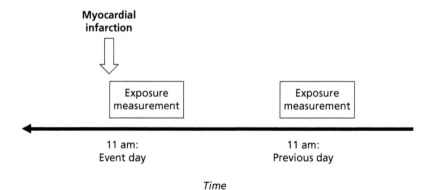

Figure 6.3 Design of case-crossover study using a reference period one day prior to the event day.

♦ The effects of exposure are transient (e.g. exposures experienced today should not exert an effect several days later);

♦ There is a crossover in exposure in some subjects (i.e. this cannot be used to examine exposures which, in individuals, are invariant).

Example 6.xii

Investigators wished to determine whether episodes of gout were related to alcohol consumption and they designed a case-crossover study. Cases were identified by having a clinically confirmed episode of gout. They were interviewed about lifestyle including alcohol consumption in the 12 hours prior to onset. The reference period chosen was the same 12-hour period 7 days previously. Alcohol consumption was compared in both exposure periods.

Issues to consider in planning a case-crossover study include what control period or periods are appropriate, confounding factors, and 'exposure opportunity'. Although confounding factors are less of an issue than when comparing two different populations (cases and controls), risk factors for the disease of interest (whose pattern of exposure is associated with the exposure of interest) can potentially confound the relationship and do need to be taken into account. These issues are discussed further in Chapter 18. Exposure opportunity refers to the ability to have the exposure of interest in the reference period. For example, if a study is considering the relationship between motor vehicle accidents and use of mobile phones while driving, then a participant will definitely have been driving in the exposure period which ended with a motor vehicle accident but may not have been driving in the reference exposure period. These issues are discussed further in articles in the 'Further reading' section.

6.5.2 **Case–cohort study**

The use of the case–control study nested within a cohort was introduced in Section 6.3. However, if a cohort has several nested case–control studies conducted within it, it seems inefficient that separate control groups need to be sampled, approached for a substudy, and then have data collected. In this situation a case–cohort may be a more efficient alternative design: here a sample of participants in the cohort are selected at baseline and all the detailed and/or expensive exposure assessment conducted in this group. In addition, cases (when they occur as the cohort is followed-up) for each of the substudies will have the relevant detailed exposure assessment carried out. The design is essentially an unmatched nested case–control study. This study retains the major advantage of the cohort study in that exposure assessment is carried out before the development of the disease of interest. Although the analysis is slightly more complicated than a case–control study, there are some practical advantages including that all the detailed assessment on 'controls' can be achieved at the beginning of the study, whereas in the case–control study one needs to wait to cases develop before a control is selected. In contrast, some of the controls selected will subsequently develop one of the diseases of interest in the substudies and therefore the number of non-cases available will be less than the number of controls originally selected. Thus, if it is estimated that at most 10% of the controls would develop one of the diseases of interest for the substudies, then the number of controls selected originally would have to be increased accordingly.

6.5.3 **Migrant study**

In animal studies, investigators have the possibility of directly controlling the environment, personal behaviour (e.g. diet), and even genetic factors which are hypothesized as being important in disease occurrence. In contrast, in free-living populations, individuals are free to decide on their diet and to choose, for example, whether they smoke, drink alcohol, or take regular exercise.

Intervening to effect changes in such lifestyle factors within controlled studies is possible, but is challenging and usually very expensive. Another option is to take advantage of 'natural experiments' where a change in lifestyle is being made by a large group of individuals. One such example is migrants moving from one country to another. This can provide the epidemiologist with important information on the influences on disease occurrence if the country of origin and new host country have different rates of the disease(s) of interest. This is particularly true when considering the relative roles of genetic and environmental factors on disease. The process of migration involves no change to the genetic make-up of an individual but is likely to result in changes to climate experienced, work, diet, and the psychosocial environment (Example 6.xiii).

Let us assume that large groups of individuals have migrated from country A to country B and that these countries have low and high rates of disease X, respectively. If the migrants manifest high rates of disease in their new country, it may be assumed that some environmental factors are important in determining disease risk. In contrast if the group maintains a low risk of disease X, there are several possibilities, including (a) genetic factors are the principal influence on disease risk; (b) although environmental factors are important, the migrants have maintained a lifestyle that is very similar to their country of origin; (c) lifestyle factors are important but the migrants were exposed to them at too old an age for them to have an important influence on disease risk. Further information may be obtained by studying not only the migrants themselves, but successive generations of migrants in the new home country. However, in such subjects there may be changes not only in environmental factors but also genetic factors.

Example 6.xiii

Breast cancer incidence in the United States is relatively high in comparison to other countries. Investigators examined the incidence of breast cancer in recent migrants to the United States. Those who had come from countries with lower incidence rates, exhibited incidence rates that were higher than their country of origin, but not as high as those of the United States. Those migrants who had come from countries with higher incidence rates still experienced rates that were higher than those in the whole United States population, but not as high in comparison to their country of origin. It was concluded therefore that the migrants' new environment in the United States did alter the risks of them developing breast cancer. Factors which could contribute to this may include lifestyle factors such as diet.

In any study of migrants, however, one concern is how representative the migrants are of their original country. Intuitively, it seems likely that those who are ill, have poor levels of general health, or low educational levels would be less likely to migrate. They may also differ in other individual ways (e.g. personality) and their lifestyle. Such factors complicate the direct comparison between disease rates in their old and new home countries. The studies can also be difficult to conduct. Effective ways of identifying the migrants in their new home country is necessary and following them prospectively to determine disease onset. It obviously becomes easier if the information is collected on a routine basis (e.g. death information or cancer occurrence) with information on their country of birth.

6.5.4 **Mendelian randomization study**

One of the main issues in interpreting an association between an exposure and a disease, is to what extent the association is confounded. For example, if a prospective cohort study finds that persons with low levels of vegetable consumption have an excess risk of dying in the 10 years after study enrolment—to what extent could that be explained by other lifestyle factors which may be more common in persons with low vegetable consumption? Such factors might include low fruit intake, high fat consumption, high alcohol intake, low levels of physical activity and smoking—and the

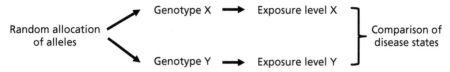

Figure 6.4 Mendelian randomization study design.

more strongly that these factors are associated with low vegetable consumption, the more difficult it is to disentangle their effects.

Mendelian randomization is a study design which takes advantages of genetic differences between individuals which affect their level of exposure to a specific factor under study. It takes advantage of the fact that inheritance of a trait is independent of inheritance of other traits and its major strength is that associations between genetic variants and disease are not generally confounded by other exposures. Indeed, individuals will usually not be aware of their genetic variant and its influence on exposure. The design has therefore been likened to a randomized controlled trial where the randomization to treatment is the genetic variant which an individual inherits (Fig. 6.4).

In order to undertake a Mendelian randomization study, one needs to identify a genetic variant which is related to the exposure under study. An alternative is to determine a genetic risk score based on a combination of genetic variants (Example 6.xiv). The effects observed in such studies from genetic variants are likely to be small and thus large sample sizes will be required.

There are assumptions made in undertaking a Mendelian randomization study. Firstly, that the effect of the genetic variant(s) chosen is (are) assumed to be through the pathway under study rather than an alternative pathway. For example, if a genetic variant is linked to level of alcohol consumption it is assumed that it does not have effects on other, potentially relevant pathways such as influencing the likelihood of smoking cigarettes, for disease occurrence (i.e. that pleiotropy does not exist). Secondly, it is assumed that the genetic variant under study is inherited independently of other genetic variants (i.e. it is in linkage disequilibrium with other genetic variants).

Example 6.xiv

Investigators wished to investigate whether high body mass index (BMI) is associated with knee osteoarthritis (OA). They recognized that high BMI was strongly associated with poor diet, smoking and low levels of physical activity and felt that the independent contribution of high BMI would be difficult to establish. Instead, information from genetic association studies, had demonstrated several genetic variants (single nucleotide polymorphisms (SNPs)) which were associated with a high BMI, allowing them to construct a genetic risk score for individuals. Using participants in a large cohort study of knee OA who had provided biological samples for genetic analysis, they confirmed that their genetic risk score was associated with the likelihood of having a high BMI. They also demonstrated that this genetic risk score was related to the likelihood of developing knee OA in the study. This suggested that BMI was causally related to developing knee OA. In such a study design there is no concern about reverse causality (knee osteoarthritis resulting in a high BMI) nor does knee OA result in changes to genes. However, it is assumed that the identified genetic variants do not increase the risk of knee OA by a mechanism other than through a high BMI (Fig. 6.5).

6.5.5 **Ecologic study**

The aforementioned studies have all collected information at the level of the individual, however, in an ecologic (also called a correlation) study, information is analysed not at the individual level but at group level. The unit on which measurement is made may be, for example, schools, towns, or countries (Example 6.xv).

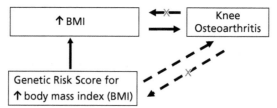

Figure 6.5 Mendelian randomization study design to investigate relationship between high body mass index (BMI) and knee osteoarthritis.

Example 6.xv

Testicular cancer rates have been increasing worldwide. Animal studies have suggested that cocoa can have toxic effects on the testis and cocoa consumption has also been increasing globally. A study was conducted to determine whether there was a relationship, at country level, between levels of cocoa consumption and the incidence of testicular cancer. The results demonstrate a strong positive correlation (Fig. 6.6). Therefore, the results are consistent with a hypothesis that cocoa may have toxic effects on the testis. However, the results cannot suggest a causal relationship—particularly when information is not available on potential confounding factors (risk factors for testicular cancer the prevalence of which is related to levels of cocoa consumption).

Example 6.xvi

Fluoride has been shown to be preventive for caries and therefore investigators wished to determine whether areas with fluoride in the water supply had lower prevalence of caries in children. They assessed the prevalence of caries in each region and also tabulated whether they had fluoride added to their water supply, and if not, what the natural level was of fluoride in the water. This showed that areas with fluoride added to their water had lower prevalence of caries and among those without fluoride added, the natural level was inversely related to the prevalence of caries.

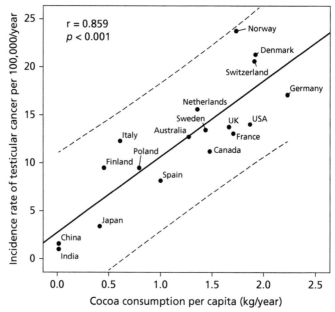

Figure 6.6 Correlation between testicular cancer incidence rates for 20–34 years-olds (1998–2002) and per capita cocoa consumption (1965–1980) in 18 countries.

Reproduced from Giannandrea F. (2009) Correlation analysis of cocoa consumption data with worldwide incidence rates of testicular cancer and hypospadias. *International Journal of Environmental Research and Public Health*. Vol 6 Issue 2, pp. 568–78. Open Access.

The advantage of this type of study is that it is generally inexpensive and quick to conduct. This is especially true if the data on disease and exposure is available from routine sources. Even if, for example, the information on level of exposure is not available, the effort to collect this on the aggregated units will generally be less than collecting exposure information on a much larger number of individuals (Example 6.xvi).

The outcome of such a study will be to conclude only that the study either supports or does not support a hypothesis about a specific exposure-disease relationship. It may also provide some information on the potential type and strength of any relationship which is found. However, it does have serious weaknesses. There is very rarely information on factors which could potentially confound an observed relationship between exposure and disease (see Chapter 18 for a discussion of confounding), and this is the greatest drawback to such studies.

If an association is demonstrated in an ecologic study, and even if information is available on potential confounding factors, it does not, however, guarantee that the relationship holds at the level of the individual. For example, there may be a positive association between per capita fat consumption and the incidence of a disease across countries, but *within* each country it is possible that a higher level of fat consumption results in a lower risk of disease. Drawing inappropriate conclusions about the relationship between an exposure and disease in individuals from ecologic studies has been termed the *ecologic fallacy*.

6.6 **Randomized controlled trials**

All the study designs previously discussed in this chapter are observational (i.e. they are studying free-living populations who make a choice about their lifestyle, work, and so on). As discussed this means that certain habits tend to cluster in individuals such as alcohol drinking, cigarette smoking, aspects of diet, and this means it is difficult to disentangle their individual effects. More formally the apparent effect of an exposure on disease risk is likely to be confounded. One way to address confounding is in study design, namely to randomly allocate exposures to individuals. Participants enter a study and then their allocation to an arm of the study is determined randomly, although there may be stratification to ensure certain key characteristics are balanced between studies (Example 6.xvii, Fig. 6.7).

Example 6.xvii

An investigator wished to determine whether regular physical activity was related to good mental health. Persons who did not regularly exercise were invited to take part in the trial. Participants were allocated at random either to a group exercise programme conducted over 12 weeks or not and were followed-up at 12 weeks and 24 weeks post-randomization. Randomization was stratified by sex and age group to ensure that these were evenly distributed between study arms. At follow-up, the mental health of both groups was measured.

This design provides very strong evidence, all other things being equal, about the causal role of an exposure on outcome. However, it is not suitable or feasible to answer many questions:

◆ these studies are very expensive and are conducted within stringent governance procedures, particularly because of the possibility of causing harm;

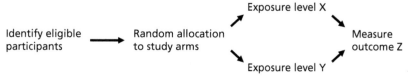

Figure 6.7 Randomized controlled trials.

◆ they assess the effect of one exposure, usually over the short-term;

◆ for many exposures it is either not feasible or ethical to consider a randomized controlled trial (e.g. cigarette smoking or alcohol consumption).

There are also practical issues which may make a randomized controlled trial less ideal than it seems:

◆ Not all persons allocated to a study arm will actually 'receive' the level of exposure intended. For example, in Example 6.xvii, people allocated to an exercise arm may not attend all of the sessions and those not randomized to the exercise arm may decide to organize to attend such a class, thinking it may be beneficial.

◆ Unless there is a placebo arm, an intervention will consist of specific effects (such as an exercise class) as well as non-specific effects (the social effect of participating in a group activity). For many non-pharmacological exposures there will not be an obvious placebo.

◆ Persons agreeing to take part in a trial may not be representative of the wider population either because of eligibility criteria (e.g. through concern about safety in certain groups of people) or through choice (e.g. persons who take part in a trial examining exercise may only be those people who believe exercise to be beneficial).

6.7 **Choice of study design**

It is apparent that many questions can be addressed by several different study designs and thus the decision has to be made as to the most appropriate design to answer a particular question. The choice is often between feasibility, that is, obtaining an answer within a required timescale, and validity (i.e. obtaining the most accurate answer). Common sense dictates that one without the other negates the value of undertaking the study and also that the two are not mutually exclusive. The decision is normally based on an appraisal of both scientific and logistic considerations. An overview is provided in Table 6.1. There are several broad considerations:

◆ Ecologic and migrant studies are primarily used to generate hypotheses about the aetiology of disease. If appropriate information is routinely collected, they can be conducted quickly and at low cost.

Table 6.1 Factors influencing choice of study design

Consideration	Study choice
Disease rare	Case–control
Investigating multiple exposures on single disease	Case–control
Investigating multiple outcomes from single exposure	Cohort
Accurate assessment of exposure	Prospective cohort
Anxiety about stability of exposure status	Prospective cohort
Register exists of person with relevant exposure	Retrospective cohort
Short-term effect of exposure and time of disease onset easily measurable	Case-crossover
Genetic variant identified strongly related to exposure	Mendelian randomization
Evaluation of exposure strongly affected by confounding, has short-term effects, no major harms and there is a comparison 'placebo'	Randomized controlled trial

- The cohort approach allows identification of multiple disease outcomes from a single exposure, whereas the case–control approach allows identification of multiple exposures associated with a single disease entity.

- The lack of quality control of data from a retrospective cohort study, particularly on exposure status, would support a prospective approach. Similarly, data may be sufficient for the primary exposure of interest, but may be lacking on possible confounders (see Chapter 18) that need to be considered.

- The prospective cohort approach, in theory, also permits setting up systems to notify change in exposure status during the follow-up period, an option that may be lacking in a retrospectively derived cohort with only 'point' data on exposure.

- Prospective cohort studies suffer from the problems of potential and unknown loss-to-follow-up rates: it is increasingly difficult to track down individuals after a time interval. Assessment of disease status may then be impossible from within the study.

- Cohort studies are substantially more expensive than the smaller case–control approach. The rarer the disease the more impracticable the cohort approach becomes. Studies that involve population screening to derive either current or future cases are more expensive than those that can utilize an existing morbidity recording system, such as a population-based cancer register.

- Time is relevant in so far as public health questions that require an immediate answer, for example, regarding risks from current occupational exposure, might not be able to wait for the 10 years it might take for a prospective cohort study to reach an answer.

Chapter 17 has information on the statistical analysis of the study designs considered.

Next are several examples of studies, with suggested designs, as a guide to how a choice is made.

Example 6.xviii

Several persons who worked on the same production line within a factory had reported that they had developed colon cancer—and worried that their disease was linked to their occupational exposure. Excellent occupational records existed going back over several years. The most obvious approach to the study was to use such records to establish a retrospective cohort and determine persons who worked in different production lines within the factory and then identify who had developed cancer subsequently. This would give results far quicker than mounting a prospective study. The latter strategy would, however, have permitted the additional collection, at 'baseline', of other potential confounding factors such as diet, smoking, and family history.

Example 6.xix

A researcher considered that a particular serum marker early in pregnancy might predict the future development of a relatively rare congenital anomaly. It was decided to mount a 'nested' case–control study storing serum from a large number of pregnant women at their first antenatal visit. Subsequently, the sera from all babies born with this anomaly would then be assayed together with sera from a sample of normal infants, matched according to date of delivery. This approach made efficient use of an expensive assay technique.

Example 6.xx

It had been observed that babies born during winter months had lower bone mass than those born at other times in the year. It was hypothesized that this may be due to lower levels of vitamin D in the mothers. However, there was a concern that in an observational study it would be difficult to identify the effects of vitamin D from other nutrients to which it was closely related and intake of which also varies according to season. A randomized controlled trial was therefore designed, whereby mothers were randomized to either receive vitamin D supplements during pregnancy or not. The outcome measured was maternal vitamin D and infant bone mass.

Example 6.xxi

A gynaecologist wished to examine the effectiveness of cervical cancer screening in reducing the incidence of invasive carcinoma. She approached this by undertaking a case–control study comparing the history of cervical smears (the exposure) in a series of women presenting with invasive carcinoma (the cases) to that in a series of normal women from the population (the controls). The hypothesis was that the cases would be less likely to have been screened. In this example, a case–control study was being used to examine the effect of a therapeutic or preventive intervention. Although such questions are more ideally addressed by a randomized prospective trial, as suggested earlier the case–control study can give a quick answer for relatively rare events, particularly for studies in which, for ethical or other reasons, randomization may be difficult.

Example 6.xxii

A government department of health had been lobbied about making it illegal to use mobile phones while driving, on the basis that they might increase the risk of a motor vehicle accident. The government requested further evidence of an association: they were not persuaded the association was causal and that it could be that persons who use mobile phones were generally persons who took greater risks. It was decided to adopt a case-crossover study where motor vehicle accidents reported to the police were identified and, using mobile phone records, use was measured in the 30 minutes prior to the accident. Comparison periods were (a) the same 30 minutes on the last working/non-working day and (b) the same 30 minutes seven days previously. These were used to determine whether mobile phone use was more common in the period before the 'crash' and whether risk was greater in the minutes close to the accident.

Example 6.xxiii

A psychiatrist wished to examine the influence of strong family support on reducing the suicide rate after hospital discharge with acute schizophrenia. He felt that the measurement of family support had to be prospective and opted for a prospective cohort study. The option of a case–control study—by comparing the family support (the exposure) in a series of schizophrenic patients who had committed suicide since hospital discharge (the cases) with that in a series of schizophrenic patients who had survived (the controls)—was dropped, given the problems in retrospectively assessing family support in the face of a recent suicide.

Example 6.xxiv

A cardiologist wished to examine the influence of the severity of angina on the subsequent risk of first MI. He decided to undertake a prospective cohort study following up two groups: an 'exposed' group with anginal attacks occurring on walking on level ground, and an 'unexposed' group whose attacks occurred only on walking up an incline. In this example, the prospective cohort approach was used to assess the influence of specific risk factors on disease prognosis, rather than on disease development per se.

Example 6.xxv

A general practitioner wished to examine the effect of salt intake on hypertension. In a pilot study, she reached the conclusion that a randomized trial was impracticable as the compliance in subjects allocated to a low-salt diet was likely to be low, and further, a proportion of subjects in the normal diet group, at their own instigation, attempted to reduce salt. She therefore conducted a case–control study and found that those whose measured blood pressure, on each of three measurements, satisfied criteria for hypertension (cases) had higher salt intake, measured using a three-day food diary, than those who did not (controls).

Example 6.xxvi

The hypothesis was proposed that there was an increased risk of MI following the death of a spouse. A case–control study was a potential strategy given the relative ease of verifying the exposure (i.e. death of a spouse). However, this exposure was likely to be rare. It was therefore necessary to undertake a more expensive and time-consuming prospective cohort study.

Example 6.xxvii

A research group was investigating the role of certain medications in the aetiology of head and neck cancer and cancers of the œsophagus, colon, and rectum. They had access to a large prospective cohort study which was measuring several outcomes (including cancer). It was too labour-intensive and expensive to conduct a full record review of medications for all persons in the cohort. They therefore conducted a case–cohort study. A medical record review was conducted for 20% of the cohort at the time of recruitment and then a record review for each person developing one of the outcomes of interest.

Example 6.xxviii

A psychiatrist wished to examine the relationship between anxiety and depression and persistent headache. He hypothesized that any observed relationship was because headaches may lead to anxiety and depression, rather than the converse. He therefore conducted a prospective cohort study, measuring levels of anxiety and depression among people who did not report headaches and followed them over one year to determine who developed symptoms. Having high levels of anxiety and/or depression resulted in an increased risk of reporting headache at follow-up.

Further reading

Case–control studies

Case–control studies (assessing differential recall)

McBeth J, Morris S, Benjamin S, Silman AJ, Macfarlane GJ (2001). Associations between adverse events in childhood and chronic widespread pain in adulthood: are they explained by differential recall? *J Rheumatol*, **28**(10), 2305–9.

Rugbjerg K, Harris MA, Shen H, *et al.* (2011). Pesticide exposure and risk of Parkinson's disease—a population-based case-control study evaluating the potential for recall bias. *Scand J Work Environ Health*, **37**(5), 427–36.

Case–control studies (temporality of association)

Goodman R, Gledhill J, Ford T (2003). Child psychiatric disorder and relative age within school year: cross-sectional survey of large population sample. *BMJ*, **327**(7413), 472.

Skinner HG, Gangnon RE, Litzelman K, *et al.* (2012). Telomere length and pancreatic cancer: a case-control study. *Cancer Epidemiol Biomarkers Prev*, **21**(11), 2095–100.

Nested case–control studies

Andersson L, Bryngelsson IL, Ngo Y, Ohlson CG, Westberg H (2019). Exposure assessment and modeling of quartz in Swedish iron foundries for a nested case-control study on lung cancer. *J Occup Environ Hyg*, **9**(2), 110–19.

Cohort studies

Enstrom JE, Kabat GC (2003). Environmental tobacco smoke and tobacco related mortality in a prospective study of Californians, 1960–98. *BMJ*, **326**(7398), 1057.

Case-crossover studies

Maclure M (1991). The case-crossover design: a method for studying transient effects on the risk of acute events. *Am J Epidemiol*, **133**(2), 144–53.

Mittleman MA, Maclure M, Tofler GH, *et al.* (1993). Triggering of acute myocardial infarction by heavy physical exertion. Protection against triggering by regular exertion. Determinants of Myocardial Infarction Onset Study Investigators. *N Engl J Med*, **329**(23), 1677–83.

Zhang Y, Neogi T, Chen C, *et al.* (2012). Cherry consumption and decreased risk of recurrent gout attacks. *Arthritis Rheum*, **64**(12), 4004–11.

Case–cohort studies

Bernatsky S, Joseph L, Boivin JF, *et al.* (2008). The relationship between cancer and medication exposures in systemic lupus erythematosus: a case–cohort study. *Ann Rheum Dis*, **67**(1), 74–9.

Mittleman MA, Maclure M, Tofler GH, *et al.* (1993). Triggering of acute myocardial infarction by heavy physical exertion. Protection against triggering by regular exertion. Determinants of Myocardial Infarction Onset Study Investigators. *N Engl J Med*, **329**(23), 1677–83.

Mendelian randomization studies

C Reactive Protein Coronary Heart Disease Genetics Collaboration (CCGC), Wensley F, Gao P, *et al.* (2011). Association between C reactive protein and coronary heart disease: mendelian randomisation analysis based on individual participant data. *BMJ*, **342**, d548.

Smith GD, Ebrahim S (2004). Mendelian randomization: prospects, potentials, and limitations. *Int J Epidemiol*, **33**(1), 30–42.

Ecological studies

Giannandrea F (2009). Correlation analysis of cocoa consumption data with worldwide incidence rates of testicular cancer and hypospadias. *Int J Environ Res Public Health*, **6**(2), 568–78.

Migrant studies

Zhang H, Chen Z, Cheng J, *et al.* (2010). The high incidence of esophageal cancer in parts of China may result primarily from genetic rather than environmental factors. *Dis Esophagus*, **23**(5), 392–7.

Randomized controlled trials

Lippman SM, Klein EA, Goodman PJ, *et al.* (2009). Effect of selenium and vitamin E on risk of prostate cancer and other cancers: the Selenium and Vitamin E Cancer Prevention Trial (SELECT). *JAMA*, **301**(1), 39–51.

Chapter 7

Quantifying the association between exposures and diseases

Which measure?

7.1 Introduction

Much epidemiological endeavour is directed towards attempting to discover the aetiology (i.e. the causes) of particular diseases, with a view to prevention. Chapter 6 discussed the options available in terms of epidemiological study design. In practice, most diseases do not have a single identifiable cause, such as infection with a specific microorganism or exposure to a particular toxin or physical trauma. By contrast, it appears that the aetiology of most common diseases globally are multifactorial and represent the effects of a combination of genetic, constitutional, and environmental factors. Thus, most exposures investigated are neither sufficient (i.e. they will not cause disease on their own), nor necessary (i.e. the disease can occur in the absence of that exposure). A simple example is that although smoking is common and is a risk factor for the development of lung cancer, not all individuals who develop lung cancer smoke and not all smokers develop lung cancer. This is discussed in greater detail in Chapter 20.

Epidemiological studies, and in particular their subsequent analysis, are therefore aimed at quantifying the level of increased risk when exposed to a particular factor, as this chapter explains. The effect measure which can be obtained to quantify the strength of the association, varies according to the type of study conducted.

7.2 Prevalence ratio

In Chapter 2 the concept of disease prevalence was introduced and in Chapter 6, how this could be measured by means of a cross-sectional study was discussed. Although primarily cross-sectional studies are for measuring disease burden and healthcare planning, in Chapter 6, it was included as one study design which can evaluate potential aetiological factors of a disease. The effect measure used to assess association in this context is prevalence ratio (sometime referred to as prevalence rate ratio, although we previously noted that prevalence is not actually a rate) (Example 7.i).

Example 7.i

A cross-sectional study in a small town collected information from individuals on gastrointestinal (GI) symptoms during the past week and also details of the company which supplied their household water. Of the 2,000 persons whose water was supplied by 'Spring Water', 150 persons reported severe GI symptoms, while among the 5,000 persons supplied by 'Still Clear', 370 persons reported GI symptoms. The prevalence of severe GI symptoms in the two groups was 0.075 and 0.074, respectively, giving a prevalence ratio of 1.01. This demonstrated that prevalence was almost identical in the two groups and severe GI symptoms were not related to household water supply.

7.3 **Risk ratio**

Risk is the probability that an individual develops a disease of interest within a specified time period and, over a population, is estimated by the cumulative incidence (average risk) in that time period. Such a measure could be derived from following up a cohort over time in which no new cohort members enter and no existing members leave (a 'closed' cohort). Comparing the risk of disease in two cohorts with different exposure experiences would allow one to derive a risk ratio (Example 7.ii). This is sometimes referred to also as 'relative risk'.

Example 7.ii

A cohort study was conducted of students in a university hall of residence during the academic year 2017–2018. Students who were not overweight or obese at the start of the university year were eligible for study. In terms of their risk of being overweight or obese at the end of the academic year, those who registered to receive vegetarian or vegan meals in the hall of residence (risk = 0.09) were compared to those who did not (risk = 0.12). This allowed a risk ratio 0.75 (i.e. 0.09/0.12) to be calculated comparing the two groups. It demonstrated that the risk of students becoming overweight or obese was relatively small, but was lower in those who opted to receive vegetarian or vegan meals.

7.4 **Rate ratios**

A cohort study measuring incidence (density) rates allows the rates in two or more subcohorts to be calculated and compared directly. Given that the comparison is of two rates, this ratio is referred to as a rate ratio. If a cohort study was examining the effect of diet on health, analysis may focus on comparing rates of cancer, for example, in vegetarians, vegans, and persons eating meat.

Example 7.iii

A prospective cohort study at a single medical centre identified all strokes which occurred among registered patients. The incidence rates among those who were and who were not diabetic were 4.7 and 1.6, respectively, per 1,000 person–years of follow-up. The rate ratio of 2.9 (i.e. 4.7/1.6) indicates that that those with diabetes had almost three times the rate of strokes in comparison to those who were not diabetic.

Analogous to the interpretation of risk ratios, when comparing the rate of disease in population A against population B, rate ratio (i.e. rate in A/rate in B) values above 1 indicate a higher rate in A, values below 1 indicate a higher rate in B, while a value of 1 implies equal rates in both groups.

7.5 **Odds ratios**

Ratios of prevalence, risk, or rates derived from cross-sectional and cohort studies are attractive measures to estimate since they reflect what the epidemiologist generally wishes to know and are intuitive to interpret. What is the change in rate/risk/prevalence of disease associated with being exposed to a particular factor? They are also easily communicated to a wider audience (e.g. 'persons who drink more than 20 units of alcohol per day double their risk of disease X' or 'those persons who report no regular exercise are twice as likely to be overweight').

In a case–control study, two groups of subjects are selected according to disease status—a group with disease and a sample of those without disease. In some instances, cases and controls are derived from a population study or the sampling fractions of cases and controls is known and, thus, the rate ratio, risk ratio, or prevalence ratio cannot be calculated. Typically, however, case–control studies have not recruited these groups from a known population base. Thus, it is not possible to determine the prevalence of disease among subjects exposed to a particular factor in comparison to those not exposed.

Instead one can calculate the odds of exposure among the cases and compare this to the odds of exposure among the controls. The odds of exposure in a group is simply the number exposed in a group divided by the number not exposed. If the odds of exposure among subjects with disease (cases) is determined and similarly the odds of exposure among subjects without disease (controls), then the ratio of these two odds ratio can be calculated as:

Odds of exposure among cases/odds of exposure among controls.

If this ratio is above 1, the odds of cases being exposed is greater than the odds of controls being exposed, and if the ratio is less than 1, the opposite is true. If the ratio is close or equal to 1, it implies that the odds of exposure are very similar in the two groups.

Example 7.iv

Among 200 patients with acute appendicitis (cases), 40 had a recent history of urinary tract infection (UTI). The odds of exposure (to UTI) were therefore $\frac{40}{160}$ or 0.25. By contrast in 120 persons without acute appendicitis (controls), only 12 had a recent history of UTI: an odds of exposure of $\frac{12}{108}$ or 0.11. The odds ratio of 2.25 indicates that the odds of those with appendicitis of having a recent UTI was more than twice those without appendicitis (Table 7.1).

Table 7.1 Odds of exposure

	UTI	No UTI
Cases	40	160
Controls	12	108

Normally, given that most of an underlying population will not have the disorder under investigation, the odds ratio will be a good approximation to the risk ratio or rate ratio calculated from cohort studies (see 'Further reading').

7.6 **Risk or rate differences**

Although epidemiological studies, most commonly, consider ratios of risk and rates in groups because of their statistical properties, it can also be important to consider risk or rate differences. It is possible, for example, for there to be large ratio of rates between two groups, but for the difference in rates to be very small (Example 7.v).

Example 7.v

A cohort study followed-up women to determine the consequences of oral contraceptive use. An analysis of use in relation to invasive cervical cancer found that among 121,362 non-users, 76 developed cervical cancer by the end of the study while among 17,533 users, 22 had developed cervical cancer. There was therefore a doubling in risk associated with use:

$$Risk\ ratio = \frac{22/17,533}{76/121,362}$$

$$= 2.0$$

However, the risk difference is very small:

$$Risk\ difference\ =\ \frac{22}{17,533} - \frac{76}{121,362}$$
$$=\ 0.00125 - 0.0063$$
$$=\ 0.0062$$

In this example the absolute risk of invasive cervical cancer is very low and therefore even when the risk is doubled, the absolute risk is still very low. This risk or rate difference is also known as the excess risk (rate) or attributable risk (rate).

7.7 **Attributable fractions**

The public health physician may wish to estimate the proportionate contribution made by an exposure to explaining ('explain' does not necessarily infer causation) the cases of a disease of interest in a given population. This depends on:

- how strongly an exposure is related to the risk of disease; and
- the proportion of the population who are exposed.

This measure is known as the population attributable fraction. It seems obvious that an exposure which is strongly related to risk of disease and which is common would have a high population fraction, whereas an uncommon exposure only weakly related to disease risk would have a low population attributable fraction (Example 7.vi). The approach to the calculation of this is given in Chapter 17.

Example 7.vi

Researchers in Australia estimated the percentage of cancers attributed to tobacco smoking as 13%. So assuming a causal relationship, this would be the percentage by which the number of cases of cancer would decrease if no-one in Australia smoked. The highest population attributable fraction was 81% for lung cancer (which is strongly associated with smoking) but was 6% for colorectal cancers, which are much less strongly related to smoking (see 'Further reading').

7.8 **Precision of measures of association**

Obviously, the robustness of the estimates of all the measures of association discussed earlier are related to the size of the study. As studies are normally undertaken on samples, any estimate of association derived from a sample is subject to error in its ability to describe the effect in the populations from which the sample was derived. For example, an estimate of the error around a sample mean is obtained firstly by calculating the standard error (SE). Obtaining a range produced by adding and subtracting twice the SE (or, more precisely, 1.96 times the SE) to the mean obtained from the sample provides the 95% confidence interval. The basis for its calculation can be found in standard textbooks of medical statistics. The interpretation of a 95% confidence interval is that if the experiment was repeated 100 times, then the true value for the measure under study would be contained in the derived interval 95 times. Confidence intervals can also be calculated for each of the measures of association discussed here. The actual formulae used to calculate the 95% confidence intervals for the epidemiological measures of association and notes on their interpretation are given in Chapter 17.

7.9 **Categorization of exposures**

Epidemiological enquiry attempts to assess the association between exposure to a risk factor and disease. For the sake of simplicity epidemiological textbooks, begin by considering exposures which are dichotomous (i.e. have only two forms, e.g. yes/no). In practice, questions of interest often relate to change in the size of risk with increasing exposure. The available choices for considering exposures are shown in Table 7.2. Most exposure variables in practice are not easily dichotomized; and indeed, adopting such a split risks losing information and does not permit analysis of the crucial 'dose–risk' effect. There may be some exposures which are categorized, but there is no 'order' inherent to the categories such as region of residence or ethnicity. Some exposure variables have natural or recognized categories.

Many exposure data collected are of the continuous type, such as age, number of cigarettes smoked per/day, or body mass index (BMI). For classical analyses the exposure could either be classified according to some predetermined categories (such as World Health Organization categories of BMI for underweight, normal weight, overweight, and obese). For some exposures these might not exist and instead exposure levels could be split into strata, with equal numbers of individuals in each strata, typically thirds (tertiles), fourths (quartiles), or fifths (quintiles). This approach of forcing equal numbers in each category is also efficient from a statistical viewpoint. In more sophisticated statistical modelling the actual values themselves can be considered and risks calculated, for example, per one-year increase of age, or per 1 mmol/L increase in serum cholesterol. In many ways such an approach is better as it 'uses all the data', but most statistical methods of generating these risks would assume that the risk is linear, which may not be the case. Persons new to interpreting such data can often be misled in that the increase in risk per one-year increase

Table 7.2 Categorization of exposure

Exposure type	Exposure sample	Possible categorization
Dichotomous	Smoking	Ever/Never
Ordinal	Region of residence	Regions: A, B, C, D, and E
Quantiles	Social class	1 (high)—5 (low)
Continuous (stratified based on standard classification)	Body mass index (kgm^{-2})	World Health Organization classification Underweight (<18.5)/Normal (18.5–24.99)/ Overweight (25.0–29.99)/Obese (≥30)
Continuous (stratified based on equal groups)	Body mass index (kgm^{-2})	Tertiles: Lowest third/Middle third/Highest third
Continuous (stratified based on hypothesized biological effect)	Smoking	Never smoker Ex-smoker Currently smokes <1/1–5 cigs/6–10/>10 cigs/day
Continuous (treated as continuous value in statistical model)	Age (years) Serum cholesterol (mmol/L)	Actual age Actual cholesterol value

in age is often very small—but this can translate into a much larger effect, for example, by 10-year age increments.

Further reading

Population attributable fraction

Pandeya N, Wilson LF, Bain CJ, *et al.* (2015). Cancers in Australia in 2010 attributable to tobacco smoke. *Aust N Z J Public Health*, **39**(5), 464–70.

Odds ratios

Vandenbroucke JP, Pearce N (2012). Case-control studies: basic concepts. *Int J Epidemiol*, **41**(5), 1480–9.

Selection of populations and samples to study in studies of disease aetiology

Chapter 8

Studies of disease causation

8.1 Introduction

This chapter focuses on the practical issues in selecting subjects for epidemiological studies, with a particular emphasis on delivering as far as possible bias-free classical case–control and cohort studies in the real world. There are other study designs, such as case–cohort and crossover studies discussed in Chapter 6 but the principles in terms of selection of subjects for study are the same as discussed next.

8.2 Case–control studies: overview

In simplest terms, the issues are who should be the cases and, given that, who should be the controls. In each instance the needs are to identify the sampling frame and then what should be the process for selecting the specific sample or subsamples needed for study.

8.2.1 Recruitment of cases

The task typically is to identify subjects with a disorder or a health state suitably defined. There are two major issues to be addressed. These are:

1. what type of cases to include—existing (prevalent) cases or only newly occurring (incident) cases, and
2. whether attempts are made to recruit all eligible patients from a target population.

These two issues are interlinked. A flow chart for considering the options is shown in Figure 8.1. A major factor underlying the choice is the rarity of the disease. It is clearly necessary for the investigator to have an idea of the likely incidence and/or prevalence of the disorder in order to make the appropriate choice.

The approach for calculating the number of cases required is described in Section 8.2.14.

8.2.2 Incident or prevalent cases?

The choice exists either to recruit only new—or incident—cases, or to include all those with current 'active' disease or prevalent cases. One benefit of the former is that the cases are not selected for disease chronicity, whereas selection of prevalent cases will exclude those whose disorder has become inactive, totally remitted. In addition, there is the paradoxical problem that if a disease, such as some forms of cancer, is associated with a rapid mortality in an important proportion of cases, then selecting prevalent cases will skew recruitment to those surviving. It is entirely plausible that the association between a possible risk factor and a disease may be different in those who survive from those who die. Further, in attempting to investigate aetiological factors for a disease, in subjects who have had the disease for several months or years it is difficult to distinguish risk factor exposure prior to and after onset of the disease.

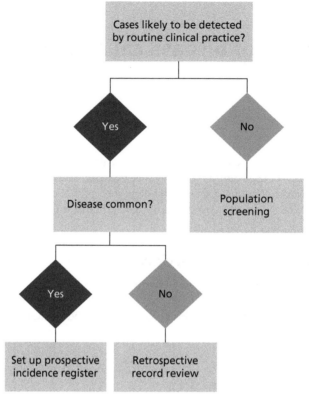

Figure 8.1 Strategies for case selection.

Example 8.i

A case–control study aimed to investigate the relationship between cigarette smoking and stroke, selecting as cases those who had been admitted to hospital, who would be interviewed about their prior smoking habits shortly after discharge. If there was an increased risk of sudden death in stroke patients who also were smokers, then restricting study to surviving cases would bias the estimate downwards of the risk from smoking.

Example 8.ii

A psychologist wanted to assess the frequency of significant life events in patients admitted to emergency departments with an attempted suicide attempt. Although ideally he would have liked to have identified subjects fairly soon after the attempt, this would have been ethically and practically difficult. He was able to identify from emergency department records a register of all such admissions and he then interviewed these patients 3–6 months after admission using an interview schedule that had been shown to be valid.

It may be possible to identify cases that have remitted or died by a trawl of medical records or from a contemporary disease register. Indeed, it may be possible to use proxies to obtain data, for example, by interviewing surviving relatives of deceased cases. (Consideration must be given also whether to adopt a similar strategy for the controls.) As suggested in Figure 8.1, if contemporary registers of new cases do not exist, it may prove impossible to prospectively recruit a sufficient number of new cases within a reasonable time. The inclusion of all available prevalent cases is the only option. This situation is particularly likely for rare disorders.

8.2.3 **Population-based or 'hospital-based series'**

Ideally, the cases selected, whether incident or prevalent, should be either all or, depending on the number required, a random sample of all cases from a target geographical population. In that way one can be sure that there has been no selection bias. In some situations, this may not be possible or practicable. If the disease is not likely to be detected by routine clinical practice, that is, a substantial proportion of cases are asymptomatic, then population screening may be the only available option.

Example 8.iii

A study was undertaken to examine occupational influences on osteoarthritis of the hip. Given that a substantial proportion of osteoarthritis cases are pain free, at least at a single point in time, the decision was taken to screen, using X-rays, a random population sample. This would thus not rely on identifying symptomatic individuals who had sought medical attention for their hip. Another advantage of this approach was that the controls could be chosen from among the disease-free individuals from the same population, ensuring their comparability.

For many rare diseases, population screening is too expensive, and may not be necessary if cases are likely to come to clinical attention anyway. In such circumstances, it may be possible to ascertain most or all incident cases within a population if:

◆ the investigator can identify all the clinical facilities serving the target population;

◆ there are a few cases, resident in the study area, who use clinical facilities outside the area;

◆ it is possible to identify (and therefore exclude) cases that live outside the study area.

The approach used is identical to that for measuring incidence (see Section 5.1).

Example 8.iv

For a proposed case–control study of acute appendicitis, an investigator chose a local government boundary as the population base. The operating theatre records and surgical admissions were reviewed for both the two local hospitals serving that population, as well as from the hospitals in four adjacent areas to which some patients, from within the target area, might attend. Only cases who normally resided within the target area were eligible for study.

A frequent and convenient source of cases is the patient population of one or more physicians with an interest in a particular disease. There are many such active 'clinical networks' of specialists, one of whose main functions is to provide a pooled database of cases for study. There are considerable advantages in terms of accuracy of diagnosis and high participation, but the question should be posed as to whether the cases seen in their practice are representative of the population at large.

8.2.4 **Recruitment of diagnosed cases: Using existing databases**

It is often appropriate to recruit cases, either incident or prevalent, from several physicians because it is rare for one physician to have a sufficiently large number of cases 'on the books'. Computerized databases will often permit the identification of patients attending other physicians and indeed other hospitals. However, as discussed in Chapter 23, access to a computerized register would typically require this to be undertaken by those responsible for the patient(s)'s care.

Example 8.v

To recruit cases for a case–control study of genetic factors in pre-eclampsia, the investigators used the local hospitals' obstetrics databases to identify all pregnancies in the previous two years with a positive entry for pre-eclampsia.

There are problems that frequently occur with this path:

◆ In most countries, routine hospital databases include diagnostic data on inpatients only, and thus disorders that do not routinely result in an inpatient admission are missed.

◆ In countries such as the United Kingdom, there are several available databases for primary care with access to a complete health record, and such databases are perfect for sampling comparator groups. However, securing access for more in-depth study can be complex and may result in a low response rate.

◆ Both hospital and primary care databases are set up for wider purposes than the more focused demands of a proposed study. Thus, there will have been little obligation for those who enter the data to be particularly aware of the needs of a study in terms of data quality and completeness for what may amount to be a tiny fraction of all cases entered.

◆ The reliance on these routine databases may also be problematic because there may be considerable diagnostic errors. It is always good practice to undertake pilot studies to assess the validity of diagnosis *before* starting a major study.

8.2.5 Recruitment of diagnosed cases

Ad hoc recruitment from colleagues can be adopted and is of value particularly in rare diseases. It is necessary to set up a special system for recruiting cases from interested colleagues. This is always easier in theory than in practice, however. Colleagues invariably overestimate the number of cases they have available and their compliance with prospective notification is variable.

Example 8.vi

A study wanted to recruit cases of children with a rare endocrine disorder. The investigators approached all their colleagues in paediatric endocrinology units and asked them to notify new attendees by sending out a monthly text message as a reminder. Recruitment was slow, and many specialists admitted they forgot to recruit even when such a patient attended.

It is, however, preferable to rely on prospective recruitment rather than ask for notifications of all previous attenders. Similarly, the recruitment phase should be restricted. Compliance is enhanced by the knowledge that this is only to be done for a fixed period, (say) three months. The notification process should be as simple as possible with clear eligibility criteria provided. A suitable communication for colleagues is shown in Box 8.1 followed by an example of a patient notification form (Box 8.2). One key task is to make sure that all those who contribute will be recognized, for example, an acknowledgement in manuscripts of the role played in recruitment or, if appropriate, offering the possibility to contribute to published articles and be an author. It may be a worthwhile investment to offer a prize to those notifying the greatest number of potential cases, or a payment per patient recruited to the study.

8.2.6 Advertising for cases and use of social media

It is always possible to go beyond healthcare resources and go directly to the public. Advertising in the media, such as newspapers, magazines, use of local radio, and increasingly social media platforms such as Facebook and Twitter. The response can be overwhelming and resources may be needed to sift through the answers received. It will then be necessary to set up a process whereby suggested cases are indeed true cases (see Section 8.2.7, 'Case verification'). Recently there has been a trend for many individuals to proactively seek involvement in research. Thus, websites such as SHARE provide a point of access to such individuals' medical records where researchers

---

Box 8.1 Example of a letter inviting recruitment of cases

Disease Research Clinic
St Anywhere's Hospital

Dear Colleague,

I am planning a case–control study to examine the hypothesis that exposure to pets may be linked to the subsequent development of Von Sturmmer's syndrome. Unfortunately, as you know, this is a very rare syndrome and I am writing to all the neurologists locally to help in case recruitment. I would be grateful if you would be willing to participate.

I am looking for patients with Von Sturmmer's syndrome. They should have:

- a positive serological test

- a disease duration of less than 2 years

Any patient who agrees to take part would be interviewed by my research nurse, Mary Jones, about pet ownership and other aspects of lifestyle. The interview would take place at the patient's home.

I enclose a copy of our enrolment form, which I would be grateful if you could complete and return for all eligible patients. The most practical approach is to arrange for the nurse in charge to make sure that there is a supply of these forms in your clinic room.

The study has the approval of St Anywhere's Ethical Committee and, of course, on the interview forms there will be no identifying personal information. The study will be fully explained to eligible patients prior to requesting their written consent to participate. I also enclose an outline protocol, a copy of our interview schedule, a photocopy of the ethical approval, and a patient information sheet.

I look forward to hearing from you.

Yours sincerely

---

can check eligibility criteria. A general point is that in all the aforementioned cases, responders, depending on the media used, will be a very non-representative sample of the notional total population with the disease. By contrast, recruitment can be very rapid and cheap. Many disease societies, especially those which are patient support or patient education groups, are often keen to use their membership as a willing source for *bone fide* research studies. Providing proper attention is paid to verification of the diagnosis and consideration in analysis to potential sources of bias, it might prove to be the most practical approach.

8.2.7 Case verification

The principles are the same as those discussed in Section 5.3.2 in relation to population prevalence and incidence surveys. It is necessary to state very clearly the rules used that allowed potential cases to be considered as cases.

It may be difficult, particularly if the cases were diagnosed at some stage in the past, to verify the diagnosis with absolute certainty. Contemporary medical records are not normally sufficiently comprehensive. A hierarchy of desirability in case verification is shown in Table 8.1. Thus clinical/pathological/radiological or similar confirmation using standard criteria, depending

---

Box 8.2 Example of a patient registration form for possible recruitment (hard copy or web based)

Von Sturmmer's Syndrome Study

Patient name ....

Address ....

....

....

or patient Identification label

Date of birth ....

Hospital number ....

This patient has agreed to be contacted for further discussion about taking part in this study and is willing to be contacted for an appointment with the recruitment nurse.

Telephone number ....

Signed .... Date ....

---

on the disorder, is the gold standard. Ideally, the investigator should have access to the actual diagnostic data, but for independent validation a contemporary report is normally acceptable. Standardization of diagnostic verification is very difficult in practice and therefore if all the histology slides, X-rays, or even physical findings, and so on, can be reviewed by a single expert, then so much the better.

Table 8.1 Hierarchical list of possibilities for case verification

Most ideal	Diagnostic confirmation using agreed criteria by investigator, including physical examination and results of investigations where relevant
	Diagnostic confirmation using agreed criteria by investigator based on contemporary records
	Diagnostic confirmation using agreed criteria by recruiting physician based on contemporary records
	Diagnostic status based on clinical opinion as judged by experienced physician
	Self-reported diagnosis by subject

Example 8.vii

In a case–control study of liver cirrhosis, it was decided to use histology as the defining criterion for acceptance as a case. The microscope slides were gathered from all potential cases and were reviewed by a single expert histopathologist.

For many disorders, pathological or similar confirmation is impossible and sets of clinical criteria have been formulated with the aim of standardizing disease classification internationally. This approach is of particular relevance in mental health but is also the main approach used in several organic disorders. Again, ideally, the investigator should clinically review all the cases.

This may be impractical, or the patients may be currently in remission and thus reliance must be placed on contemporary clinical records. These again may provide insufficient data for the purposes of applying a standard disease classification scheme. Ultimately, the investigator has two choices: either exclude those cases for whom diagnosis may not be proven, or include them but undertake, at the analysis stage, a separate analysis to determine the influence of including unconfirmed cases. This choice depends on the number of cases available and the proportion with missing data.

Finally, although self-reported diagnosis is listed in Table 8.1 as the least ideal, in certain circumstances self-reporting is the only option available. This is true, for example, when studying symptoms (e.g. pain). Only the individual subject knows whether they have a headache or not!

In addition to specifying rules for which cases are to be included, it is necessary to state at the beginning the rules for those cases to be excluded. Examples of such criteria, often necessary for practical or ethical purposes might include:

- disease status not verified
- emigrated
- significant physical/psychiatric comorbidity
- not fluent in the language of the country in which the research is conducted

Besides a lack of diagnostic data, another reason for a case being excluded could be the unavailability of the patient, for geographical, medical, psychological, or other reasons. It is important for the reader of any publication to have a feel for what these exclusion rules are, again because the results can only be extrapolated to those who are studied. If the study method involves an interview or completion of a questionnaire, familiarity with the native language is required and those who are illiterate may need to be excluded. Sometimes unexpected exclusion criteria are forced on the investigator. In a collaborative study that one of the authors was undertaking in a Mediterranean country, many of the young males were unavailable for study because of military service duties—this was not an exclusion criterion that had been planned!

8.2.8 **Recruitment of controls: overview**

This is probably the most vexed issue in case–control study design. In broad terms, the controls should be representative of the population from which the cases have arisen. In other words, if a subject chosen as a control had become a case, then they should have had the same chance of being included in the study as did the cases. For population-based case–control studies, when all cases in a defined population area are selected, the source for the controls is obvious. It is a greater problem deciding how to recruit controls when cases have been selected from a hospital or clinic.

8.2.9 **Strategies for control selection: Population-based**

The optimal situation, as just stated, is where a whole population has been screened to detect the cases and a complete list or sampling frame exists. Then the only requirement is to take a true random sample of those who do not meet the criteria for being a case.

Example 8.viii

A general practitioner used a standard questionnaire and screened his female registered population, aged 45–64 years, to detect those with probable depression. He then undertook a case–control study comparing their lifetime history of hormonal use gleaned from records in the cases detected with an equal number of randomly selected women aged 45–64 years from his practice who had a normal depression score on screening.

Frequently, a population sample of cases is based on ascertainment from the relevant clinical facility or facilities, but the population from which such cases attend is not a fixed one as patients may choose which medical facility in their area they attend and may even travel some distance to receive such care. It is thus impossible to take a map and draw a line around which one can be certain that all eligible cases had been recruited. An alternative approach to be used in these circumstances is to take another population-based listing approximately covering the population concerned, such as the list of individuals registered to receive medical care at one or more general practices. In this example, the controls should be as closely representative as possible of the population from which the cases were selected. Thus, the general practices selected should be the same as those from which the cases arose. If the cases are selected from a very wide area (i.e. no single target population is identifiable), selecting controls individually from the general practice list of each case is appropriate.

Example 8.ix

In Example 8.iv on acute appendicitis, the general practitioner for each case of appendicitis ascertained was asked to identify, as potential controls, the name of the next three individuals on the age–sex register of the same sex and age (within 1 year). The general practitioner then approached these persons on behalf of (and using materials provided by) the study investigator and those who agreed had their details passed on to the research team.

8.2.10 **Other sources of population controls**

The registers of individuals listed here may not be available for all populations and access may be denied to the investigator. There are other sources of population controls.

Population registers without ages

In the United Kingdom, local electoral registers (lists of eligible voters) are available to the public. They are reasonably up to date but exclude those under the voting age (or, in reality, those who will not reach the voting age in the period in which the register is valid), those who do not register, or those not eligible to vote in any elections (e.g. nationals of some other countries). They cover perhaps 90–95% of the population. Their major drawback is the absence of information on age, and the fact that individuals can opt out of the publicly available register.

Example 8.x

In a case–control study, an investigator undertook the role of assessing reproductive factors in the aetiology of rheumatoid arthritis; the cases were women with the disease attending several hospitals in the London area. The controls were selected from random samples of people with possible female names from three local electoral registers. Electoral-register responders who were outside the age range of the cases, or who declared themselves to be male, were subsequently excluded from the analysis.

Neighbour controls

One little used option, given its expense, is to use local street maps to obtain a near neighbour. This approach will at least ensure that the controls are from the same sociogeographical population as the cases. If the street layout is appropriate, rules can be established.

Example 8.xi

In a case–control study of home factors (lighting, ill-fitting carpets, and so on) related to fractured neck of femur in elderly females (over the age of 75), the investigator identified the address of all eligible cases from hospital registers who were non-institutionalized at the time of injury. For each case a researcher visited the household on each side and all female residents aged over 75 were eligible for inclusion as controls.

8.2.11 Strategies for non-population-based control selection

In some situations, the strategies we've just detailed will not be appropriate. Firstly, the population base from which the cases arose may be impossible to determine. This may be true when cases are recruited from hospital. The selection factors that resulted in an individual with a particular disorder attending and being diagnosed by a particular hospital are complex. Secondly, response rates from randomly chosen population controls are often very low. There is a greater personal incentive for cases to participate than controls. There are, however, several choices for controls that address these problems. The first two attempt to select what aims to be a 'random' sample of the non-disease population.

Telephone recruitment

In populations with good telephone coverage, it may be possible to purchase population lists of telephone numbers for 'cold calling'. Many people opt out of such schemes and such calling is often resented and the approach can result in a low response rate. It is often a two-stage process, with the initial call identifying the presence within the household of a suitable individual (e.g. with regards to age and sex), and a follow-up call to obtain participation. This is a very popular method in the United States and several commercial companies undertake the background calling. Telephone recruitment is now very unusual partly because landlines are much less common compared to mobile phones now and also because many people now 'block' telephone numbers they don't recognize. Partly as a result of 'cold-calling', people have generally become less receptive to this mode of communication.

Social media

Social media platforms such as Facebook are an increasingly used approach to identify people who may be willing, and often are, to provide information about themselves. This is clearly a restricted population subject to many biases, but the reach is substantial and recruitment can be achieved quickly and cheaply.

Disease controls

One widespread approach in the literature, often in rare diseases recruited from several centres, is therefore to use cases attending the same clinical facilities with a different disease. The presumption being that the controls were drawn from the same base population as the cases and by choosing other disease groups, it is allowing for health behaviour and factors associated with attendance at a particular health facility. The problem is—which disease to choose?

Example 8.xii

A hospital-based case–control study of acute myocardial infarction was conducted using patients admitted to the hospital with myocardial infarction as 'cases', while age- and sex-matched 'controls' were selected from those attending the emergency department on the same day (without myocardial infarction). The study showed that cases consumed much less alcohol than controls, despite the fact that most other studies showed that heavy alcohol consumption was a risk factor for myocardial infarction. The result was explained by the fact that many of the conditions presenting in the emergency department were related to heavy alcohol consumption.

Although such an example in theory drew from the same population base, there were so many selection factors leading to emergency department attendance that makes their selection as a control group inappropriate

This is also a particular problem if one relies on choosing controls from a single disease group. It is therefore preferable to choose several conditions, which the investigator has no *a priori* reason to believe has an association with the major risk factors under study, and to select controls from these groups. Using such methods will ensure that one disease group will not dominate the control group and have undue influence on the results.

Example 8.xiii

In a case–control study of rheumatoid arthritis, women with other musculoskeletal conditions attending the same clinics were chosen as controls. Both cases and controls were approached in the same manner ('We are interested in looking at the relationship between arthritis and hormonal/gynaecological factors') and the presumption was that if the controls had developed rheumatoid arthritis instead, they would also have been ascertained as cases.

Family/friend controls

This again can be a useful strategy for two reasons: (i) personal knowledge of the case will aid recruitment and encourage compliance; (ii) relatives and friends (which could include visitors of hospital recruited cases) are likely to be from a socioeconomically similar population. As household contacts will share the same environment, it is appropriate to choose a non-household relative. A non-blood relative, if appropriate, can be useful if genetic factors may be of relevance. The typical strategy for friend (e.g. US 'buddy') controls is to ask the case to supply the names of three friends of the same age and sex, from whom the investigator then selects one at random for study. One potential problem with either friends or family is one of overmatching, that is, the case and controls are too similar with regard to the exposure under investigation. For example, smokers tend to have friends who smoke and the same applies to alcohol consumption, aspects of diet, level of physical activity, and other lifestyle factors. Despite the expectation of a high response, many cases may be reluctant to involve friends or relatives and tend to select unrepresentative super-healthy and cooperative individuals. One final example of control selection illustrates these difficulties.

Example 8.xiv

In a case–control study of women with a chronic disease, the investigator proposed to study, as controls, sisters-in-law of the cases on the basis that, unlike friend controls, the cases did not have to make the selection, only provide the names. These middle-aged women should have been very likely to have at least one sister-in-law as the term encompasses wife/wives of the brother(s), sister(s) of the husband, and indeed wife/ wives of the husband's brother(s)! In the event, the investigator was able to obtain data on sisters-in-law for only 20% of the cases, unknown whereabouts of what had been presumed to be close relatives were more common than expected!

8.2.12 **One or two control groups?**

If no single control group is ideal, then there is an interesting question, 'Is it a reasonable to re-cruit two dissimilarly drawn control groups, with different selection factors, in the hope that the comparison of the case group with either group will reveal the same broad answer as regards as-sociation with the risk factor under study?'. In these circumstances it would be more difficult to argue that control selection had explained the results obtained. By contrast if there are differences in results between the two comparison groups, that would indicate that differences in the methods employed did affect the results and hence the conclusions. In the absence of a methodologically obviously superior control group, interpretation of the results can be difficult. It is a fine balance, as with a less-than-perfect control group inappropriate confidence can be placed in the results.

Example 8.xv

In one study of a rare connective-tissue disease, cases were recruited from the national membership list of a patient self-help group. Two control groups were selected. The first was from the members of a different disease self-help group, with a disorder thought to be unrelated to the exposure being investigated. The second was chosen from primary care registers. The aim was to distinguish factors associated with disease from those associated with self-help group membership.

8.2.13 **Matching**

This refers to the process by which the investigator attempts to ensure that the cases and controls are similar with respect to those other variables that are risk factors for the disease and are (or may be) associated with the exposure under study, the so-called confounding variables (see Chapter 18). This will reduce an imbalance between groups. Although typically each case would be matched with one control, for it may be necessary to compensate for a limited small number of cases to match with two, three, or even four controls per case to retain sufficient statistical power (see Table 8.2).

Example 8.xvi

In a case–control study investigating the risk of smoking for chronic lung cancer, the cases had both higher smoking rates and lower consumption of fruit and vegetables than the controls.
Note: It is difficult to disentangle whether there was a true effect of smoking, independent of the level of fruit and vegetable consumption.

In this example diet is a potential confounder for the effect of smoking. There are three pos-sible approaches to confounding variables. The first is to match controls so that they have the same exposure to the confounding factors as the cases. This can either be done on an individual case–control pair basis (individual matching) or on a group basis, that is, ensuring overall that the case and control groups have a similar distribution of fruit and vegetable consumption (frequency matching). However, collecting information on diet from potential controls would involve a sub-stantial amount of work. The second is to recruit controls, to measure the confounding factor of interest, and to deal with this issue in the analysis stage (see Section 18.4). The third approach, used increasingly where there is a large database, is to use *propensity matching*. This is more relevant to cohort studies and is discussed further in Chapter 20.

Problems with individual matching

There are also several specific practical problems with matching individual cases to one or more controls:

◆ It is subsequently impossible to examine the influence of any of the matching variables on disease risk.

◆ There is a danger of overmatching (i.e. controls are selected to be so similar to the cases in respect of their risk of exposure that they end up with an almost identical exposure frequency).

◆ One can only match if data on matching variables are available, in advance, to the investigator. Apart from age and sex (and perhaps proxy measures of social class), this is rarely the situation. Thus, to match for smoking status would require a prior survey to determine the smoking status of the potential controls!

◆ It may be impossible to find a perfect match if several different variables are being controlled for at the same time. The search for controls then becomes expensive and time-consuming.

◆ Matching may also be inefficient: if no controls can be identified for a case, or the controls chosen refuse to participate, the case also has to be excluded from the analysis.

Before leaving the discussion of matching it is important to mention the use of the twin study: in the classical example of a disorder whose aetiology is presumed to lie in the influence of specific environmental susceptibility factors on a particular genetic background. In this instance, a case–control study examining environmental factors in disease-discordant identical twins is a clear way of matching for the genetic factors.

An approach which retains the advantages of matching but which overcomes some of the problems associated with individual matching is 'frequency' matching. This ensures that overall the groups are similar even if individual matched pairs cannot be identified

Example 8.xvii

In a case–control study on the effect of various environmental exposures on the risk of a relatively rare congenital malformation, the investigators recruited cases from the obstetric registers of four large maternity units. The investigators wished to ensure that the cases and controls were similar in relation to maternal age, parity, and calendar year of birth, each of which might be a potential confounder. They used the facilities afforded by the obstetric databases to group their non-affected births by these variables and take random samples within each group in proportion to the number of cases from each group. This ensured that the distributions of these key variables were similar between cases and controls. This also proved a substantially easier option than attempting individual matching.

The problem with frequency matching is the lack of ability to look for *interactions,* both between the confounders and between the potential confounders and the exposure of interest. For instance, in Example 8.xvii the cases and controls might have the same distributions of maternal age and parity but they were different in their relationships—for example, there may have been more cases with an older maternal age who had had multiple pregnancies—which in combination might substantially increase the risk of the malformation under study.

8.2.14 Study size

The final consideration in setting up a case–control study is deciding on the appropriate sample size. This is a crucial step to ensure that the study has a reasonable expectation of being able to produce a useful answer. If the calculations suggest that more cases or resources are needed than are available to the investigator, the study should not proceed. Conversely (and very rarely) it may be that the number needed to be studied is smaller than expected and that expense and effort can be saved.

The major effects on sample size are:

♦ the expected frequency of exposure in the controls (which requires either prior knowledge or a pilot study to determine);

♦ the size of the effect that the investigator would not want to miss.

Indeed, it seems intuitively likely that the rarer the exposure, the larger the number of cases required. Indeed, the case–control approach is inefficient in the face of a rare exposure. Secondly, if the investigator wishes to be able to detect an increased risk of, say, 1.5-fold, this would require a larger study than if only large increases in risk were being sought. (There are many simple-to-use software programs available that make sample size calculation easy.) As an example, the data in Table 8.2 were obtained from the Open Source Epidemiologic Statistics for Public Health, an easy to use online calculator for sample size and related epidemiological calculations (see further reading). The table covers a broad range of exposure frequencies and risks. The table shows the substantial influence of the control exposure frequency on sample size. The emerging sample size figures also show how much easier it is to detect large increases in risk than small ones. If exposure is being stratified into several different levels, a greater number of individuals will need to be studied. Similarly, if interest is in the interaction between two risk factors then a large increase in the required sample size is inevitable.

The figures obtained should be taken as a guide rather than the exact number to be recruited. Although software programs will provide seemingly 'accurate' sample size requirements (e.g. 429 cases), it should be remembered that uncertainty in the parameter's input (e.g. proportion of exposure in controls) will be reflected in uncertainty of the sample size required. For this reason, it is often best, rather than carrying out a single sample size calculation, to conduct calculations under several assumptions.

Example 8.xviii

In a study (with the sample size calculations shown in Table 8.3) the 'best estimate' for the proportion of controls exposed is 0.15. It was therefore decided to conduct a study with 225 subjects to give 80% power to detect an odds ratio of 2.0. If, however, the proportion exposed is only 0.10, the study would not even have power of 70%, while if the proportion exposed is 0.20, power will be greater than 90%.

The previous calculations assume that equal numbers of cases and controls will be obtained: this is the most efficient approach. However, when the number of cases is limited (i.e. when the disease is rare) it is possible to compensate by increasing the number of controls (Table 8.4). As shown in this example, there is little gain beyond having four times as many controls as cases.

Table 8.2 Sample size for case–control studies

Estimated proportion of exposure in controls	Number of cases required for minimum odds ratio to be detected				
	1.5	2	3	4	5
0.05	1,774	559	199	116	81
0.10	957	307	112	67	48
0.20	562	186	72	45	33
0.30	446	153	62	40	31
0.40	407	144	61	41	32

Note: Assume power 80%, 95% confidence level, and one control per case.

Table 8.3 Power calculations for case–control studies

Estimated proportion of controls reporting	Power of study (%)				
	70	75	80	85	90
0.10	246	274	307	347	402
0.15	181	201	225	255	295
0.20	150	166	186	211	244

Note: Odds ratio to detect 2.0, 95% confidence level, and one control per case.

Finally, a word of warning: these figures assume that the numbers stated are the numbers actually studied. Ineligible and unconfirmed cases, together with deaths, wrong addresses, refusers, and other non-respondents, will need to be taken into consideration. Thus, for example, with a typical final participation rate of 60%, the numbers stated must be multiplied by approximately 1.7 to provide the number of cases that need to be approached.

8.3 Selection of subjects for cohort (longitudinal) studies

The central issue in setting up a cohort study is the selection of the population(s) to be studied according to their exposure status. As discussed in Chapter 1, the issues are the same whether the aim of the study is (i) to determine the development of a disease in those exposed or not exposed to a suspected particular disease risk factor at baseline, or (ii) to determine the development of a specific outcome in individuals with or without the presence of a disease state at baseline.

The main questions that influence the approach to be used for population selection are:

i) Should the study ascertain the exposure status from historical data and the outcome currently (the retrospective cohort approach), or should exposure status be ascertained currently with the outcome determined by future follow-up (the prospective cohort approach)?
ii) Should the exposure be considered as just present or absent, or at multiple levels?
iii) Should the exposure be measured at a single point of time or should change in exposure be captured?
iv) Should the different exposure groups studied be derived from a single target population?
v) How many subjects should be studied?

Table 8.4 Influence on sample size of increasing the number of controls per case

Number of controls per case	Required number of:		
	Cases	Controls	Total
1:1	307	307	614
2:1	223	446	669
3:1	194	582	776
4:1	180	720	900
5:1	171	855	1,026
6:1	166	996	1,162

Notes: Estimated proportion of controls exposed 0.10. Odds ratio to detect 2.0. Power 80%.

8.3.1 **Retrospective or prospective study cohorts?**

The choice of retrospective or prospective cohort design was discussed in Chapter 6. At a practical level, the choice is determined by the availability of high-quality historical exposure data on the one hand, and the practicality and costs of a prospective study on the other. If a retrospective study is being considered, the following questions need to be addressed:

i)   Are data available on a sufficiently large number of individuals?

ii) Is the quality of the exposure data sufficiently high to permit accurate allocation to different exposure category groups?

iii) If the exposure changes over time, does the information available allow the investigator to assess this?

iv) Are there any data on potential confounding variables?

v)   Are there sufficient data available from follow-up to determine the disease status of the population, both in terms of being able to ascertain completely the presence of disease and to verify the diagnosis in those ascertained?

Two examples illustrating the use of retrospective cohorts may be of help here.

Example 8.xix

In a study designed to quantify the relationship between body weight at age 20 and subsequent risk of non-insulin-dependent diabetes, an investigator discovered the availability of army medical records giving details of body weight and height in male conscripts in the late 1970s. In a pilot study using general practice and other record systems, he was able to trace around 40% of the original cohort, whose diabetic status was then easily assessed by questionnaire. The investigator decided that the study was practicable and that the body weight and height data had been gathered using appropriate methods. There was also good data on potential confounders such as parental health and socioeconomic factors. He was however concerned about this loss to follow-up given that those who had developed diabetes might be more likely to respond to the questionnaire. Clearly, this would need to be taken into consideration when interpreting and extrapolating the results.

Example 8.xx

A paediatrician wished to investigate the relationship between weight gain in the first year of life and subsequent intellectual development. She used records from community child health clinics to identify a group of children born 10 years previously on whom there were data available on birthweight and weight around the first birthday, and was able to link these to subsequent school records.

By contrast, recruitment of a prospective cohort will require knowledge of current exposure status. Depending on the question to be asked, the decision needs to be made between using existing data sources or setting up a special survey to determine exposure status. The former is cheaper and quicker. However, the latter permits the investigator to document exposure accurately and to collect data on other important variables. One advantage of the prospective approach is, even if existing data sources are being used, the investigator can influence the collection of the exposure data.

Example 8.xxi

An occupational-health physician wished to investigate the association between certain industrial exposures and the risk of skin rashes in an industry. The quality of the exposure data available from the employment medical records was poor and the employees themselves were unaware of their exposure history in sufficient detail. He therefore set up a prospective cohort study and provided the personnel department with a specially designed pro forma on which they could record both current and future exposures in a structured way.

In this example there was no alternative to the rather expensive and lengthy recruitment procedure given the exposure data required, and the results would thus take some time to accumulate. By contrast using historical data, even if there had been an accurate source, may not have been relevant to current day exposures in that industry.

Example 8.xxii

A proposed investigation on risk factors for falling in older people required the investigators to recruit a population sample that were then surveyed by trained interviewers on possible risk factors for subsequent falls. The interviewers also undertook a limited examination of visual acuity and postural stability.

8.3.2 How should exposure be categorized?

The categorization of exposure depends on the main question(s) to be addressed, as discussed in Chapter 6. This decision will influence the choice of populations to be studied and the size of the study (see next).

Example 8.xxiii

In the occupational exposure example (Example 8.xxi), the research questions were concerned with several dimensions of exposure related to average intensity, maximum intensity, and duration in months. The researcher had no prior belief which of these dimensions would be more important and whether the relationships would be linear, threshold, or more complex. He designed the study to be capable of answering many of these attributes, though he was aware of the problem of multiple hypotheses testing leading to false positive results

Example 8.xxiv

In an epidemiological study of the influence of height on the subsequent risk of back pain, the investigator considered that it would be appropriate to consider the risk by dividing the population into five equal groups, or quintiles, by height. The risk of back pain could then be assessed separately in each of the groups. In planning the study, she needed to ensure there would be a sufficient number in each of the five groups to permit valid comparisons.

In such an approach, the groups do not necessarily have to be equal in size but may be divided into biologically more coherent groups. The advantage of having equal-sized groups is that it is often statistically more efficient (i.e. the comparisons would have greater power). The decision about the approach to be used in considering the exposure can be (and frequently is) left until the analysis stage.

8.3.3 Studying the effect of multiple exposures

For the sake of simplicity, many introductory epidemiological texts imply that cohort studies are best applied to single exposures, and preferably those that can be categorized into present or absent. In practice, the analytical software available for cohort studies permits multiple exposures to be studied simultaneously and their separate risks assessed.

Example 8.xxv

An investigation was planned to determine the risk factors for premature death in elderly women admitted to hospital with a fractured neck of femur. Multiple exposure data were gathered at baseline assessment, including mental test scores, indices of body mass, presence of related disorders, and haemoglobin level. Thus, this cohort study did not consist of a single exposed population, but, rather, a single study population from whom the various exposures could be ascertained for subsequent analysis.

8.3.4 Ascertainment of exposure status

Given the information just given, the most obvious strategy is to select a 'whole population' and investigate the exposure status of every individual, perhaps by a screening survey. The population is then divided into two or more exposure groups depending on their exposure status at screening. The advantage of this approach is that both the 'exposed' and the 'non-exposed' groups are truly representative of the exposed and non-exposed individuals from the population under study. Indeed, many of the large multiexposure, multioutcome population-based cohort studies referred to in Chapter 6 are very much designed for that purpose.

The anxiety is that when the exposed and non-exposed groups are selected from different 'parent' populations, it may be impossible to separate the influence on disease risk of differences in other disease-related variables in the two populations. This strategy, however, is unavoidable if the exposure is relatively rare and the investigator needs to use an 'enriched' sample to obtain sufficient numbers of exposed individuals.

Example 8.xxvi

A gastroenterologist wished to investigate the hypothesis that being a vegetarian was associated with a reduced risk of developing large-bowel cancer. In order to obtain sufficient numbers, he recruited his 'exposed' cohort from the membership of local vegetarian societies and compared their risk with populations drawn from general practice who had been surveyed about their meat-eating habits. He obtained data on other variables such as alcohol consumption in both groups as he recognized that members of the vegetarian societies might have differed in other ways in regard to their risk of developing bowel cancer.

In this example, the investigator attempted to collect data on possible confounders (see Chapter 18) that could be adjusted for in the analysis, with the hope that if a protective effect was seen in the vegetarians it could be determined whether this was due to having a vegetarian diet. The problem is that there may be unknown variables associated with being a member of vegetarian societies that are thus impossible to measure. In these circumstances, rather than not do the study, the best option is to do what is reasonable and practicable, but note in the report that it is impossible to exclude the possibility of a selection effect.

8.3.5 Study size

In all epidemiological studies, recruitment of sufficient sample sizes for study is of crucial importance. As with case–control studies, the sample size is determined by the statistical power considered appropriate to detect stated increases in risk, traditionally at the 95% confidence level. The determinants of sample size are thus the increase in risk to be detected, the background risk in the unexposed or lowest exposed group, and the frequency of exposure. The calculations are readily done with widely available software packages. Table 8.5 provides some typical sample-size calculations under a variety of assumptions. The first half of the table assumes either that the population can be split equally into two, based on their exposure status, or that the investigator aims to recruit an enriched exposed cohort and an equal-sized unexposed group. The second half of the table is based on the desire to investigate a rare exposure (approximately 10%) of the population. The figures are based on the cumulative occurrence of the disease outcome by the end of follow-up. In an analogous fashion to Table 8.3 it is often prudent not to rely on a single power calculation. Having established the order of magnitude of certain parameters (e.g. cumulative disease risk in unexposed), it is useful to examine the effects on power of variations around this estimate (Table 8.6).

Manifestly, the rarer the disease the greater the number that need to be studied. Similarly, to uncover a largish effect (risk ratio >3) it requires a substantially smaller sample size than it does to detect a smaller effect of (for example) 1.5.

Table 8.5 Sample-size calculations for cohort studies based on the frequency of exposure and presumed disease risk

Frequency of exposure (%)	Cumulative disease risk in unexposed (%)	Risk ratio to be detected	Number of subjects to be recruited	
			Exposed	**Unexposed**
50	10	3	71	71
		2	219	219
		1.5	725	725
	5	3	160	160
		2	475	475
		1.5	1,550	1,550
	1	3	865	865
		2	2,510	2,510
		1.5	8,145	8,145
	0.1	3	8,800	8,800
		2	25,000	25,000
		1.5	82,000	82,000
10	10	3	35	305
		2	110	990
		1.5	380	3,410
	5	3	75	665
		2	235	2,115
		1.5	810	7,260
	1	3	400	3,580
		2	1,240	11,170
		1.5	4,230	38,060
	0.1	3	4 000	36,400
		2	12,500	113,000
		1.5	43,000	385,000

If the exposure is rare, the number of exposed subjects that need to be studied can be reduced by increasing the number of the non-exposed. Conversely, using an enriched exposure sample, to give equal-sized exposed and non-exposed cohorts, can clearly reduce the overall size of the study.

The decision is therefore a compromise between cost and the difficulty in obtaining a sufficiently large exposed group. The sample size can be reduced by continuing the follow-up for longer *if disease (outcome) risk remains constant or increases over time*. Thus, if the disease risk is a uniform 1% per annum, the longer the period of study the greater the number of cases that develop and thus the smaller the numbers to be followed up. The balance between long follow-up of a relatively small cohort compared with short follow-up of a relatively large cohort depends on

Table 8.6 Power calculations for cohort studies

Cumulative disease risk in unexposed	Power of study (%)				
	70	75	80	85	90
12	142	158	176	199	230
10	176	196	219	247	286
8	227	253	282	319	369
6	313	347	389	440	509

Notes: The number of cases required is shown assuming: ratio of exposed: unexposed, risk ratio to be detected = 2.0, 95% confidence interval, frequency of exposure 50%.

the cost implications, the requirement to obtain a quick result, the problems with loss to follow-up with increasing time, and the pattern of disease risk among other factors.

For example, a short follow-up may also be inappropriate if the latency between exposure and disease is long. This is, for example, particularly true in relation to cancers, where too short a study may fail to detect a real effect. It also must be remembered that the sample size calculations assume no loss to follow-up and they will need to be weighted accordingly to take account of the estimated losses. The sample size calculations would also be based on the open source software mentioned earlier (see 'Further reading'). The number of cases required would need to be shown, assuming ratio of exposed:unexposed, risk ratio to be detected = 2.0, 95% confidence interval, frequency of exposure 50%.

Further reading

Selection of controls

Wacholder S, McLaughlin JK, Silverman DT, Mandel JS (1992). Selection of controls in case-control studies. I. Principles. *Am J Epidemiol*, **135**(9), 1019–28.

Wacholder S, Silverman DT, McLaughlin JK, Mandel JS (1992). Selection of controls in case-control studies. II. Types of controls. *Am J Epidemiol*, **135**(9), 1029–41.

Wacholder S, Silverman DT, McLaughlin JK, Mandel JS (1992). Selection of controls in case-control studies. III. Design options. *Am J Epidemiol*, **135**(9), 1042–50.

Registers of people interested in participating in health research

SHARE http://www.registerforshare.org

Sample size calculation

Open Source Epidemiologic Statistics for Public Health http://www.openepi.com/Menu/OE_Menu.htm

Chapter 9

Use of secondary data

9.1 **Introduction**

Traditionally, much of the published epidemiological research has been based on new (primary) data collection. Samples of subjects, selected from different sources, are investigated, often requiring direct subject contact to obtain the necessary information. Even when such direct contact is not required, there is often the need to extract necessary information from individual subject records such as medical files. There is often no alternative source of information although, as discussed in this chapter, the greater digitization of information is changing that scenario with the potential that the availability of such information might preclude the need for primary data.

Primary data collection will always have the advantage of being able to collect all the required data items and can build in quality assurance for each item. The disadvantage is that epidemiological studies requiring primary data collection are increasingly expensive, time-consuming, and subject to several hurdles to success, including ethical and regulatory approval. Furthermore, high levels of patient and public participation are hard to achieve and loss to follow-up is a real problem. These can impact on even the most optimally designed study, constraining the *internal* validity of the conclusions.

Resources and practical issues can also constrain the nature of the target population and thus, depending on sampling frame, may be of limited *external* validity.

Example 9.i

A group of clinicians interested in a rare autoimmune disease had established between them a register of their current cases to be used for a variety of studies. Although possibly the only practical way of assembling an appropriate size sample, the patients recruited were only a subsample of a wider population of patients, many of whom would have been under the care of less specialized clinicians.

The alternative is to exploit data gathered for other purposes (*secondary data*), often for statutory or administrative reasons, but often based on whole populations. In many countries and regions, at all levels of healthcare, health databases can be searched for diagnostic and treatment codes. Not only are such data available but, depending on their source, they are accessible by the internet.

The same applies to data gathered from large population epidemiological surveys when the funders of such studies are keen to ensure the widest possible access to the resource.

Example 9.ii

The Research Data Center of the National Center for Health Statistics is the body responsible in the United States for providing access to the data collected in their very large population studies such as the National Health and Nutritional Examination Surveys (NHANES). Bone fide researchers can obtain data extracts to perform their own analyses (see 'Further reading').

The other growing potential is to link routine data sources of various types to answer almost an infinite range of questions.

Example 9.iii

A researcher was able to obtain permission to link, in an anonymized fashion, past data on school absences and examination performance in girls of school leaving age with their subsequent outcomes of pregnancy.

These types of data, and the potential of linkage, are often referred to as 'Big Data'. There are clearly research benefits in their use but also legitimate public concern as to the potential for abuse. This chapter will consider the spectrum of the data available to researchers, how they can be accessed and used, and their limitations.

9.2 **Types of data available**

The data available to researchers will vary between country and region and is also changing over time, so this chapter can only provide an outline of what might be available. As with the example of NHANES mentioned here (Example 9.ii), data are available to researchers from other countries and not only (as in that instance) to those resident in the United States. This is not a lone example.

Example 9.iv

The United Kingdom has a system of collecting routine data from many primary care practitioners which provides access to the complete health record. This data source, formerly known as the General Practice Research Database (GPRD), now has links to secondary care data as the Clinical Practice Research Datalink (CPRD) and has provided researchers across the world with access to data, particularly on the outcomes following the use of prescribed medication in primary care.

The main sources of data are considered next.

9.2.1 **Census data**

Every major country collects detailed data on the entire population typically every 10 years. The data on health and illness are limited but vary from census to census. Tabulations are available online and, for example, in the United Kingdom, it is possible to request specific analyses.

Example 9.v

Researchers in Leicester in the United Kingdom were able to obtain data on the prevalence of self-reported long-term health conditions by ethnicity, tabulated by age and gender, to examine different needs within their multiethnic population (see 'Further reading').

Access to individual data is normally barred for a substantial period of time (e.g. 100 years), although older data may be of interest for historical purposes.

9.2.2 **Birth and death data**

Statutory requirements to notify births and deaths, including the cause in the latter case, have provided much useful information, particularly on patterns of severe disease. The available data allow for examination by time and place. Linkage of data from population surveys can be useful to provide information on outcomes.

Example 9.vi

The USA-based Longitudinal Study of Ageing with its rich list of baseline data items is linked to the National Death Index, which provides researchers with ongoing information on the fact of, and cause of, death.

9.2.3 **Disease registers**

Disease registers have the triple value of firstly being a source of information in their own right, without further need for study, on the incidence of different disorders: again, analysis by age, gender, geography, and time are normally available, as well as (in some cases) by socioeconomic indicators and ethnicity. Secondly, they can be linked to other routine data sources, for example, such as national death data to obtain information on survival. Thirdly, as shown next, it may be possible to access such registers for recruitment of cases for study.

Most countries do not have many nationwide disease registers, with the exception of cancer. Often such registers that do exist are for public health purposes, for example, registers of specific communicable diseases (see 'Further reading').

Cancer registers have been a key tool in monitoring trends in cancer incidence and survival both within and between countries. The quality of the information collected, for example, on histological type and stage, being fundamental to examining trends in survival. Cancer registers have the power to address questions on possible risk factors.

Example 9.vii

Local regional incidence rates of lung and respiratory tract cancers were correlated with publicly available data on particulate atmospheric pollution. This allowed an analysis of the relationship between the two. Obviously, such an ecological analysis cannot allow for the effects of important confounders such as smoking.

9.2.4 **Healthcare utilization registers**

Data systems utilized by healthcare providers are available and cover an individual's total health record. Such data can provide access to a population database on those diagnosed with any of the disorders that are likely to be covered by that healthcare system. For systems based in primary care this in effect covers all disorders apart from those self-managed by the individual. Thus, for CPRD in the United Kingdom, similar systems in many European countries as well as records from those enrolled in health plans in North America and elsewhere provide such information. In some instances, it is possible to go back to the healthcare provider for further information to confirm the diagnosis.

Some examples illustrate this.

Example 9.viii

Inhabitants in Olmsted County Minnesota receive all their healthcare at the Mayo Clinic in Rochester and its associated affiliates. These providers have a unique record system that provides access to the records of all patients with any diagnosis made over the past several decades. These data have been used for several studies of disease incidence, severity, and outcome (see 'Further reading').

Example 9.ix

Finland has a national system of recording the diagnoses of persons eligible to receive welfare payments for a large range of long-term disorders, ranging from depression to rheumatoid arthritis. This resource can be used to assess incidence, and also by linkage to death and cancer records other adverse health outcomes.

Example 9.x

The CPRD from England and Wales (discussed earlier in Example 9.iv) can provide researchers with a list of patients recorded under a list of diagnostic codes. A sample of the participating general practitioners have agreed to allow researchers to contact them for further information that can be used to confirm the diagnosis.

The other major role of such data sources is to provide access to cohorts based on specific health interventions such as drug use for pharmaco-epidemiology studies as in Example 9.iv.

Indeed, with the increased availability of advanced medicines which have profound biological activity (both monoclonal antibodies and small molecules), licensing is dependent on the company supporting a post-marketing surveillance study to assess long-term risks and benefits.

Example 9.xi

The authors of this book have been involved in setting up registers of patients treated with biological drugs for rheumatoid arthritis and ankylosing spondylitis. These registers have the capacity to provide all stakeholders with information on the long-term benefits and harms from these drugs. Ideally such registers can be linked to the subjects' electronic health record, where such records exist, which then precludes the necessity for direct patient follow-up.

The concept behind drug registers has spread to surgical interventions with, for example, registers of patients receiving a new hip or knee joint existing in most major countries, see further reading.

9.2.5 **Normal population surveys**

The examples so far in this section have focused on data available from health sources. Much epidemiology requires access to information from population samples and their follow-up. In many countries, there have been very large studies, some focused on people of specific age groups, for example, children or older people, others on broader population groups. For example, in the United Kingdom, the Million Women Study encompasses over one million normal women, recruited when attending for breast cancer screening, providing a rich source of epidemiological data on predictors of women's health. Such studies are widespread and many use similar methodologies across different countries to allow both within and between country comparisons. As already mentioned, the funders, often national public bodies, demand that the data collected from such surveys should be made available to epidemiological researchers for wider exploitation.

9.2.6 **Biobanks**

Although the term 'biobank' is used in many different contexts, in an epidemiological sense it refers to the collection of biological samples such as DNA and serum to sit alongside questionnaire and interview data to enhance the value of the latter. Such material allows researchers to access biological samples to test biomarkers and genetic associations, which otherwise might not be available.

Such samples might also provide useful biomarkers to validate or replace data items that would otherwise require detailed questionnaire. Examples include:

◆ Serum cotinine as a validation of (non) smoking response

◆ Serum vitamin D as a better marker of vitamin D status than dietary intake

Other population surveys include data from physiological measurements, such as blood pressure and data from imaging. As mentioned in Example 9.xii, the UK's Biobank study holds a very broad range of data items, collected on numbers that otherwise would have been impossible to achieve.

Example 9.xii

A summary of the data collected at the UK Biobank Assessment Centre follows here (see 'Further reading' for more information on the full list of data):

> *All participants in UK Biobank were recruited through assessment centres, designed specifically for this purpose (a map of the 22 assessment centres is provided in the Essential Information section of the Showcase). Data collected at the assessment visit included information on a participant's health and lifestyle, hearing and cognitive function, collected through a touchscreen questionnaire and brief verbal interview. A range of physical measurements were also performed, which included: blood pressure; arterial stiffness; eye measures (visual acuity, refractometry, intraocular pressure, optical coherence tomography); body composition measures (including impedance); hand-grip strength; ultrasound bone densitometry; spirometry; and an exercise/fitness test with ECG. Samples of blood, urine and saliva were also collected.*

9.3 **Linkage**

As suggested here earlier, the maximal enhancement of routinely collected data is the ability to link to other data sets. Thus, a prospective cohort study can be undertaken by linking a data set with 'baseline' variables to routinely captured data on clinical outcomes, as suggested in many of the examples in this chapter.

Linkage may be built in from the start (e.g. the UK CPRD was designed to link primary care records to hospital data). Alternatively, linkage can be undertaken on a case by case basis, depending on the needs of the researcher.

Example 9.xiii

In Sweden researchers were able to link a register of prescriptions for the use of certain drugs with data on sickness benefits paid out when individuals were unemployed. They were then able to examine one of the possible health economic benefits of the proposed treatment.

Example 9.xiv

In another example from Sweden, researchers were able to link questionnaire data on self-reported recreational drug use reported by conscripts to the army with subsequent admissions to a psychiatric facility with schizophrenia.

Linkage obviously requires an identifier that is common to the data sets. This may be a single national identification number available in some countries. Alternatively, a collection of readily available variables such as date of birth and gender, with current residence, might allow matching with an acceptable degree of accuracy.

The real challenge is the protection of the public and their agreement to allow linkages. If used inappropriately, there is a real danger of serious breaches of confidentiality and consequent individual harm.

Individuals might agree to linkages with identifiable information if they can be reassured about the *bone fide* use of the data, that the researcher, although being potentially able to identify the individual subject, would not attempt to do that but only use the linkage to provide aggregated data.

Increasingly in many jurisdictions, the potential that a researcher could identify a specific individual is precluded by having a system of 'pseudonymization' of data. This means replacing any identifying characteristics of data with a pseudonym, or, in other words, a value which does not allow the data subject to be directly identified. There would always be the possibility of the custodian of the data sets being able to identify the subjects, but the researcher would in theory only have the false identifier.

By contrast, 'anonymization' of data, as defined by European Data law means

> *processing it with the aim of irreversibly preventing the identification of the individual to whom it relates. Data can be considered anonymised when it does not allow identification of the individuals to whom it relates, and it is not possible that any individual could be identified from the data by any further processing of that data or by processing it together with other information which is available or likely to be available.*
> (Data Protection Commissioner, 2018)

Of course, 'irreversibly preventing the identification' cannot always be assured. It would not be impossible, for example, knowing from a survey response, that there was an individual of a certain age and occupation living in a small town, from being identified, if there was a strong desire to do so. The point is that such identification is against the law in most countries.

9.4 **Accessing routine data**

The reason why the future of epidemiological research is likely to be embedded increasingly in the use of routine data is based on the ease of availability. In this chapter, we have provided links to websites of some data sources, there are several others where the data are available online.

In other instances, application must be made to use the data and depending on the data sets, the researcher might be provided with the raw individual data to undertake their own analysis or the data custodians might undertake specific tabulations as requested. The term 'custodian' refers to the individual or organizations that manage the data and oversee its quality, storage, archiving, and release. Custodianship does not mean that they *own* the data, which is a more complex legal issue. Unrestricted access to publicly available data sets is rarely allowed and researchers will often have to complete an application, analogous to a research grant application, to justify the question(s) they are going to ask, and their proposed approach to analysis. *Thus, users of such data sets should be prepared to submit what can amount to a full protocol in the same way as might be necessary for a grant application, except if access is permitted the funding is for the user.* Those who provide access to data, while wanting to ensure maximal exploitation, are concerned about reputational risk and would wish to reassure themselves that the data will be used appropriately.

One issue is that access to data means that other researchers have the same access. Consequently, most large publicly available data sets are not restricted to those who ask first. The identity of the recipients of the data, and often the purpose to which they are planning to use the data, are also publicly available. In a competitive research environment, it is thus possible that different groups may be working on the same data set at the same time. Further an increasing condition of access is that the analyses undertaken are also made publicly available and add to the value of the originally stored data.

A final issue is that when raw data are provided, their format and nature is variable. The data may need 'cleaning' to remove errors, duplicates, and so on. There are often substantial needs for sophisticated data manipulation skills and utilization of anonymized raw data can be challenging to researchers. Researchers are strongly advised to seek advice and input from those with experience in handling data from the targeted sources. It is easy not to allow enough time or resource to adequately generate the data in a form that the formal statistical analysis can begin.

9.5 **Combining primary data collection with the use of secondary data**

This chapter has presented the use of secondary data as an 'either/or' with primary data. In fact, the situation is more nuanced, and the existence of existing data sources can be used as a population base to recruit subjects for more intensive primary data collection. Conversely, such sources can be used to gather follow-up information using routine health data sources from subjects that had been recruited and studied for a primary data-based project. Examples from both retrospective case–control and prospective cohort studies illustrate that researchers can use the existence of secondary data sources either to enhance the value and breadth of their original primary data directed study, or to render it more efficient in terms of time and resources.

Example 9.xv

In a study aiming to look at genetic influences on the risk of a relatively rare disease, the researchers used the existence of a large population based epidemiological study to identify cases and controls, and then obtained access to the stored DNA samples to undertake a candidate gene association study in their own laboratory.

Example 9.xvi

In a study aiming to examine the effect of childhood nutrition on bone density in early adult life, researchers were able to access the nutritional data collected in early infancy from a large epidemiological study undertaken previously which had also collected information on several possible confounders. They then obtained permission to sample some of the cohort at age 18 and seek their consent to measure the current bone density.

Example 9.xvii

A study of patients recruited from hospitals who had all received the same surgical implant were then followed up by linking to their subsequent hospital record and the regional cancer register to ascertain future morbidities without the need for further contacting the patients themselves. Not only did this reduce costs but mitigated against high levels of subject non-response had follow-up been based on direct patient contact.

9.6 **Conclusions**

There is a clear shift in epidemiological research away from academic researchers undertaking primary data collection towards spending more effort exploiting available data sets and the possibilities afforded by linkage between them. This leads to a debate as to what strategy a researcher should choose (i.e. how to decide between primary data collection and analysis of secondary data).

The advantages of using secondary data can be summarized as:

◆ Access to large and very large national and even international samples and populations

◆ Substantial savings in costs and time

◆ Possibility to undertake replicate studies over time, and between geographical areas

◆ Possibility of linkage to very broad sets of predictors and outcomes, far more than what could be achieved in a single funded epidemiological study

The disadvantages of using secondary data can be summarized as:

◆ Data collected may not be ideal in terms of instruments used or timing of collection, for the study question

◆ Quality of data (such as amount missing or way in which it was collected) is limited to the standards used by the specific data collection process and may be inadequate for the desired purpose

◆ Rules regarding data access and indeed publication may be restrictive

◆ Costs and resources are not negligible

◆ Others analysing the same data may publish their work before you

As public funds support large national data collections, the pressure on epidemiologists to better use such existing data sources and resources for individual primary data collection is likely to be harder to justify. In addition to the issue of resources the balance is between gain in extent and type of data against loss in control on quality and detail of data. Finally, in a world where data protection is an ongoing concern, societal acceptance of the use of data (whether anonymized or not) could limit its availability for research. The balance between individual privacy and the greater public good will always be a live issue.

Further reading

Access to data from large population studies
The Research Data Center of the National Center for Health Statistics https://www.cdc.gov/rdc/

Biobanks
http://biobank.ctsu.ox.ac.uk/~bbdatan/ShowcaseUserGuide.pdf

Communicable disease registers
https://www.gov.uk/government/publications/notifiable-diseases-weekly-reports-for-2017

Data linkage
Douglas A, Ward HJT, Bhopal R, *et al.*; **SHELS researchers** (2017). Is the linkage of census and health data justified? Views from a public panel of the Scottish Health and Ethnicity Linkage study. *J Public Health (Oxf)*, **25**, 1–6.

McDonald JT, Farnworth M, Liu Z (2017). Cancer and the healthy immigrant effect: a statistical analysis of cancer diagnosis using a linked Census-cancer registry administrative database. *BMC Public Health*, **17**(1), 296.

Surgical registries
Sedrakyan A, Campbell B, Graves S, Cronenwett JL (2016). Surgical registries for advancing quality and device surveillance. *Lancet*, **388**(10052), 1358–60.

Smith AJ, Dieppe P, Howard PW, Blom AW; **National Joint Registry for England and Wales** (2012). Failure rates of metal-on-metal hip resurfacings: analysis of data from the National Joint Registry for England and Wales. *Lancet*, **380**(9855), 1759–66.

Reference

Data Protection Commissioner. *Anonymisation and pseudonymisation*. Portarlington, Co. Laios, Ireland. Copyright © 2018, Office of the Data Protection Commissioner. Available at: https://www.dataprotection.ie/docs/Anonymisation-and-pseudonymisation/1594.htm

Part E

Information from epidemiological studies

Chapter 10

Collecting information

10.1 Introduction

A major activity of any epidemiological study necessitates gathering the information in a format and of a quality and completeness that are appropriate for the analysis planned. As discussed in Chapter 9, much of epidemiological activity is directed towards the analysis of data gathered for other purposes, such as routine health records. This chapter therefore focuses on the issues surrounding the collection of information that otherwise would not be available: *primary data collection.*

10.2 Role of primary data collection

Epidemiological information comes from a variety of sources. These may be conveniently divided into those that are available from previously documented data and those that require the gathering of new information. Examples of the former include extracting information about individuals from their medical records, occupational records, and similar data sources. However, if such individual information is not available in such sources, then obtaining information direct from the subject is required. The most frequent approach is to use a questionnaire to obtain data direct from the subject. It may be necessary to obtain data about the subject from a proxy respondent if, for example, the subject is a child, is too ill, is dead, or is otherwise incapable of answering. The questionnaire poses several methodological challenges. This chapter is therefore focused on the methodological aspects of questionnaire development and design. Outside the scope of this chapter, given the infinite number of sources of information from measurement, is the requirement to have information gathered from patient measurement including physiological measures (such as blood pressure), blood and other tests on body fluids or tissues, and imaging. Issues relating to the validity and consistency of these types of data are, however, the same as for questionnaires and are discussed in detail in Chapters 11 and 12.

10.3 Interview or subject completing questionnaire?

There are several ways of approaching subjects to provide information. Often, and most ethics committees would expect this, the approach is a two-stage process; the first is for the investigator (or the person who legitimately holds their information, such as the general practitioner) to contact the subject asking if they would like to participate, and the second stage involves collecting the specific information required. There are options of course for going back to subjects for additional information if required.

Example 10.i

A study of the risk factors for certain birth outcomes involved handing out letters at an antenatal clinic, seeking permission for the mothers to be interviewed during the twentieth week of pregnancy. At that interview they were asked if they could be contacted by telephone for a short interview after the birth.

Table 10.1 Options for collecting information from subjects

Contact with the subject	Examples of methods to collect information
Direct	◆ Face-to-face interview in public or private setting
	◆ Telephone, Skype, or similar interview
Indirect	◆ Postal survey
	◆ Collection by mobile app
	◆ Email/mobile request with link for web-based questionnaire

There are several ways that information can be obtained direct from subjects and these are listed in Table 10.1.

The clear advantage of the indirect approaches is that they can cover a large population, at little cost, in a short period of time. With direct methods, appointments must be arranged and this is particularly time-consuming. In addition to the issue of resources, the choice may be determined by factors such as the literacy of the target population, the availability and take-up of the chosen medium, and the sensitivity of the questions.

The key considerations in deciding between these two broad approaches are listed in Table 10.2.

1. The response rate may be higher in the interview approach, which necessitates a direct contact (including by telephone) to the subject. The main reason for non-participation is apathy rather than antipathy, and it is the experience of many that direct personal contact frequently ensures a greater response. However, telephone equipment often now allows the receiver to see the number calling and if it is not recognized it is less likely to be answered. This is a result of 'cold calling' becoming more common among sales companies. This advantage is lost, however, if the subject does not answer unknown numbers or if the initial request for interview is sent by post, requiring a positive response.

2. The completeness of the answers can be more assured by the direct approach. In self-completed hard copy questionnaires, questions may be ignored either deliberately or by accident. A useful ploy to minimize this in postal questionnaires is to add at the bottom something to the effect of, 'Can you please check that you have filled in all the relevant questions before returning this questionnaire?' With electronic-based instruments this is not an issue, as the design of the

Table 10.2 Direct or indirect approaches to information gathering

	Direct	Indirect
Cost	High	Low
Response rate	May be higher	May be lower
Completion of questions	High	May be lower
Complex questions	Can be included	Should be minimized
Interviewer bias	May be present	Not relevant
Interviewer variability	May be present	Not relevant
Sensitive questions	May be difficult	May be easier
Recall	May be different	

form can preclude going to the next question if the previous question is either ignored or an incomplete answer is given. This is familiar in all web-based instruments in normal life.

3. Questionnaires can have a fairly complex structure, for example, requiring routings of the type 'If *you answer 'no' please go to question 7, otherwise go to question 11'*. Such instructions, although relatively simple, can result in confusion. The best answer is as far as possible to avoid these internal routings, otherwise an interview-administered instrument or a web-based questionnaire may be better approaches.

4. A related issue is that complex questions in subject-completed questionnaires may be misinterpreted and answered inappropriately. By contrast, the interviewer can guide the answers and explain those that are more complex. Some areas, such as details of medical history and occupational exposure, are difficult to encapsulate in simple, easily answered questions, whereas the trained interviewer can separate the relevant from the irrelevant and obtain a more useful product.

5. By contrast, some issues, such as those relating to sexual and family relationships, substance injection may be better addressed by an indirect questionnaire, where the subject does not have to confront the interviewer. Typically, adolescents, for example, may be more willing to fill in an anonymous questionnaire about various aspects of their lifestyles than relate them to 'an adult in authority'. There are also some tactics in interviews which can preserve some blindness of the interviewer to the answers received and expertise in such approaches should be sought.

6. Interviewers are also subject to bias, particularly if they are aware of the hypothesis under investigation. They may, for example, probe more deeply in investigating cases than controls for a particular premorbid exposure, or may inadvertently give a direction on how to respond.

7. A related issue is that in studies involving more than one interviewer, there is scope for variability due to differences in the approach used by the interviewer and in the interpretation of any replies. Some of this may be overcome by training and standardized methods of administering the questions. In large surveys, the interviewers are frequently given a scripted text to read to ensure that they are presenting the material in a similar manner. It is difficult to exclude the possibility of interaction between the subject and the interviewer, with subjects responding differently to different personality types, however standardized the delivery of the questions.

8. Recall by the patient subject may be different when given the same question by an interviewer and in a self-completed questionnaire. The setting for completion is different between the two. In the interview situation there may be no time for the subject to consider his or her answer and/or to change it after an initial response. By contrast, given the greater time for completion of a self-completed questionnaire, a motivated subject may enquire of close family members and look for other supporting information for previous events.

Example 10.ii

A study asked individuals what travel immunizations they had had in the past 5 years. A telephone interview elicited a much lower frequency of certain immunizations than the same questions administered via a web-based survey. The assumption was that with the latter the subjects were able to look through their own records.

In summary, there is no single best approach. Financial and time constraints may exclude an interview-administered survey. If that is not the situation, the decision has to be made taking account of the points just mentioned. Ultimately, it is the nature of the information requested that will determine which of these imperfect approaches is the preferred option.

10.4 **Face-to-face and telephone interviews**

The use of the telephone is an attractive compromise between the face-to-face interview and other indirect ways of obtaining data. Compared to the former it is cheaper, saving in time and travel costs. Many subjects, reluctant either to attend for an interview or to invite a stranger into their home, may be content to answer questions over the telephone. Similarly, the face-to-face approach requires an initial contact either by telephone or post, to establish an appointment whereas, with permission, the telephone interview can be a 'cold call' although this can also result in a higher non-response. The telephone option also permits the initial contact and the information gathering in a single act. Internet-based video interviews using 'Skype', 'FaceTime', or similar can also be useful in establishing a better rapport than just voice calls. However, there are several disadvantages of telephone or internet phone contacts and these are:

◆ population selection is restricted to those with a telephone, leading to underrepresentation of lower social groups in some countries;

◆ telephone numbers may not be listed in directories;

◆ contact will need to be made outside normal office hours to maximize participation;

◆ multiple attempts may be necessary to reach a given subject;

◆ a direct refusal must be accepted, whereas in a postal survey a second or subsequent mailing may be issued to initial non-responders.

10.5 **How to formulate a questionnaire**

This is one of the most difficult tasks in survey research and there can be few investigators, despite the strenuous attempts at piloting and pretesting their questionnaire, who would not change their instrument if they were to repeat the study. The most common mistake is to ask too many and too detailed questions that are never analysed. The authors' experience, of sending out a questionnaire for comment from colleagues, is to receive numerous suggestions for additional topics ('Then while you are asking about x, why not ask about y?'). The computer files of many epidemiologists are littered with answers to questions never to be analysed!

10.5.1 **Open or closed questions?**

An important issue in survey research is the choice between 'open' and 'closed' questions. Unlike social science, most epidemiological surveys adopt the closed question approach as being the most efficient approach for data handling and analysis. This is best illustrated by example.

Example 10.iii

A researcher wanted to assess the amount of exercise subjects participated in during an average week. At the simplest level the choice between an open and a series of closed questions is shown in Table 10.2.

In the first situation, the subject is being asked to consider what activities he or she undertakes that would fit in with this description and to write them down. In the alternative formulation, the subject is presented with a list of options to make a decision (yes or no) about each one. Not surprisingly, the decision about the better approach is not absolutely clear (Box 10.1). Subject recall may be enhanced by the closed approach. Thus, in the example given in Table 10.2, walking and cycling may not be considered by some subjects as 'physical activities' and thus are ignored. By contrast, the open question can detect an enormous number of activities, which would be impossible in the 'closed' approach without an overlong survey form, much of

Box 10.1 Open and closed questions on physical activity

Option 1 'Open'

What sports and other physical activities do you undertake each week on a regular basis (at least 30 minutes)?

Please list each form of exercise and the length of time you spend doing it.

Activity   Length (in minutes/week)

1. ....

2. ....

3. ....

Option 2 'Closed'

For each of the following sports tick the box if you regularly spend more than 30 minutes each week undertaking that activity.

☐ Walking
☐ Jogging
☐ Working out at gym
☐ Exercise class
☐ Dancing
☐ Cycling
☐ Swimming
☐ Racket sports

which would be left blank. The open question allows the subject to address and describe complex issues which the investigator had not considered: thus, if the subject is a football referee, he or she may be reluctant to tick against playing football, yet the investigator may wish to detect this activity. Results from open questions are more difficult to handle analytically. The design of the database to handle the answers will need to take account of the material received. Similarly, the material will need to be carefully reviewed to determine how it fits in with the planned analysis. If one is undertaking a survey of 10,000 people a considerable amount of time would need to be set aside for processing just this single question. The most useful approach, in the absence of any previously available off-the-shelf questionnaire, is to use an open approach in developing and piloting the questionnaire and then to use closed questions formulated on the basis of the answers received. A modification of the closed approach which may be appropriate is to provide a list of options which includes 'Other'. If respondents tick this box, they can be invited to 'Please specify'.

10.5.2 Questionnaire design

The rules of questionnaire design are straightforward. Questions should:

- be simple;
- cover one dimension;

- have a comprehensive choice of answers; and
- have a mutually exclusive choice of answers.

To expand on these: first, the questions should be simple and cover one dimension only. It is better to ask separate questions, which should be closed rather than open (Table 10.3).

Example 10.iv

Rather than ask the complex question 'If you have ever regularly smoked cigarettes (at least once per day), how many years was this for?', it is preferable to separate out into a series of simpler questions that does not require the subject to perform calculations with the risk of error or lack of precision. Such questions could be:

1. *Have you ever smoked cigarettes at least once a day Yes No*
2. *If yes:*
   a. *What age did you start regularly smoking Age (years)*
   b. *Do you regularly smoke now Yes No*
   c. *If not smoking regularly, what was your age when you stopped Age (years)*
   d. *What was the average number of cigarettes smoked per day Number*

This latter approach is simpler to complete and then it is the researcher's task to do the calculations, for example, of number of years and intensity smoked (in this example smoking is often described in 'pack years', i.e. 10 cigarettes smoked for 10 years is equivalent to five 'pack years'.)

Secondly, in any closed question with a choice of answers, the choice should cover all possible answers including 'don't know/can't remember' which is different from 'no'. The choice of answers should be mutually exclusive, and it should not be possible for a respondent to tick more than one choice unless this is specifically requested.

Some examples of poor question design are shown in Table 10.4. Among other items, they display the problems that subjects may have in recall and the problem of lack of mutual exclusivity. Thus, in the second question the 'it varies' option may be the most accurate answer for all but the teetotal, ruling out any useful information emerging.

There are numerous research studies discussing colour, size, layout, and length of questionnaires produced for self-completion, whether electronically or in hard copy. Some are inevitably more 'user-friendly' than others, enhancing response (see 'Further reading'). Certainly, desktop publishing techniques have enhanced the appearance of questionnaires, but it is not clear whether these aspects substantially improve either the response rate or the quality of the answers; ultimately it is the quality of the questions that is the crucial factor. Some design features seem useful. A front page just with a study title and a few lines of instructions seems to be preferred, as there is a perception that the answers are kept 'under cover'. The print should be large enough and sufficiently widely spaced to be read with ease.

Table 10.3 Open and closed questions

	Open	**Closed**
Subject recall	Reduced	Enhanced
Accuracy of response	Easier to express complex situations	Difficult to investigate complex situations
Coverage	May pick up unanticipated situations	Will miss areas not anticipated
Size of instrument questionnaire	May need fewer lines of text	May need many pages of text
Analysis	More complex	Simpler

Table 10.4 Examples of poor question design

Question	Problem
What was your height at age 25?	Subject may have difficulty in recalling height. No option for 'can't remember', and thus the subject may be forced into an inaccurate response.
How many days a week do you drink alcohol? ☐ Never ☐ 1–2 ☐ 3–4 ☐ 5–6 ☐ Everyday ☐ It varies	The 'It varies' option is difficult to follow. As no subject is likely to have an identical pattern every week, then expect a substantial proportion completing this non-informative option.
What is your current occupation—if not currently employed, please put your most recent job?	The question is too vague concerning the amount of detail required. The questions need to be very specific, requesting the name of organization/firm and exact job title.
Do you take any of the following drugs or medicines? ☐ Painkillers ☐ Antidyspepsia ☐ Diuretics	Subject may not understand medical terms. Better to ask an open question to list names of current medication.
Have you ever taken the oral contraceptive pill? ☐ Yes/No If yes, how long did you take it for? _____ _____years	A superficially simple question that is full of problems. Does taking one tablet count as 'ever taken'? More problematically, it is very difficult—if not impossible—to aggregate cumulative consumption over a lifetime, taking into account breaks for pregnancies, and so on.
How many times a week do you eat cheese? _____ times	One of the problems with this type of question is asking about a theoretical time period; far better to ask about a real time period (e.g. last week).

Complex words should be avoided, as should long sentences. Shading may be used to highlight where the answers should be inserted. Instructions should always be given on what to do with the questionnaire after completion, including provision of prepaid envelopes for return.

Further reading

Questionnaire design

Edwards P (2010). Questionnaires in clinical trials: guidelines for optimal design and administration. *Trials*, **11**, 2.

Edwards PJ, Roberts I, Clarke MJ, *et al.* (2009). Methods to increase response to postal and electronic questionnaires. *Cochrane Database Syst Rev*, **8**(3), MR000008.

Marcano Belisario JS, Jamsek J, *et al.* (2015). Comparison of self-administered survey questionnaire responses collected using mobile apps versus other methods. *Cochrane Database Syst Rev*, **7**, MR000042.

Chapter 11

Obtaining valid information

11.1 Introduction

The information obtained in any study should be valid (i.e. the 'truth'). The limitations imposed on studying 'free-living' populations, as opposed to studying volunteers who may be willing to undergo invasive procedures or laboratory animals, is that indirect methods frequently must be used to obtain the data required, often by interview or questionnaire. The answers obtained may not represent the true state of the individual.

Example 11.i

A questionnaire is widely accepted as a simple means of screening a population for the presence of angina (the Rose Angina Questionnaire). It relies on self-reports of exertional chest pain. Clearly, there will be errors in its use in classifying coronary artery disease, but the alternative of coronary artery angiography is not appropriate for an epidemiological study.

Example 11.ii

As part of a study, it was necessary to investigate the dietary intake of vitamin D. The most valid approach would be for the subjects to weigh all food consumed during the period of study and provide duplicate portions for biochemical analysis. The approach chosen was 24-hour recall, where the subject recalls his or her total dietary intake during the previous 24 hours. This approach was substantially more acceptable and less costly.

The issue, at a practical level, is therefore not which is the valid method, but what is the size of the error in adopting the feasible option, and, by implication, does an error of this size alter the interpretation of the data obtained?

11.2 Sensitivity and specificity

The reader will probably be aware of the application of validity tests in assessing the performance of diagnostic and screening tests. In this situation, the objective is to evaluate the ability of a test to distinguish correctly between true disease-positive and true disease-negative individuals. It is conventional to evaluate this performance in terms of the two indicators, as shown in Table 11.1, *sensitivity* and *specificity*.

- *Sensitivity* is the proportion of subjects who truly have disease, who are identified by the test as 'disease positive'.
- *Specificity* is the proportion of subjects who truly do not have disease, who are identified by the test as 'disease negative'.

These proportions are often multiplied by 100 and expressed as a percentage.

When the result of a diagnostic test is dichotomous (positive or negative), the investigator simply needs to calculate the sensitivity and specificity of the test and decide whether they are

Table 11.1 Classical assessment of validity

Test result	'The truth' +ve	–ve
+ve	TP	FP
–ve	FN	TN
	TP + FN	FP + TN

Notes:

TP: true positives, correctly identified

FN: false negatives—true positive but test negative

FP: false positives—true negative but test positive

TN: true negatives, correctly identified

Sensitivity = Proportion of persons with disease correctly identified as disease positive = $\dfrac{TP}{TP + FN}$

Specificity = Proportion of persons without disease correctly identified as disease negative = $\dfrac{TN}{TN + FP}$

satisfactory for the purposes intended. Often, however, the result of a test may be a category or a reading on a continuous scale. In these cases, the investigator will need to evaluate the specificity and sensitivity at each (or a sample of) possible cut-off definitions for positive and negative. Thereafter a choice will need to be made of the cut-off that optimizes sensitivity and specificity for the purposes intended.

Example 11.iii

A study measures the concentration of substance X in the urine as a screening test for disease Y. In practice, during a population study all those screened have a concentration between 6 and 92 mg/l. There is an overlap between the distributions of concentrations between those with and without the disease. At the extremes, if the cut-off for disease is taken as a score of more than 0 then the sensitivity of this cut-off will be 1 (i.e. everyone with the disease will be labelled as disease positive). It is clearly not a useful cut-off, however, since the specificity is 0 (i.e. no-one without the disease is labelled as disease negative). Conversely if the cut-off is over 95, the disease sensitivity is 0 and the specificity 100. The challenge will be to find a cut-off value between these extremes that satisfactorily optimizes the values of sensitivity and specificity.

There is no 'magic figure' for either sensitivity or specificity above which a test can be said to perform satisfactorily. If the test result is a score then the investigator, by making the cut-off less stringent, will be able to increase the sensitivity. However, specificity is also likely to fall. One approach to choosing a cut-off is to plot a graph of sensitivity v. 1-specificity—a receiver operating characteristic (ROC) curve (Fig. 11.1).

The diagonal (dotted) line in Figure 11.1 represents the results from a hypothetical test that was no better than random at distinguishing positive from negative. The more discriminatory a test, the steeper the initial upper portion of the curve, and the greater the area under the curve. One possible 'optimal' cut-off is to choose the value corresponding to the shoulder of the curve (the point nearest the top left-hand corner of the graph).

The most suitable cut-off point will depend on its intended use. If screening for cancer one may wish to choose a cut-off other than the so-called optimal point. By increasing the sensitivity of the test, the number of false negatives would be reduced. This would likely be at the expense of decreasing the specificity (i.e. the number of false positives would rise).

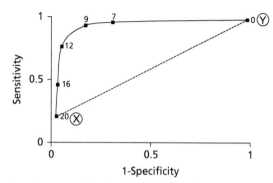

Figure 11.1 Example of receiver operating characteristic (ROC) curve: results of an interview questionnaire to determine presence of clinical depression

Notes:

• The 20-item questionnaire yields a score between 0 and 20. The values for sensitivity and specificity are calculated from a sample of 200 individuals, all of whom were interviewed with the use of the questionnaire and, additionally, clinically evaluated by a psychiatrist.

• At cut-off point X (equivalent to a cut-off of 20), very few individuals score positive, hence detecting few cases (sensitivity 0.2) but also few false positives (specificity 0.95). At cut-off point Y (equivalent to a cut-off of 0), all individuals are positive and hence the entire population is detected as a case (sensitivity = 1) with all true negatives classified as positive (specificity = 0).

• The results from five of the potential cut-offs are shown. At a score of 9 or more, the interview score would appear to be at its most discriminatory. A higher cut-off (e.g. 12) would miss too many true cases. A higher cut-off would result in a steep drop in sensitivity with only a small improvement in specificity, and vice versa for a lower cut-off.

Example 11.iv

In a large prospective cohort study of the possible long-term hazards from the use of the oral contraceptive pill, the aim was not to miss any possible morbid event. In seeking, therefore, to maximize their sensitivity by the ascertainment of all subsequent cases with a stroke, the investigators included a very broad range of neurological signs and symptoms that would be considered as positive.

Alternatively, in other circumstances high specificity will be important.

Example 11.v

In a case–control study of hypertension, the decision was made to restrict recruitment of cases to those individuals who had an untreated diastolic blood pressure of greater than 100 mmHg, sustained over three readings taken at weekly intervals. The desire was to have maximal specificity and not include individuals with a transient rise in blood pressure due to anxiety.

The previous discussion has focused on determining the validity of disease classification. However, the same principles apply to the classification of exposure in epidemiological studies. If it is appropriate to consider the exposure as dichotomous (exposed/not exposed) and the results from a gold standard are available, then the sensitivity and specificity of the method used can be determined as just explained.

Example 11.vi

In a large prospective study aimed at determining whether a particular trace-element deficiency was linked to the development of stomach cancer, deficiency was defined on the basis of a simple 'dipstick' test on a random urine sample. The validity of this approach had been previously investigated by comparison with the more cumbersome and costly collection and analysis of 24-hour urine samples collected from 25 volunteers.

11.3 **Validity for variables that are not dichotomous**

More typically, particularly in relation to exposure, a state may not be dichotomous, and then the question at issue is not whether the survey method got the right answer, but how close the value obtained was to the true value. The consequence of any impaired validity is misclassification of either disease or exposure status. The investigator therefore needs an estimate of the extent of any misclassification. One approach is to grade misclassification, based on the comparison of the answers to a survey with the 'true' grade.

Example 11.vii

The validity of self-reported levels of alcohol consumption was assessed by comparison with presumed 'true' data derived from a sample of spouse interviews. In this example, one can distinguish minor misclassification (one grade out) from more major misclassifications (Fig. 11.2). The weighting given to the misclassification depends on the investigator.

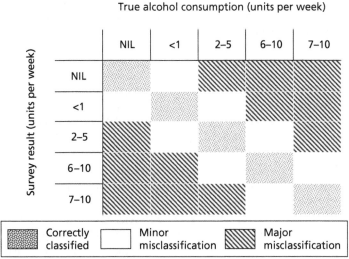

Figure 11.2 Assessment of validity in more complex situations

11.4 **Possible approaches for independent validation**

In the situations described in Examples 11.vi and 11.vii, the assumption is made that there is an independent gold standard measurement that will give the truth and allow an evaluation of validity and the size of the potential problem of misclassification. In reality, this is frequently neither available nor practical. Survey methods are often based on uncorroborated subject recall, and validation of the answers appears elusive. There are, however, several approaches that can be used to attempt to measure validity:

♦ validate in other studies;

♦ contemporary documented data (e.g. medical records, pregnancy/birth records, occupational/ personnel files);

♦ reports from spouse or close household contact or other close contact;

♦ in-depth investigation of random sample of respondents.

Note the following:

i) It is always worthwhile to use a method that has been validated in other studies of similar populations. Thus, the questionnaire to detect angina, mentioned in Example 11.i, has been validated against clinical diagnosis. No further validation is necessary unless it is thought that the characteristics of the questionnaire are such that there may be differences in sensitivity between populations, perhaps due to variation in language. There are many other examples where standard questionnaires have been validated against an independent gold standard, for example, on medication use or dietary intake. Unfortunately, secular, social, and geographical differences between populations mean that it may not be possible to assume that if a survey method has been shown to be valid in one group, it is necessarily valid in another.

ii) Where possible, the investigator should obtain contemporary collected information to validate recalled responses by using such sources as medical and occupational records.

Example 11.viii

A self-completed questionnaire was used to estimate previous oral contraceptive use. It was possible to validate the responses by checking against the respondent's general practice and family planning clinical records. Indeed, it was only necessary to study a small sample, at the start, to confirm the validity of the method used. It was also necessary to examine the records of a sample of those who denied ever taking oral contraceptives to confirm the validity of the negative response.

iii) In the absence of contemporary records, it is often possible to corroborate recalled information against that obtained from a household or other close informant. Again, this can be restricted to investigation of a sample. The problem in this situation is that when the two sources give conflicting answers, it cannot necessarily be assumed that one is inherently more accurate than the other, although, intuitively, the interpretation of such conflicts will depend on the topic investigated.

iv) If no other sources are available, then the investigator may have to find an alternative method of investigation for validating results from a sample, which might require an invasive or semi-invasive procedure. Some examples of this are shown in Table 11.2. Thus, urine cotinine is a sensitive test for cigarette smoking. A seven-day weighed-diet survey is probably the gold standard against which other dietary survey methods should be compared. In postal questionnaires using self-recording of height and weight, these measurements may be validated against the results obtained from true measurements. In surveys designed to detect clinical conditions, self-reported diagnoses, for example, of psoriasis, may be checked with evaluation by 'an experienced physician'. The hope is that, first, the survey method will be shown to be valid and, secondly, it will be necessary to undertake the validation in only a sample.

Table 11.2 Examples of validation approaches for samples from surveys

Survey variable	Validation approach
Cigarette smoking	Urine cotinine Blood carboxyhaemoglobin
Dietary intake based on food frequency	Seven-day weighed diary record
Self-reported height/weight	Standardized measurement
Self-reported disease status	Evaluation by experienced clinician

11.5 **Misclassification**

The final consideration, in relation to validity, is that it is worth remembering that the problem is one of misclassification. An imperfectly valid method will misclassify individuals, as regards either their disease or their exposure status. Perhaps surprisingly, misclassification need not be a disaster. If, in comparative studies (such as case–control or cohort investigations), the misclassification is random then the effect will be to make it more difficult to discover a real difference against this background 'noise'. Thus, if the study detects a difference (say) in exposure between cases and controls, then the fact that there is random misclassification could not explain the result, which still stands. Indeed, that true association between an exposure and disease state will be greater than that observed in the study.

Example 11.ix

A case–control study of middle-aged women examined the influence of self-reported weight at age 25 on current bone density. It was found that there was a substantial positive association between current bone density and recalled weight. The investigators, although anxious about the dubious validity of recalled weight from many years previously, thought it unlikely that those with low bone density were more likely to underestimate their recalled weight than those with high bone density.

Non-random misclassification is more serious and is based on there being differences in the validity of the survey method in its application between groups. Here the effect on the study results cannot be predicted, and depends on the direction of misclassification. Hence it may be possible to explain an observed association by non-random misclassification. These concepts are discussed further in the discussion of bias in Chapter 19.

Further reading

White E, Armstrong BK, Saracci R (2009). *Principles of Exposure Measurement in Epidemiology: Collecting, Evaluating and Improving Measures of Disease Risk Factors.* Oxford Scholarship Online (Chapter 4: Validity and reliability studies); DOI: 10.1093/acprof:oso/9780198509851.001.0001

Chapter 12

Repeatability

12.1 Introduction

The previous chapter focused on the challenges in obtaining valid information from participants within epidemiological studies in 'free living' populations. An equally relevant consideration is the difficulty in obtaining consistency of the results. Several terms are used in describing this phenomenon. They are often used interchangeably, although some authors have attempted to distinguish between them (Box 12.1).

Common sense determines that there may be a variety of reasons for failure to obtain consistent or reproducible results.

◆ First, there may be true subject variation. This is particularly relevant in physical measurements such as blood pressure, heart rate and similar variables that, in normal individuals, vary with time, even over short periods. There is also normal variation in lifestyle habits such as amount of exercise or diet, as well as physical and psychological symptoms.

◆ The greater concern, however, is that of a lack of consistency in the result obtained in the absence of true subject change. This lack of consistency may be due either to a single observer being inconsistent in the method of measurement or to inconsistencies between one or more observers. If this occurs to any major extent, data obtained from studies may be difficult to interpret because apparent differences between subjects might reflect differences in measurement.

12.2 Reducing subject variation

In any study the aim is to ascertain real individual measures that have biological meaning but exclude those that contribute random error, sometimes referred to as 'noise'. What constitutes 'noise' depends on what is the aim of the investigation.

Example 12.i

A study aimed to compare the blood pressure between adolescents from different ethnic groups. In planning the study, the researchers were aware that several factors can affect blood pressure including time of day, relationship to time of last meal and of last exercise. Thus, in addition to standardizing the approach to measurement, the participants were also measured within a narrow time of day and with limits to recent exercise and food. By contrast, if the research wished to examine time of day as a predictor of blood pressure then the participants might still need to have similar restraints in terms of time of last meal and exercise, but time of day would be a relevant predictor to record.

12.3 Reducing observer variation

As mentioned, individual observers may vary in their results due to variation in their methods of measurement, even when keeping subject level variation to a minimum. Training to assess this and continuous observation during a study can help. Ensuring observers follow a rigid protocol,

---

Box 12.1 Terms used to describe the results of epidemiological studies

Repeatability:	Strictly, given the same set of circumstances, how consistent are the results obtained?
Reproducibility:	An alternative expression for repeatability typically as applied to a measurement tool.
Reliability:	Normally reserved to determine consistency between observers or between techniques. If consistent results can be explained by true subject change, this is therefore not due to poor reliability of the measurement.
Agreement:	Typically reserved for expressing level of consistency between observers.

---

which equally applies to administering a questionnaire as it does to physical measures, is also recommended. In general, a single observer can reduce the variability compared to when multiple observers are used.

In many studies it may be impossible to use a single observer to obtain all the necessary data and therefore multiple observers are required. However, a single observer may prove to be just as inconsistent over time as multiple observers. In theory, with rigorous training and standardization of approach, it should be possible to measure and minimize inconsistencies. Training may need to be repeated during the data collection period of a study to ensure maintenance of quality. Some illustrative examples are shown next.

Example 12.ii

A study involved the use of a stadiometer to measure height. In pilot studies of a single observer undertaking repeated measurements on the same subjects, some inconsistency was noted. After extra training this inconsistency disappeared.

Example 12.iii

In the same study as in Example 12.ii, a second observer had difficulty in obtaining acceptably close results to the first observer when assessing the same test subject. Again, training removed this inconsistency. As a quality control against 'drift', the two observers were checked every three months during the study by duplicate measures on six, randomly selected subjects.

There is, however, the potential problem of subject–observer interaction such that even in response to an interview, different subjects respond differently to minor differences between observers: this requires very close attention during training.

It is not always necessary to formally test consistency within observers.

Example 12.iv

In an interview-based study that involved a quality of life assessment, a pilot study suggested that certain questions were answered differently depending on the sex of the interviewer. The answer to this was to use interviewers of one gender only.

If between-observer agreement is good, it can be assumed that within-observer agreement is also satisfactory. Clearly, the converse is not the case.

Example 12.v

In a study assessing perceived severity of eczema on a 0–4 scale, the investigator was concerned about incon-sistency in assessment by an observer. It was not sensible for the observer to undertake duplicate assessments on the same patients because it would be impossible not to be influenced by the results of the first assess-ment, given the difficulty in ensuring blindness of assessment. The investigators overcame this problem by undertaking a training session using photographs, which included repeats that showed good between-observer consistency.

12.4 **Observer bias and agreement**

These are different concepts, but both may explain inconsistencies or lack of reproducibility in re-sults between observers. Bias occurs if one observer systematically scores in a different direction from another observer, whereas poor agreement can also occur when the lack of precision by a single observer is random.

Example 12.vi

In a study that required observers to score X-rays by making measurements of the images based on specific landmarks on the images, it was found that one observer routinely measured from different landmarks on the films. This led to substantial disagreement and a systematic bias between that observer and the others. However, there was also variation due to the inherent difficulty on precisely locating the landmark on some of the films because of the quality of the images.

The possibility of bias is relatively easily assessed from differences in the distribution of meas-ures obtained. Thus, (i) for continuous variables it is relatively simple to compare the results from two observers by using a paired t-test or similar approach, and (ii) for categorical variables the frequencies of those scored in the different categories can be compared with a Chi-squared or similar test (see also Section 12.5.1).

The assessment of agreement is discussed next in detail.

12.5 **Study designs to measure repeatability**

In any study in which multiple observers are to be used, it is necessary to measure their agree-ment before the start of information gathering. The same principles apply when there is a concern about a lack of consistency within a single observer. The essence of any study to investigate this phenomenon is to obtain multiple observations on the same subjects by the different observers (or replicate measures by the same observer) done sufficiently closely in time to reduce the likelihood of true subject change. An ideal approach is to enlist some subject volunteers who are willing to be assessed in a single session by multiple observers. It is important to take account of any order effect (i.e. where there is a systematic difference in measurement response with increasing number of assessments). One strategy to allow for this is to use the so-called 'Latin square' design (Table 12.1). In the example illustrated, five subjects are assessed by five observers in a predeter-mined order. With this kind of design, it is relatively simple statistically, by using an analysis-of-variance approach, to separate the variation between different observers from that due to order and, of course, that due to the subjects themselves. A similar approach may be used when testing for reproducibility within an observer. One problem, however, particularly in assessing interview schedules, is that both the subject and the observer may remember the response. In such circum-stances the replicate interviews need to be spaced in time, but not to such an extent that the true state of the subject has changed. The particular details of individual studies will determine what an appropriate interval is.

Table 12.1 The 'Latin square' design for a study of repeatability: five subjects (1–5) and five observers (A–E) giving the order in which the observers assess the subjects

Observer	Subject				
	1	2	3	4	5
A	1st	2nd	3rd	4th	5th
B	5th	1st	2nd	3rd	4th
C	4th	5th	1st	2nd	3rd
D	3rd	4th	5th	1st	2nd
E	2nd	3rd	4th	5th	1st

12.5.1 Analysis of repeatability

The analytical approach is different for measures that are categorical and those that are continuous.

Categorical measures

For categorical measures, the kappa (K) statistic is the appropriate measure of agreement. It is a measure of level of agreement in excess of that which would be expected by chance. It may be calculated for multiple observers and across measures which are dichotomous or with multiple categories of answers. For the purposes of illustration, the simplest example is of two observers measuring a series of subjects who can be either positive or negative for a characteristic. There will be patients that both observers agree have the characteristic and similarly do not have the characteristic. There will be other subjects where there is disagreement.

The kappa statistic is calculated as follows.

Judgement by Observer B	Judgement by Observer A		
Observer B	**Positive**	**Negative**	**Total**
Positive	a	b	a + b
Negative	c	d	c + d
Total	a + c	b + d	a + b + c + d = N

$$\text{Proportion that A scored positive} = \frac{a+c}{N}$$

$$\text{Proportion that B scored positive} = \frac{a+b}{N}$$

Therefore, by chance alone it would be expected that the proportion of

$$\text{subjects that would be scored positive by both observers} = \left[\frac{a+c}{N} \times \frac{a+b}{N} \right]$$

$$\text{Proportion that A scored negative} = \frac{b+d}{N}$$

$$\text{Proportion that B scored negative} = \frac{c+d}{N}$$

Therefore, by chance alone it would be expected that the proportion of

subjects that would be scored negative by both observers $= \left[\dfrac{b+d}{N} \times \dfrac{c+d}{N} \right]$

Therefore, total expected proportion of agreement $= \left[\dfrac{a+c}{N} \times \dfrac{a+b}{N} \right] + \left[\dfrac{b+d}{N} \times \dfrac{c+d}{N} \right] = P_e$

Maximum proportion of agreement in excess of chance $= 1 - P_e$

Total observed proportion of agreement $= \dfrac{a+d}{N} = P_o$

Therefore, proportion of observed agreement in excess of chance $= P_o - P_e$

The observed agreement in excess of chance, expressed as a proportion of the maximum possible agreement in excess of chance (kappa), is:

$$K = \frac{P_o - P_e}{1 - P_e}$$

Example 12.vii

In this example two observers were asked to score X-rays of 120 subjects as to whether they thought a specific abnormality was present. The results were:

		Observer A	
Observer B	**Positive**	**Negative**	**Total**
Positive	57	13	70
Negative	16	34	50
Total	73	47	120

The two observers had the same judgement on 91 subjects (57 + 34).

$$\text{Thus, the observed agreement} = \frac{57 + 34}{120} = 0.76.$$

Just knowing the actual positive rates for each observer (73/120 for Observer A and 70/120 for Observer B) then just by chance alone it would have been expected that the product of these two proportions would give the expected number in which both scored positive. Adding in the expected number where both scored negative, the overall agreement is then:

$$= \left[\frac{73}{120} \times \frac{70}{120} \right] + \left[\frac{47}{120} \times \frac{50}{120} \right] = 0.52$$

$$\text{Thus kappa } K = \frac{0.76 - 0.52}{1 - 0.52} = 0.50.$$

The use of kappa is important, as the often-used proportion of total agreement does not allow for the fact that some agreement is due to chance. The interpretation of kappa values is subjective, but as a guide Table 12.2 may be useful.

Table 12.2 Interpretation of kappa

Value	Strength of agreement
<0.20	Poor
0.21–0.40	Fair
0.41–0.60	Moderate
0.61–0.80	Good
0.81–1.00	Very good

Mathematically kappa can range from – 1 to + 1. Values below zero suggest negative agreement (i.e. which means that if one observer scores positive the other is more likely to score it negative than positive!). This is not normally of relevance unless circumstances are bizarre. Values close to zero suggest that the level of agreement is close to that expected by chance.

Bias can be assessed by examining the marginal totals. In Example 12.vii, the proportions scored positive by the two observers were similar (70/120 vs. 73/120), excluding any serious systematic bias even though the agreement is only moderate.

Continuous measures

For continuous measures, the simplest initial approach is to determine for each individual subject the absolute level of disagreement between observers. Several measures of agreement can then be obtained. First, calculation of the mean disagreement and the standard deviation around that mean can give an estimate of the range of disagreements. Secondly, calculation of the standard error of the mean disagreement can be used to provide a 95% confidence range for the likely mean disagreement. Finally, the closer the mean disagreement is to zero, the less likely is the presence of systematic bias.

Example 12.viii

Forty subjects had their waist circumference measured by two observers. The following results were obtained.

| Subject number | Circumference (cm) measured by: | | |
	Observer A	Observer B	Difference, *d*
1	64.2	64.6	–0.4
2	71.3	71.0	+0.3
3	80.4	84.2	–3.8
.	.	.	.
.	.	.	.
.	.	.	.
.	.	.	.
40	66.2	65.4	+0.8
Mean	**70.6**	**71.0**	**–0.4**

The average difference between the two observers was (A–B) –0.4 cm (and assume the standard deviation = 0.25).

An assessment of agreement can then be calculated:

Limits of agreement

The 95% range of disagreements (observer A–B) = $-0.4 \pm (1.96 \times 0.25)$

$= -0.9$ to $+0.1$.

Thus, the disagreement between these two observers for 95% of subjects will be between –0.9 and + 0.1 cm.

In addition, the data can be plotted graphically. On the x axis is plotted the mean of the two values and on the y axis the difference (a 'Bland–Altman' plot). The plot can then display the range of agreements but also if there is a systematic bias between the two observers. The plot can also illustrate if there is a relationship between the level of the score and the amount of agreement.

Further reading

Dunn G (1992). Design and analysis of reliability studies. *Stat Methods Med Res*, 1(2), 123–57.

Landis JR, Koch GG (1977). The measurement of observer agreement for categorical data. *Biometrics*, 33(1), 159–74.

White E, Armstrong BK, Saracci R (2009). *Principles of Exposure Measurement in Epidemiology: Collecting, Evaluating and Improving Measures of Disease Risk Factors*. Oxford Scholarship Online (Chapter 4: Validity and reliability studies); DOI: 10.1093/acprof:oso/9780198509851.001.0001

Chapter 13

Participation in epidemiology studies

13.1 Introduction

Epidemiologists have traditionally considered that one of the hallmarks of a 'good' epidemiology study is a high participation rate, and indeed this is often one of the metrics used in scales which formally assess quality. In practice it can be very difficult to get an epidemiologic study which has a very low participation rate published in a high-quality journal. The main reason is that, all other things being equal, lower participation will increase the influence of non-response bias in a study (a type of selection bias which is discussed in Chapter 19). However, it should be noted that even in studies with high participation there exists a possibility of selection bias if non-participants are markedly different from participants in aspects that are key to the conditions being studied.

Nevertheless, today people are less willing to take part in epidemiological studies than they were in the past. There has been a steady decline over the past 50 years in industrialized countries, with one review estimating that between 1970 and 2003 participation rates among controls in population-based case–control studies declined at a rate of almost 2% per year (see 'Further reading'). The authors of this book, when conducting research in the United Kingdom, using population-based sampling frames and asking people to complete a paper questionnaire, have experienced this. In the 1990s, surveys would typically achieve participation rates around 70–75%, but in the 2010s this has decreased to around 30–35%. Telephone surveys have had the same experience. However, some studies achieve higher participation than others. Why is this? It will be discussed next why participation is likely to have decreased and what researchers can do in the design of their study to increase the chance of subjects responding. Furthermore, it is just as important for cohort studies that subjects continue to participate and are not lost to follow-up. This will also be considered later in this chapter (Section 13.5).

Firstly, the terms which are used to describe participation in epidemiology studies will be considered, because different studies measure this in different ways and even use similar terms to mean different things.

13.2 Measuring participation in epidemiology studies

When reporting the results of epidemiology studies, authors use a variety of terms and calculations to describe the extent to which persons took part in the study. Given that there are no absolute standards for the various terms and their calculation, this can mean that two authors use the same term to describe this but calculate it in different ways. Examples of the terms used include 'return rate', 'response rate', 'cooperation rate', and 'participation rate'. The first observation to make is that none of these are actually 'rates', they are all properly called 'proportions'. Next is to understand where potential confusion arises. If a postal survey of the adult population is undertaken and persons who are aged 25–74 are eligible, how do you deal with the questionnaires that are not delivered and marked 'return to sender', 'person has moved away', or where you are notified that the person has died? Should these persons be considered not eligible and thus removed from the denominator? Certainly that seems reasonable if a person has died, but what about the others? One doesn't know where the others have moved to—it could be to a nearby street (thus making them still potentially eligible) or to another country (probably making them not eligible). If persons do not reply at all (and there is no other notification) do you assume they were eligible or not? If your sampling frame allows you to tell the sampled person's age you might reasonably assume that they are eligible, but where you rely on information given by the respondent to determine eligibility, it is not possible to know whether a non-respondent would have been eligible.

Some studies classify 'respondents' and thus the response proportion based on everyone who has replied, whether they have given any useful information or not. If someone started to complete the study questionnaire but returned it only half-completed, they have certainly responded, but have they provided enough information to participate? In such circumstances it can be a good idea for a study to define a 'minimum data set' which subjects are required to provide in order to be classed as a participant. For example, if a respondent to a questionnaire missed out the question on gender, it is likely that they will be classified as 'missing' in most analyses.

If a study requires not only a postal questionnaire to be returned but also a biological sample to be provided (such as saliva for genetic analysis) is a study subject considered a participant if they only return the questionnaire? In such scenarios it is prudent to report participation separately for each stage of a study.

The *Dictionary of Epidemiology* (see 'Further reading') only defines *response rate* and does so as follows: 'The number of completed or returned survey instruments (questionnaires, interviews, and so on) divided by the total number of persons who would have been surveyed if all had participated. Usually expressed as a percentage'. Although this is useful, researchers will still need to make a decision on how to operationalize this definition.

The American Association for Public Opinion Research has clarified how its organization defines terms. It defines *response rate* as 'the number of complete interviews with reporting units divided by the number of eligible reporting units in the sample'. In epidemiological studies, reporting units would normally be individual people. In contrast the *cooperation rate* is defined as 'the proportion of all reporting units interviewed of all eligible reporting units ever contacted'. The difference here is that the *cooperation rate* is calculated among persons with whom contact is made and eligibility is established. This term is rarely used in epidemiology although the definition is used, but termed response rate or participation rate by many studies. Given the fact that, for ethical reasons, people are often given the option of responding with a blank questionnaire to avoid further contact, the term *participation* may grow in use and more accurately describes what is being measured.

Given the complexity of designs (such a multistage aspects of some studies) the notion of having a simple proportion describe participation is unrealistic. The main message for researchers is that it should be made clear in any publication how participation has been quantified (and at each stage of a study, if applicable). There is a tendency for researchers to try to obscure the true participation or not describe it all, particular if the participation proportion is low. Not only is this bad practice, but it can potentially lead to misinterpretation of results by readers. An example of the detail which may be given is in Figure 13.1. Using these data, it can be seen that figures could be presented in a variety of ways: participation ranges from 39.6% (of persons in the original sample) to 42.5% (of persons in the original sample who were assumed to have received the invitation to participate), or it could be expressed (although not very usefully) as 46.4% 'returned the study questionnaire' (i.e. 2,165/4,661). Giving the flow chart is the most transparent way to report the information.

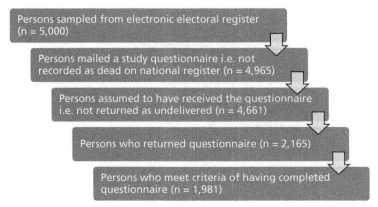

Figure 13.1 Example of a flow chart reporting participation in study.

Example 13.i

Figure 13.2 shows how a researcher might report participation in a study manuscript. This describes the process of participation from drawing of the sample from the sampling frame to identifying how many people have provided sufficient information to make a useful contribution to the main study analyses. The conservative estimate of participation in this study is 21.0% (i.e. 2,094/9,949; 9,949 is the study sample who have not been notified as dead). Some authors might report the participation rate as 21.7% (i.e. 2,094/9,656), using as the denominator, the number of persons likely to have received the invitation to participate. However, the people who have not received the questionnaire (because, for example, they had moved) were a part of the sample and may, for example, have different aspects of lifestyle and history of disease from those less likely to have moved.

Example 13.ii

In a hospital case–control study, cases were persons diagnosed with adenocarcinoma of the lung admitted to one of three hospitals on an island. The senior nurse identified 130 newly diagnosed cases within the study period and approached them to ask whether they would be willing to consider taking part and meet the study coordinator to learn more about the study. A total of 87 persons agreed to do so (the others were either not interested to take part, did not have time, or the senior nurse considered them too ill). Thereafter when they had received further information, 78 took part in the study as cases. The participation rate among cases in this study is therefore 60% (i.e. 78/130).

13.3 **Reasons for non-participation**

There are several reasons why subjects refuse to participate in research (and specifically epidemiological research), whether this involves completion of a mailed questionnaire or attendance at a clinical facility for a moderately invasive procedure such as a blood test or imaging. The major reasons are:

- lack of interest or perceived personal relevance;
- inconvenience;
- avoidance of discomfort;
- financial cost;
- antipathy to research;
- worry about confidentiality.

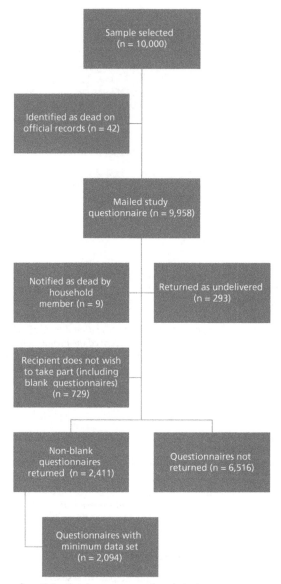

Figure 13.2 Reporting of participation in a cross-sectional study.

In practice it is often difficult and perhaps unethical to seek an explanation for non-participation. The various reasons given here for non-participation are, however, discussed next with suitable strategies for their reduction.

13.3.1 Lack of interest or perceived personal relevance

Most epidemiological studies find that the proportion of persons invited who agree to participate is higher among females and increases with older age. In reality, it is difficult to solve this differential participation by demographic factors. In sending out letters of invitation, it is often valuable to stress that there is a need to study persons without the disease of interest in order to understand

---

Box 13.1 Invitation to participate emphasizing the need for persons with and without disease under study

'... *we have therefore chosen to study individuals from the general population, selected at random from the electoral register. It is only by receiving answers from a broad section of the population that we can understand why some people develop [this disorder] ...*'

---

disease. Indeed, it is common to receive letters from those invited to take part querying whether, if they don't have the condition under study, their replies are useful. Some subjects do not participate because they do not see any personal gain. Their current health status is likely to be a key determinant. Those with the disease under study (such as cases in a case–control study) are more likely to enrol to seek a greater understanding than those who perceive themselves to be healthy (controls). Conversely, in practice, those who have poor health may, in practical terms, consider it difficult to take part.

It is useful to state clearly that it is the goal of the study, for example, to compare those with and without the disease of interest, and why a population recruitment policy has been followed (Box 13.1).

It is often a more productive strategy to use registers constructed from healthcare sources, such as those registered with a general practice, to approach general population samples. If the letter-head also includes the address of that local practice and is signed (on behalf of the study) by the general practitioner, there is a greater perceived relevance and sense of involvement, as well as approval from a trusted source. Suitable phrasing is shown in Box 13.2.

13.3.2 **Inconvenience**

This may reflect an unwillingness to spend time completing a form, a reticence to receive a home visit or a reluctance to attend a survey centre. Clearly, depending on the nature of the survey, much can be done to reduce the level of inconvenience to the subjects targeted (Table 13.1). Diaries of symptoms or of variable exposures, such as 24-hour food intake diary, are useful but they are tedious to complete. Response can be disappointing, and the mere fact of recording exposures can change them. For example, respondents may choose to have more convenient ready-made meals rather than weighing and preparing a meal *de novo*, or the recording of intake may cause them to reflect on their diet and change it. In the letters sent prior to home or survey centre visit, it is useful to cover the issues mentioned in the table. Maximum effort should be made to allow easy access and without cost, and to make the visit as short as possible. Poor organization or experience can rapidly become known, particularly through social media, hindering later recruitment.

Box 13.2 Explaining why someone has been approached to participate

'Researchers from the University of Aberdeen have asked our practice to help with a large health study. We have agreed that the attached questionnaire can be sent to a random sample of our patients ...'

Table 13.1 Strategies to reduce inconvenience

Type of strategy	Strategies
Postal survey	Clear instructions and estimate of time to complete
	Keep questions simple
	Ask the minimum number of questions to achieve study objectives
	If possible, avoid sensitive questions
	Provide reply-paid envelope
	Provide contact details for queries
Home visit	Offer choice of times, including outside working hours
	Be clear how long visit will last and keep it to a minimum
	Be sensitive to needs of elderly participants and those with dependents such as young children
Survey centre visit	Offer choice of times, including outside working hours
	Be clear how long visit will last and keep to minimum
	Provide transport costs and parking facilities
	Reduce waiting time to a minimum
	Provide contact details for cancellations/rebookings

13.3.3 Avoidance of discomfort

This is obvious and while it has not often been a feature of traditional epidemiological studies, it is more common now for studies to identify persons for further investigation with more invasive procedures which may involve imaging, receiving treatment, and so on. It may be that some techniques are not possible for some persons to undertake such as magnetic resonance imaging among persons with claustrophobia. The best approach is to be clear about what taking part in each stage involves, the commitment required (which may be over several weeks) and any risks in taking part.

13.3.4 Financial cost

As mentioned in Table 13.1, the survey should be prepared to reimburse the costs of travel and parking. The timing of visits should be done to reduce the need for time off from work or the need to obtain extra childcare. Sensitivity shown in these issues is often amply rewarded. It is becoming more common for epidemiological surveys to reimburse participants for their participation. Ethics committees usually approve of such reimbursement although not at a level which could be seen as an inducement to take part.

13.3.5 Antipathy to research

As mentioned already, though difficult to measure, probably the greatest reason for non-participation is a less than positive view about the benefits of research in general or the particular project. Mostly this is neutral, but at the extreme end there will always be some strongly worded letters or telephone calls in response to a request for participation. To the novice these can be unsettling and time-consuming to deal with. When conducting large studies, say of 100,000, even if only 0.1% are annoyed about the request, that will result in about 100 letters, which can seem like a lot!

The reality is that, provided that all required approvals are in place for the project (see Chapter 23), these inevitable but infrequent events can be easily managed without compromising the research. The most appropriate way to deal with such complaints is quickly and by a polite letter expressing regret at any distress or telephone call. It is also recommended that complainants are provided with details that all the necessary regulatory approvals are in place.

It is our perception that such complaints are becoming more common.

◆ It is easier now for people to express their displeasure through, for example, email or social media.

◆ People are aware of data protection regulations which are in place in many countries and wonder how researchers have obtained their contact details. They often believe that access may have been given to other data (e.g. medical records) without their permission. It is now standard practice therefore to have the initial approach come from the person who has legitimate access to their data (such as general practitioner) and data only to be passed on once a person has decided to take part, and with their consent.

◆ There are more demands on people's time from researchers and this is likely to contribute to lower participation.

◆ There has also been a reduction in trust in researchers. Firstly, there have been several research scandals where researchers have conducted unethical research, or commercial companies try to gain information from people, in the guise of research, and then sell the information they have gained. There are also many 'consumer surveys' conducted now masquerading as research, with little value other than to the company conducting them.

13.4 **Maximizing participation in epidemiological studies**

There is now a considerable body of evidence on strategies which increase participation in epidemiological studies conducted using a postal questionnaire (Table 13.2).

13.4.1 **Incentives**

Providing incentives to those persons invited increases participation. The most effective incentives are monetary, and larger incentives are more effective than smaller incentives. If an incentive is being offered, it is most effective if it is not contingent on receiving a response (i.e. it is given up-front with the questionnaire).

Example 13.iii

A study conducted of health among workers in several industries found, in the first few workplaces surveyed, that the proportion of workers agreeing to participate was low. The chief investigator therefore decided to include £10 with the study questionnaire. Another investigator preferred only to give £10 to those who responded but the evidence available suggested that this would be less effective, and the administration of the payments was more complex and costly.

13.4.2 **Questionnaire length, content, and appearance**

It has been consistently shown that invitees are more likely to return shorter questionnaires, when the topic of the questionnaire is interesting to the respondent and when it doesn't contain any sensitive questions. Response has been shown to increase if there is an assurance of confidentiality.

Table 13.2 Strategies to increase participation

Approach	Specific strategy increasing response
Incentives	Monetary incentive vs. no incentive; larger vs. smaller monetary incentive
	Monetary incentive vs. non-monetary incentive
	Non-monetary incentive vs. no incentive
	Incentive not contingent on response
Questionnaire length and content	Shorter questionnaire; assurance of confidentiality
	Interesting questionnaire topic; questionnaire does not include sensitive items
Delivery strategy	Advanced notification of questionnaire
	Registered mail vs. normal mail; Use of first class mail for outward posting; hand-written addresses; stamped reply vs. business reply envelope
	Postal response option only vs. postal or internet response options
	Follow-up reminder; follow-up reminder which includes copy of questionnaire vs. follow-up reminder without a second copy of questionnaire
Origin of contact	University vs. not university
Communication strategy	Personalized letter of invitation

Example 13.iv

An investigator found that a study questionnaire when all the required questions, instruments, information, and consent sections had been added resulted in it being 28 pages in length. On giving it to colleagues to answer, she found that it took an average of 45 minutes to complete. She thought it unlikely that people would be willing to spend this amount of time. Therefore, she went through the questionnaire and removed all items or instruments which were not critical for the study objectives. This resulted in a 16-page questionnaire that took 25 minutes to complete and which she considered would be more acceptable.

13.4.3 **Delivery strategy**

There is good evidence that sending advance notice of a questionnaire being delivered increases response when the questionnaire is received. The reason is not clear, but people might appreciate the advance notification and/or look out for the questionnaire arriving. It is important, however, to put clear contact details on the advance notification letter (and to be prepared to receive communications) since the receipt of this letter will potentially reveal persons who have moved away, died, are too ill to complete a questionnaire, or otherwise just don't want to receive a questionnaire. An example of such an advance notification letter is given in Box 13.3. Where investigators have the facility available, sending out the initial communication by 'priority post' (or registered) is associated with higher participation.

As might be imagined, sending a reminder increases participation and it is most effective if another copy of the questionnaire is included.

Sometimes the evidence on factors which influence participation seem counterintuitive. Generally, it is considered good practice to increase opportunities for people to respond. However, in studies which have looked at, within postal questionnaire surveys, whether giving people the additional option of replying by electronic means (web questionnaire accessible via the internet), they have found that it does not improve participation, and in some cases has even resulted in a lower overall response rate.

Box 13.3 Example advance notification letter for epidemiological study

Practice headed paper

Miss Holly Burton
77 Scotswood Road
HOPKINSTOWN
CF37 6SZ

13th July 2018

Dear Miss Burton

Health study

The University of Aberdeen has asked our practice to help with a large health study. We have agreed that a questionnaire can be sent to a random sample of our patients, and your name has been selected. You will receive the questionnaire within the next couple of weeks.

You do not have to take part in the study if you do not want to, and your healthcare will be un-affected by your decision. In fact, the practice will be unaware of whether you took part or not. Your participation would be much appreciated by the research team, irrespective of whether you think you are in good health or not.

If you should have any queries regarding the study, please contact [insert name], at the University of Aberdeen, on [insert telephone number] or [insert email].

Thank you for your help,

Yours sincerely

GP name

On behalf of [practice name]

13.4.4 Origin of contact

Studies which come from a university are associated with higher participation than those coming from other sources.

13.4.5 Communication strategy

A personalized letter of invitation has been shown to result in higher participation than a letter which is not personalized.

Example 13.v

Although it was easier to prepare standard letters that said 'Dear Sir or Madam' for all invited participants in a population survey of 20,000 persons, the investigators decided to devote time to producing individualized letters starting, for example, 'Dear Mrs Lamont'. The letter included an assurance that information provided would be treated as confidential. They also made sure that their university logo was prominent in the letter. Each of these decisions were made in order to improve the chance of invited persons participating.

Box 13.4 Example invitation letter for epidemiological study

Study no. ⬚⬚⬚⬚⬚⬚

[Insert study logo]   [Insert logo of the organization conducting the research]

The Maintaining Musculoskeletal Health Study

SURVEY QUESTIONNAIRE

(All information will be kept strictly confidential)

We would be grateful if you could complete this questionnaire which should take about 20 minutes. The study, conducted by the University of Manchester, is concerned with identifying people who have been to their doctor with pain. *However, your answers are important to us even if you do not have pain.* The questionnaire is the first step in a study to test new approaches for improving treatment of pain.

Please read through the covering letter from your general practitioner before filling in the questionnaire. Participation is, of course, voluntary. We will treat all responses as confidential. They will be used for research purposes only. As a 'thank you' for your time we have enclosed a £10 voucher which can be used in several high street stores.

If you have any questions about this study, please contact:

[insert named person, address, telephone, and email details]

If you do not want to take part in this survey, please show this by ticking the box below and posting it back in the envelope provided. This will ensure that you are not approached again.

By ticking this box, I confirm I do not want to take part in the study and do not want to be contacted again. ⬚

Taking account of these factors, an example of an invitation letter to participate in an epidemiological study is given in Box 13.4. As in this example, such an invitation is often accompanied by a letter from someone whom the recipient already knows.

On occasion, one may opt to have a very brief invitation letter but to provide relevant details of the study in an enclosed information sheet. An example of such an information sheet is provided in Box 13.5.

13.5 **Follow-up of subjects in a cohort study**

There is a specific need to maintain participation over time in cohort studies. The term 'retention' is often used to describe this. Thus, the crucial activity to enhance the validity of a cohort-based study is the follow-up of the individuals recruited after their baseline investigation. There is a requirement to keep track of the study population. Although some outcomes (such as vital status or incident cancers) may be ascertained through linkage to national records, most require contact

Box 13.5 Example information sheet for epidemiological study

[Insert study logo]   [Insert logo of organization conducting research]

INFORMATION SHEET

Study title: Women's Health Study (WHEST)

We would like to invite you to take part in a research project. We are interested in women's health, and specifically, in symptoms some women may experience. The aim of this study is to find out how common the symptoms are and how they affect the general well-being of the women. Your participation is highly important to us regardless of whether or not you experience any of the symptoms we ask about. Please take your time to read the following information carefully and please get in touch with us if you have any questions.

What will I have to do if I take part?
If you decide to take part, you will need to complete a survey questionnaire which is included in this pack.

How long will it take?
The questionnaire will take about 30 minutes to complete.

What are the possible risks of taking part?
There are no risks envisaged with taking part in this study.

Are there any possible benefits?
There are no direct benefits to you as a participant. However, by participating you will be helping to improve our knowledge of the impact of some common symptoms in women and indirectly contribute to finding ways of improving the management of the symptoms.

Do I have to take part?
No, taking part is voluntary. If you would prefer not to take part, you do not have to give a reason. If you do not wish to take part, please return a blank questionnaire and you will not be contacted again. If you take part but later change your mind you can withdraw at any time.

What happens to any information that you obtain?
The university complies with the Data Protection Act and all information will be treated with the strictest confidence.

Will you pay my expenses?
A prepaid return envelope is included therefore there is no cost to you.

Can I get any more information?
If you have any other queries, please feel free to contact [insert contact name] at:

[insert contact address, telephone number and email]

Funding: This study is funded by [insert funder's name]

This study has been reviewed by [insert name of ethics committee].

with the participant directly. It is good to keep in regular contact to learn about change of address. In many countries, for a short time, persons will redirect mail to their new address giving a time window still to contact them at their previous address.

Example 13.vi

In a study determining survival among persons receiving chemotherapy for lung cancer, the investigator sent out a postcard every six months to determine whether the individual still lived at his or her baseline address. She was concerned about identifying those who had moved and although all participants were linked to national records for vital status, it provided an alternative way to be alerted that they had died.

It may also be important to determine whether there has been a change in the exposure status since baseline assessment. The necessity to obtain this information depends on whether the study is examining the risk of 'ever exposed' or of length or other measure of exposure dose. The investigator should also consider whether those previously unexposed have become exposed.

Example 13.vii

A major prospective cohort study was undertaken to examine the risk of second-hand tobacco smoke on health. The intended follow-up was for 10 years. Participants were contacted annually to reassess their second-hand smoke exposure (since they may have changed workplace, partners, and so on) and also to learn whether they had moved address.

Any follow-up can also be used to determine change in status for other potentially important variables that might affect the analysis, such as confounders (see Chapter 18). Thus, in Example 13.vii, if someone has made changes to their lifestyle which resulted in reduction of exposure to second-hand smoke, they may also have changed their alcohol consumption and diet, and it would be important to capture this.

13.5.1 Ascertaining disease status

There are several strategies for ascertaining disease status during follow-up (Table 13.3). If the researcher is interested in deaths, then there will be national recording systems available to ascertain these. Most countries now have population-based cancer registries. For specific incident diseases for which an existing register is likely to ascertain all cases, data collection is simplified. This might be achieved using national cause-of-death registers, national morbidity registration, or hospital inpatient diagnostic or primary care registers. The success of these approaches relies on the likely

Table 13.3 Options for obtaining information on disease status in cohort studies

National registers	Will usually measure vital status, cause of death; national cancer registers are available in many countries
Disease notification registers	Information may be available from hospital or general practice registers
Continuous monitoring using specific notification methods	Either the patient could record events in diary (such as hospital admissions) or there could be continuous monitoring of general practice records
Cross-sectional surveys	General practice record review; hospital record review; subject questionnaire/interview/examination surveys

completeness and accuracy of ascertainment. It may be necessary to undertake pilot validation studies to confirm these assumptions.

Example 13.viii

In a multinational occupational cancer study, the investigators used national cancer registries to ascertain the cases that developed. In several countries, they were able to take advantage of the system where they could 'flag' all their study population at the start of the study. They then received notification of cancers when they were registered.

It is possible to use a similar approach when population-based diagnostic registers for hospital inpatients exist.

Example 13.ix

In a Swedish study, an epidemiologist was able to obtain questionnaire data on marijuana use by army recruits. He was then able to link the national identity numbers to hospital inpatient databases to obtain subsequent information on admissions with schizophrenia.

Such linking of registers has most commonly been undertaken in Scandinavia, although it is becoming increasingly possible in other countries. While the opportunities to link data sets have increased, so too has awareness and legislation concerned with data protection, that is, defining how (and by whom) data about individuals is accessed and used, specifically in relation to the consent. Thus, while access is often possible, the process can be complex, time-consuming, and increasingly costly.

Example 13.x

In a general-practice-based study of low back pain, a baseline population survey of psychological and other risk factors was followed by the continuous notification by the general practitioners of all new consultations with low back pain. This notification was achieved electronically because the reason for all consultations in these general practices was routinely logged on a computerized register, and the codes to identify consultations with low back pain were ascertained.

In most circumstances, such registers are insufficient or are unavailable, and a specific system for disease ascertainment needs to be introduced. In theory, the most appropriate tactic is to supply the subjects with a special form to post back if a specified outcome occurs. Alternatively, if a small number of clinical departments are involved, the reporting system could be via clinicians. In reality, these sorts of reporting systems often result in incomplete ascertainment. Therefore, combining these with an available records system might be the best solution.

Example 13.xi

In a study, an attempt was made to identify subsequent strokes in general practice patients who had had a baseline blood pressure measurement. An alert was placed in the electronic records of the patient to alert the general practitioner, in the event the patient had a stroke, of specific pieces of information that should be recorded (e.g. type of stroke). This approach, though fine in theory, failed in practice for several reasons including lack of time of the general practitioner and record of stroke, which almost always was diagnosed in hospital, did not make its way into general practice records.

Others have tried giving study subjects postcards to post back if they develop the disease under question. Apart from very short-term investigations, for example, an outbreak of food poisoning, it is likely that such cards will be lost or forgotten. Thus, in many prospective surveys, it is necessary for the investigator to contact the study population directly during the study to obtain the necessary outcome data. This will require a cross-sectional survey using a postal (or electronic) questionnaire, interview, or examination as appropriate. Multiple surveys are likely to be required and the timing of the surveys must be sufficiently close in order not to miss events. An example of a follow-up letter for use during a prospective cohort study is given in Box 13.6

Example 13.xii

In a large prospective study of fracture risk, the participants were sent a simple annual questionnaire enquiring about fractures in the previous 12 months. Other studies had suggested that recall of fractures over a 12-month period would be adequate.

Box 13.6 Example letter to accompany follow-up questionnaire for epidemiological study

[Insert study logo]   [Insert logo of organization conducting the study]

Julianna Kosłowska
13 High Street
ASHFOLD CROSSWAYS
RH13 6HN

12-month follow-up

Dear Miss Kosłowska,

The Maintaining Musculoskeletal Health Study

The 'Maintaining Musculoskeletal Health' study team are grateful for your continued participation in the study. We are contacting you now, 12 months into the study, to find out about your health. It is very important for us to be able to determine this and to know if your symptoms have stayed the same, worsened, or improved. This allows us to understand better what factors influence symptoms. **This is the last time-point in the study we will ask you to complete a questionnaire.**

The questionnaire enclosed is very similar to the one you filled in before you entered the study, and should take you no more than 20 minutes to complete. Once completed you should return it in the enclosed postage-paid envelope. If your contact details have changed since we were last in touch, you can tell us about this in the questionnaire. All data which you provide will remain confidential within the study team.

If you have any questions, please contact

[insert name, postal address, telephone number, and email]

Sincerely,

[Insert name of study principal investigator]

13.5.2 **Minimizing loss to follow-up**

The final issue in the study design is ensuring that losses to follow-up are minimized, both to reduce the likelihood of bias and to maintain sufficient numbers, so that the prestudy sample-size calculations remain valid.

The following strategies can minimize losses:

i) Use disease registers that do not require direct contact with subjects.

ii) Keep follow-up period to a minimum.

iii) Encourage continuing participation by regular feedback and other contacts, for example, newsletters, birthday or Christmas cards.

iv) Demonstrate to participants the value of their contributions, and a lay summary of progress (and some results) can be helpful in this respect.

v) Minimize the obligations and inconvenience to participants. Answering a questionnaire by post regularly is likely to be more acceptable than repeated requests to attend for examination or blood taking.

vi) Collect information at baseline that offers alternative approaches to contact if a subject moves or dies. Suggestions include electronic communication (email), names and addresses of non-household relatives, neighbours, or employers. Depending on where a study is conducted there may be systems for locating individuals who have moved.

vii) Provide postcards at baseline to participants in the study, asking for them to be posted back in case of relocation (although, as mentioned earlier, this may not be a fool-proof method).

Further reading

Trends in participation in epidemiology studies

Galea S, Tracy M (2007). Participation rates in epidemiologic studies. *Ann Epidemiol*, **17**(9), 643–53.

Reporting participation in epidemiological studies

Morton LM, Cahill J, Hartge P (2006). Reporting participation in epidemiologic studies: a survey of practice. *Am J Epidemiol*, **163**(3), 197–203.

Porta M (ed) (2015). *Dictionary of Epidemiology*, 6th edition. Oxford University Press, New York, NY.

Standard Definitions: final dispositions of case codes and outcome rates for surveys. American Association for Public Opinion Research (2016 Version). Available at: http://www.aapor.org/AAPOR_Main/media/publications/Standard-Definitions20169theditionfinal.pdf

Evidence in relation to maximizing participation in epidemiological studies

Edwards PJ, Roberts I, Clarke MJ, *et al.* (2009). Methods to increase response to postal and electronic questionnaires. *Cochrane Database Syst Rev*, **3**, MR000008.

Chapter 14

Feasibility and pilot studies

14.1 Introduction

Many epidemiology studies involve large numbers of participants, are conducted over a long period of time (such as cohort studies), and are very expensive. This is particularly the case in randomized controlled trials, which because of complex regulations and bureaucracy over their conduct, can be extremely expensive even if only a relatively straightforward intervention is planned. Therefore, if the study finds out that the duration of the study visit, the sensitive nature of some of the questions asked, or the distance most people are required to travel are all unacceptable and are affecting recruitment, then this will have important implications. It is likely that the study would need to be stopped, replanned, and new approvals sought. This would have a significant impact on the timescale of delivery of the project and probably also result in increased costs. For this reason, it is becoming more common to conduct pilot and feasibility studies. Both are conducted in anticipation of a future larger study or trial, and indeed grant-awarding bodies will often expect to see evidence that they have been conducted. Eldridge and colleagues (see 'Further reading') propose that *'a feasibility study asks whether something can be done, should we proceed with it, and if so, how'*, while a pilot study is a study *'in which a future study or part of a future study, is conducted on a smaller scale'*.

14.2 Feasibility studies

Feasibility studies are used to test individual components of a study. All epidemiological studies include various components and in planning it is important to list these and to decide whether any prior feasibility studies are required. Figure 14.1 gives examples of the areas which may be suitable

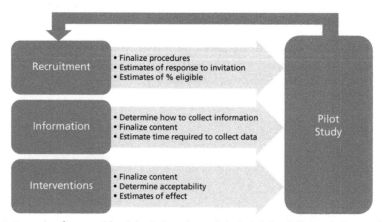

Figure 14.1 Preparing for an epidemiological study or clinical trial: feasibility and pilot studies.

for feasibility studies including recruitment, information collection, and (if applicable) interventions. The results of these feasibility studies would then allow details to be finalized, which would then inform the conduct of a pilot study.

Example 14.i

An investigator was planning a two-year cohort study to examine, among persons referred to mental health services, which persons were at high risk of attempting to take their own lives. In planning the study, the investigator made a list of issues that she considered important to determine before undertaking the study:

a) *How would eligible subjects be identified and when, in terms of their contact with medical services?*

b) *What proportion of eligible subjects would be willing to take part?*

c) *How would information be collected from each subject (from medical records, from interview, by questionnaire)?*

d) *How easy would it be to follow-up participants, how many will continue to take part, and how could information on relevant outcomes be identified?*

e) *How much researcher and administrative staff time is required to 'process' the recruitment of a subject to the study?*

She found that previous similar studies had used two named friends or relatives as a back-up approach to keep in contact with the study participant and found that together with reports from participants, general practitioner notes had been shown to be able to identify when relevant outcomes had occurred. She therefore decided to conduct two feasibility studies. One focused on points (a) and (b) earlier (identifying and contacting potentially eligible subjects) and the other focused on point (c), investigating alternative ways of collecting the necessary data.

As in Example 14.i, when assessing the feasibility of different aspects of a study, it can be informed by the past experience of the investigators or colleagues or other researchers. Published work can also provide insights into successful approaches; although written reports will often not provide detailed enough information on, for example, how in practice subjects were approached and how recruitment took place. If recruitment takes place through clinics, staff working there will be invaluable in identifying how and when patients can best be approached. Support will be needed not just from the clinician in charge but also the nursing staff working in the clinic, if a study is going to be successful. One of the biggest issues for most studies will be recruitment. Whether it be a population-based cohort study, a hospital-based case–control study, or clinical trial, recruitment will ultimately determine whether the study is a success or not. No matter how important the study, how sophisticated the design, it will fail if sufficient numbers of subjects are not recruited. It is important to be extremely cautious when estimating likely recruitment. Clinicians have a tendency to overestimate the number of persons who they actually see with a specific condition!

An example of the useful range of information which may be obtained from feasibility studies is given in Examples 14.ii and 14.iii.

Example 14.ii

An investigator planned to conduct a case–control study of Parkinson's disease and to recruit cases through a local clinic. The clinician in charge estimated that approximately 20–30 cases were seen per month in the clinic. The investigator took this as an initial estimate but decided to (a) ask clinic staff to record prospectively the number of persons seen over a three-month period who could be eligible, and (b) approach them to tell them about the planned study and whether they would consider taking part if asked. Over the three-month period the staff found 30 unique people with Parkinson's disease (others were repeat attenders) but estimated that 20 would be potentially eligible. The others did not meet specific diagnostic criteria or were taking part in other studies. Of those approached eight said they would probably agree to take part. The others considered that the additional clinic visits required to take part in the study would mean that it was not possible for them to easily take part. This feasibility study allowed the investigator to have much more realistic estimates of recruitment to her study.

Example 14.iii

A prospective cohort study on respiratory health involved a clinic assessment at the time of recruitment. The assessment lasted two hours and therefore slots were set aside at 09:00, 11:00, 13:00, and 15:00 to accommodate participants. There were enough time slots provided to accommodate all the participants. A feasibility study of the baseline assessment visit found that the visit was almost always completed within two hours. However, the 09:00 and 15:00 slots were very unpopular with study participants and were frequently unfilled. Therefore, it was decided that instead of having two full-time nurses working on the assessments, four part-time nurses would work on the project and only the 11:00 and 13:00 visit slots would be offered.

Sometimes feasibility studies may be undertaken at an earlier stage of a study, even if it is not clear whether a study is actually required (Example 14.iv).

Example 14.iv

There was concern in a US community that there were higher rates of cancer than could be expected and that this may be a result of pollution of groundwater supplies with agricultural or industrial chemicals. Community leaders called for a study to examine whether there was an excess and, if present, the cause. The local health institute felt that a comprehensive evaluation would be extremely expensive, and they did not consider that there was enough evidence to launch such a major study. Instead they proposed a feasibility study, which would allow them to evaluate the currently available evidence and to determine the possible approaches for its study. This would allow officials to make a more considered decision on how to proceed. However, the work itself would reassure the community that the officials were taking the issue seriously (see 'Further reading').

Example 14.v

A major epidemiological study invited all adults aged 18–89 years in a defined geographical area to take part. Persons agreeing to do so were required to attend a clinic visit. During the visit they completed a questionnaire. One of the items required them to list their current medications: drug name, dose, and frequency. Many participants were unable to remember this information and responded 'don't know' to the item. In the revised study procedures, therefore, participants were asked to bring their current medication with them to the clinic visit and the research nurse recorded this information on the system.

Researchers often wonder whether they can collect information on a likely size of effect from feasibility studies. This might mean the size of association in a case–control study or effect of intervention in a randomized controlled trial. In reality, a small feasibility study is not going to provide estimates of effect (that is, of course, the reason the main study or trial is being conducted). However, if one was piloting the intervention in a group of people who would be eligible for a future trial, then one might expect to see positive effects at least consistent with those being used to inform the sample size calculations.

14.3 **Pilot studies**

In contrast to feasibility studies, which are looking at individual aspects of studies, pilot studies are putting all the individual components of a study together and testing the 'whole system'. Figure 14.1 emphasizes the role of the feasibility studies in informing details of the pilot study. However, the pilot study can also provide information which then results in aspects of the study being redesigned (see Examples 14.vi and 14.vii).

Sometimes the pilot study is carried out as an 'internal pilot' i.e. the study is commenced but with the intention, for example, that the first wave of mailings is 'testing the system' and built in to the study timetable will be an opportunity to make small changes. This approach can be suitable and less costly, but it is unlikely to be able to accommodate major changes to a study. This may be valuable, particularly in instances of rare diseases where all identified cases may need to be used to give the study sufficient power. Instead it is more common for there to be a stand-alone pilot study which is conducted and then an evaluation takes place on whether it was successful and/or what elements need changing.

Example 14.vi

A prospective cohort study was planned to examine predictors of outcome for persons undergoing a knee replacement operation. Recruitment was arranged to take place during patients' preoperative assessment. Feasibility studies established that the method of recruitment was acceptable to patients and nurses, that the questionnaire was easy to understand, and that it could be completed in 30 minutes. When a pilot was designed, however, in practice it was found that there was not enough time to complete the questionnaire while waiting for their assessments. Many patients took the questionnaire home but failed to return it, leading to many patients recruited having to be excluded. The preassessment visit was reorganized to allow a dedicated 30 minutes time slot for completing the questionnaire prior to the participant being called for their first assessment.

Example 14.vii

A 2 × 2 factorial randomized controlled trial designed for persons with poor sleep (affecting their health) involved them being randomly allocated to either six sessions of cognitive behaviour therapy and/or a group-based exercise programme. Feasibility studies had determined how best to recruit people, tested the instruments to be collected in the study, and a small number of patients were given 'taster' sessions of one of the interventions. When the pilot study was conducted, however, feedback indicated that patients allocated to exercise and cognitive behaviour therapy felt that there was a lot of overlap between the interventions, while some advice was contradictory. Therefore, the investigators had to work on a minor redesign of both interventions to rectify this issue for persons assigned to both interventions.

The sort of questions which can be addressed in a pilot study are given in Tables 14.1a–c. They have been divided into scientific, process, and resource issues. Some of them could be addressed in

Table 14.1a Possible 'scientific' issues which can be addressed in pilot studies

Scientific issues
Are the eligibility criteria for entry to the study clear to the research nurses?
Can recruitment be completed within the time available during the clinic visit?
Do potential participants have concerns (a) about participating in some parts of the study? (b) not covered in the patient information sheet?
Were there questions which participants had trouble completing on the questionnaire?
Did any participant notice any errors in the questionnaire?
What proportion agreed to follow-up in six months' time?
What was the missing item rate on the clinical information which nurses recorded through the medical notes?
(In a trial) how many of the treatment sessions do participants engage with, on average?

Table 14.1b Possible 'process' issues which can be addressed in pilot studies

Process issues
What were the most popular day and times for persons to request their clinic visit?
Was the participation rate similar across all researchers? How did those with the highest recruitment rate achieve this?
What was the distribution of times to complete recruitment for an individual in the clinic? What did those who recruited subjects more quickly do differently?
Considering the various 'activities' that participants needed to complete for recruitment, were there any 'bottlenecks' in the system? If so, how could it be arranged differently to avoid this?
Two different types of recruitment letter were used—was there any difference in participation rate or feedback on the letters?
By how much does recruitment have to be slowed if one of the recruitment nurses who undertake clinical measurements is not available?
What rate of mailing invitation letters generates a flow of potential participants that the research nurses can deal with, without having a large backlog?

feasibility studies, however, in reality it is not possible to conduct feasibility studies on all aspects of a study and thus they may be addressed in the first instance in the pilot study where all aspects of study preparations come together. As discussed earlier it may be that the pilot study only highlights some minor issues, which can easily be rectified and thus one can progress to the main study or an application for funds for the main study, backed up by the appropriate feasibility and pilot data. Alternatively, it may be that substantial issues are highlighted at the feasibility stage, such that a substantial rethink of the approach to recruitment is required and a further feasibility study is warranted.

In summary, the pilot study (or pilot studies) is an essential component of preparing to conduct an epidemiological study. Ample time and resources invested at this stage will be rewarded with a greatly enhanced chance of a successfully conducted main study.

Table 14.1c Possible 'resource' issues which can be addressed in pilot studies

Resource issues
How many clerical staff are required to mail out 5,000 invitations and to process the returns?
How many telephone queries does a mailing of 5,000 invitations generate and how long do these take to deal with?
What is the most efficient way of processing the returns: e.g. (a) entering all questionnaires as they return; (b) enter eligibility information and only continue to enter information if they are confirmed as eligible; (c) visually look at the questionnaire eligibility responses and put as low priority for data entry those identified as not eligible?
How many research nurses are required to deal with all persons potentially eligible, from a 5,000-person mailing, and which doesn't result in a backlog of recontact of more than two weeks?
(In a trial with group therapy) what is the longest waiting timing for a person before the treatment group is complete and ready to start?

Further reading

Bender AP, Williams AN, Sprafka JM, Mandel JS, Straub CP (1988). Usefulness of comprehensive feasibility studies in environmental epidemiology investigations: a case study in Minnesota. *Am J Public Health*, **78**(3), 287–90.

Eldridge SM, Lancaster GA, Campbell MJ, *et al.* (2016). Defining feasibility and pilot studies in preparation for randomised controlled trials: development of a conceptual framework. *PLoS One*, **11**(3), e0150205.

Pilot studies for randomized controlled trials

Thabane L, Ma J, Chu R, *et al.* (2010). A tutorial on pilot studies: the what, why and how. *BMC Med Res Methodol*, **10**, 1.

Analysis and interpretation of epidemiological data

Chapter 15

Preparation of collected primary data for statistical analysis

15.1 Introduction

Although increasingly epidemiological studies are based on the analysis of existing data sets (including linked data sets), many studies still require primary data collection. Such data may come from patient questionnaires, interviews, abstraction from records, and/or the results of tests and measures such as weight or blood test results. The next stage is to analyse the data gathered from individual subjects to provide the answers required. Although statistical analysis is a necessary, and conceptually perhaps the most difficult, part of the task, most of the work in the analysis of any epidemiological study is in the preparation of the data. Indeed, the availability of modern software means that the statistical analysis stage often requires much less time than that required for the preparation of the data. Although reviewers and readers of epidemiological reports may comment on the dexterity of a statistical analysis, the painstaking and laborious work in ensuring that the data is in the appropriate form and free of errors is often taken for granted.

This lack of emphasis is also true for those planning studies. In many grant applications, resources are requested for data collection and for statistical and computing expertise, but no provision has been made for the more resource-consuming tasks of data preparation.

15.2 Hard copy or electronic means of data capture

Studies will vary as to whether the primary data is collected directly into a computer application that can then be analysed using software programmes, or whether the data is in some other 'hard' form and would need to be entered into a suitable data collection package.

Table 15.1 gives several options for how data can be gathered, which will depend on the nature of the data required and the resources available.

There is no 'best buy' and the method will need to be determined by the scale, study population, resources, and context of the study. Data preparation tasks will need to be adjusted accordingly. A hard copy of data can be useful to allow checking for quality and errors but adds an extra stage to the process, which increases both costs and the possibility of errors transcribing from one format to another.

Example 15.i

A study in an antenatal clinic required the midwives to complete a form for each patient visiting with weight, blood pressure, and so on. Although it would have been much easier for the researchers and minimized errors if the midwives could have entered the required data directly onto computer screens during the consultation, this did not fit easily in their pattern and location of work, and they preferred to complete paper forms and send these to the study team.

Table 15.1 Typical options for data collection

Options for collecting data
Patient/subject completed paper form
Interviewer completed paper form
Patient/subject completed electronic form using tablet or phone app
Patient/subject completed electronic form using a web-based system
Extraction of individual subject items from electronic database for separate study

15.3 **Hard copy data collection direct from subjects**

On receipt of the data, the first stage is a manual review of the data gathered. This may involve checking of self-completed questionnaires or a review of data forms used to obtain interview or other data. Self-completed questionnaires are prone to several errors. Questions may have been missed, multiple answers given when only one was required, inconsistencies emerging such as a subject responding negatively to 'ever pregnant?' but then giving the age of first child. Another problem occurs when the subject ignores the choices given and writes a small (or even a long!) note giving a detailed answer relevant to that particular question. Piloting and field testing may reduce the likelihood of such problems but cannot eliminate them altogether. Decisions should be made on how to deal with such errors. The counsel of perfection is to contact the subject again for clarification, although this is often not feasible or indeed ethical. Otherwise rules must be adopted based on common sense.

Example 15.ii

In a large population-based survey covering different lifestyle factors, several subjects had answered negatively to the consumption of specific pharmaceutical preparations including the oral contraceptive pill, but had then gone on to give a starting date and duration of exposure. The decision was made to convert the initial negative answers to those lifestyle exposures to positives on the assumption that the subject had made an error.

Example 15.iii

In the same population-based study as that just described, respondents were asked if they had 'experienced pain during the past month which had lasted at least one day'. If they responded positively, they were asked to indicate on a manikin the individual sites at which they had experienced pain. A small proportion of subjects had indicated pain on the body manikin, but had answered negatively to the first question about pain. Here it was decided to take the answer to the first question as 'true', assuming that if persons had pain in some body sites, it did not meet the definition required (i.e. 'had lasted at least one day').

Frequently, though, it is difficult, if not impossible, to work out the 'correct' answer, and the data on that particular question for that subject has to be considered as missing.

Example 15.iv

In a survey on pregnancy-related factors, one woman had ticked 'yes' to the question asking about ever having a successful pregnancy, but crossed out the subsequent question dealing with dates of pregnancies. There may have been reasons for that woman not wishing to provide the data, or the initial 'yes' might have been wrong. Without further information, it is not clear which of these alternatives was most likely to be true.

15.4 **Hard copy data collection information by trained interviewers**

For interviewer-obtained data, the interviewers can be trained to check the interview form carefully, before leaving the subject, in order to pick up omissions, obvious errors, and common transcription problems such as inserting the current year instead of year of birth. Often within such a short time, the interviewer can recall the correct answer and at the very worst it may be possible to recontact the subject if the time interval is short. Frequently interviews are conducted over the telephone and the same checking process should be allowed, and time made available at the end of the interview. When the interview involves collection of information such as recording of physical findings, it may be possible to collect material that could be used for validation purposes.

Example 15.v

In a survey involving home visits, trained nurses were asked to examine and score the subject for psoriasis (among other items of physical examination). In cases of doubt the nurses were asked to take pictures on a mobile phone, with the patient's consent, and their findings were discussed soon after the interviews with an experienced clinician, who could then make a judgement as to the likelihood of psoriasis being present.

15.5 **Preparing hard copy data for indirect computer entry**

It is not always possible for the data collected to be in the appropriate format required for data analysis. It is therefore necessary to modify the data before entering it on to the computer database. This modification is referred to as *data coding*, the 'coding' implying that a simple 'language' is developed to facilitate data entry and analysis. Data that are already in numerical form, such as year of birth or number of children, can be entered directly and do not require coding. Other simple categorical variables such as sex may be modified for ease of data entry. Typical codes might be 'm' for male and 'f' for female. The layout of the typical computer keyboard with a separate number keypad accessed via the 'Num Lock' key means that data entry is often physically easier if only numbers are used. Thus, one can easily substitute '1' for male and '2' for female. Multicategory answers can be coded similarly (e.g. '1' for never smoker, '2' for ex-smoker, and '3' for current smoker).

Decisions can also be made about missing or inappropriate answers. If an answer is missing, one option is to leave that field blank for that subject; alternatively, a standard number such as '9' can be used. A separate code may be used for questions that are inapplicable. It also might be scientifically important to distinguish between individuals who, after consideration, answer 'don't know' from answers that are missing.

Example 15.vi

In a survey of women's health, a series of questions were asked about the age at last menstrual period. A coding scheme was devised such that if an age was given this was entered as a two-digit number. For other possible answers the following codes were applied: questions unanswered, code '00'; if a woman was still menstruating, code '88'; if a woman had recorded a surgical menopause (i.e. hysterectomy), code '77'; if a woman had indicated that she was menopausal but could not recall when she had her last period, code '99'. The advantage of this scheme is that it allows separation of these very different groups of women.

The task can be made simpler if the hard data-recording instrument, such as a questionnaire, is precoded at the design stage. A very simplified version of how this might look is shown in Box 15.1.

Using this approach, the answers can be entered directly. In this example, a subject ticking 'single' for question 2 would be automatically coded and could be directly entered onto the database as a '1'. The numbers under 'Office Use Only' refer to the place on the database where the answers are to be entered. The use of such instruments does not reduce the need for careful checking before data entry.

This approach may not be appropriate if the coding scheme is complex. It is also sometimes necessary to design the coding scheme once the answers have been reviewed. Box 15.2 shows an example of a coding scheme that was used to apply codes after data collection. In particular, the subject was asked about current medication in question 7, but the researcher was interested only in certain categories of drugs as indicated in the coding schedule.

It was thought easier to ask an 'open' question about drug use rather than rely on the subject accurately ascribing their own medications to a particular class of drug. Note also in this example that the researcher converted heights from imperial to metric before data entry. This is not strictly necessary or indeed desirable, as a computerized routine can be used after data entry to achieve such a conversion, minimizing the possibility of human error. In this example the coding schedule to question 7b permitted a separation between those not taking any prescribed medications (code '8') and those who were, but could not remember the number of different preparations (code '9').

Box 15.1 Example of a precoded questionnaire

| Subject number | 4 | 2 | 1 | | 1–3 |

1. What is your date of birth?

    day   month year   4–3

2. Please tick in the appropriate box your current marital status

Single	☐	1
Living as married/Married	☐	2
Separated	☐	3
Divorced	☐	4
Widowed	☐	5

10

3. Have you ever smoked cigarettes regularly (i.e. at least once a day for a month)?

☐ 1
☐ 2

11

12–13

If YES, what age were you when you first started smoking regularly?

year

Box 15.2 Example of a questionnaire and accompanying coding schedule

Questionnaire

OFFICE USE
ONLY

6. What is your current height without shoes?

☐ ☐☐ ☐☐☐
feet   inches   7–9

7a. Are you taking any prescribed medicines or tablets currently?

☐ YES   a) ☐
☐ NO   10

7b. If YES, how many different drugs are you taking?

B) ☐
   11

7c. If YES, can you give us the names as stated on the container?

c) ☐ 12
   ☐ 13
1. _____   ☐ 14
2. _____   ☐ 15
3. _____   ☐ 16
4. _____
5. _____
6. _____
7. _____

Coding schedule

6. Height: use the attached table to convert to metric to the nearest centimetre

7a. Yes = 1
No = 2
If missing leave blank.

7b. If Yes, enter the number of different drugs.
If more than '7' put '7'
Enter '8' if not applicable.
Enter '9' if missing

7c. Column 12 Any antibiotic   Yes = 1 No = 2
Column 13 Any analgesic   Yes = 1 No = 2
Column 14 Any sedative/hypnotic   Yes = 1 No = 2
Column 15 Any diuretic   Yes = 1 No = 2
Column 16 Any beta-blocker   Yes = 1 No = 2

15.6 **Indirect computer data entry**

In many studies optimal use of resources would use some form of electronic data capture but, for reasons already stated, manual data entry may be required although effective scanning hardware may substitute. Scanning still requires human interaction to ensure that errors in transcription are not made or there are no other technical difficulties. Raw data can be entered either: (i) indirectly from the coded data forms; or (ii) directly from the uncoded data, with the data entry clerk coding simultaneously. If the coding schedule is simple this is an easy matter, otherwise it is better to separate the tasks of coding and entry. Data entry is a skilled task and, given its repetitive nature, mistakes are inevitable for the expert as well as the novice. Data sets can also be entered by professional agencies, who by their speed and accuracy can work out to be a cheaper option as well. 'Double data entry' is also to be encouraged, although as the name suggests it doubles the effort. With this approach data is entered twice and straightforward software will highlight inconsistencies between the two sets of data entry. This procedure substantially reduces the likelihood of data entry errors.

Example 15.vii

As part of a large population study the investigators built in quality assurance checks. It was estimated that the error rate of the data entry clerks was approximately 1 per 100 key strokes. Assuming that the errors of each clerk were independent of each other, then using double data entry would reduce the error rate to 1 per 10,000 keystrokes (i.e. $1/100 \times 1/100$). It was decided the extra cost was worth the substantially decreased error rate.

15.7 **Direct electronic data entry**

Increasingly, primary data, gathered either from subjects or by trained interviewers, is entered direct onto a tablet or smartphone using touch screen or similar technology. Indeed, voice-activated responses are also often sufficiently accurate. Direct entry has the advantages of minimizing transcription errors and increasing speed. Conversely, though, the lack of a hard copy record may be discomforting to some. It is also easier on hard copy to scribble some marginal notes for later consultation, whereas entry at the time of interview means a rapid decision must be made as to the single best answer.

Example 15.viii

A psychiatrist handed out tablets to a series of patients to gather sensitive information which had proved difficult to collect in face-to-face interviews. At the end of the survey, the application provided a summary of the answers which the interviewee ticked as being correct. The data collection provided sufficient security that no identifiable information would be stored.

15.8 **Missing data**

One of the major problems in the analysis and interpretation of epidemiological surveys is that of missing data. This might arise for several reasons. In self-completed questionnaires, and even interview-administered surveys, data may be missing because of:

(i) poor recall by the subject
(ii) a question not understood
(iii) the lack of a suitable category for an unexpected answer

(iv) genuine error in missing out a question

(v) concerns about confidentiality

Thus, in addition to the problems posed by total non-response by a subject, important data may be missing from some of those who do participate, hindering the interpretation of the study as a whole. If important items are missing, such as variables that are essential in disease or exposure classification, that subject may need to be excluded completely from analyses. A more frequent problem is the absence of more minor items. This results in different totals being used in the analysis as well as opening up the possibility of bias; for example, in a survey of women's health, those for whom no age of menopause is available may be more likely to have an irregular menstrual history than responders to that question.

There is little, however, that can be done at the stage of data preparation. It is important, as mentioned earlier, to distinguish in the design of the study instrument between, for example, those who are unable to recall and those for whom no suitable category is available. If missing data are identified soon after the time of the survey, the subject can be contacted, or a proxy source of information used to fill in the gaps. If the missing item is part of a standard instrument, there may be accepted rules for estimating the value of the missing item.

Example 15.ix

A 10-item questionnaire was designed to measure the extent of disturbance of a set of symptoms with aspects of everyday life. In this questionnaire, each item was scored from 0 (no interference) to 10 (maximum interference) to give a total score of 0–100. Pilot studies showed that for whatever reason some questions were not completed. Rather than discard the whole questionnaire for that subject, the scoring system allowed substitution of any item missing a response score, with the average score of all other items answered, provided that the total number of missing items was 2 or less.

Example 15.x

In a long-term outcome study following a femoral neck fracture, 30% of patients could not recall the month of their fracture. They were each assumed to have fractured in June of the recalled year of fracture (i.e. mid-year), thereby allowing person-months of follow-up to be calculated for each subject, with the error for an individual subject being limited to six months.

In preparing the data for analysis, therefore, the possible reasons for data absence should be entered if likely to be of relevance. It is then possible to undertake some preliminary analyses comparing the frequencies of other important variables between those with and those without missing data.

Example 15.xi

In a case–control study of cervical cancer, 20% of those who were interviewed declined to answer the question about the number of sexual partners. These non-responders were not, however, different from women who answered this question in relation to other variables of sexual activity gathered, such as age at first intercourse. In presenting their data on the number of partners as a risk factor, the investigators commented that they had an incomplete data set to address this question but from the data available there was no reason to believe that the results from those answering the question could not be extrapolated to the study population as a whole.

Outside the scope of this chapter, it should be noted that there are several analytical techniques now in widespread use to fill in gaps in data by *imputing* their likely values based on the other information available, both from the individual subject and from the results of the data set. It is often relevant to consider if results are missing by an unrelated event (e.g. if an interviewer was ill) or if the missing data might be related to some key aspect (e.g. the subject was ill on the date of survey). In prospective studies, with multiple time points, consideration can be given to a missing result, whether or not to use the previous result, or calculate an estimate based on the data that is present.

Expert statistical guidance should be taken on any imputation techniques to be used and how they should be interpreted. It is important that on any stored data set, it should be made clear what data items are true collected information and which are imputed.

15.9 **Data errors**

Missing data is often the major threat to data quality but errors and inaccuracies in data collection and manipulation are also important to consider. When data are entered either directly or indirectly onto a computer, it is possible to instigate some processes to minimize the likelihood of errors.

One simple step is to put *range checks* into what can be entered. Thus, if an investigator decides *a priori* that any weight of under 35 kg or over 110 kg is likely to be erroneous the computer system can reject weights outside this range being entered. Although such errors may be detected in the initial manual data check, with large surveys it provides an additional and more watertight procedure.

In a similar manner, an investigator will set up the database to prevent the entry of any answers that are clearly inconsistent with other data, for example, pregnancy details being recorded for males or an age of an event given which is older than the subject's current age. Other examples of prior consistency checks are given in Tables 15.1 and 15.2.

Other consistency checks should be constructed, perhaps with expert advice.

Example 15.xii

An occupational exposure study collected information on different job titles and some specific exposures. As a check, individuals who within that workplace indicated they had spent time in a particular role should have

Table 15.2 Examples of common range and consistency checks

Range	
Age	Within expected range
Adult height	Between 1.45 m and 1.95 m
Adult weight	Between 35 kg and 100 kg
Age at menopause	Between 40 and 55
No. of cigarettes/day	Below 60
Consistency checks	
Males	Not pregnant
Non-smokers	Not giving number smoked per day
Age at menopause	Not given before age at birth of youngest child
Unemployed	Not giving details of current occupation

also indicated in response to a separate question that they had been exposed to high levels of noise. Where there were inconsistencies it was possible to check the employment records.

15.10 **Recoding of entered data**

Often the data are collected in formats that are not relevant for addressing the questions behind the study. Thus, before the main statistical analysis the actual data may be recoded into more meaningful categories.

Example 15.xiii

In a study each subject's actual weight and height was recorded but as the analysis was only concerned with subjects who were within a normal body mass index/mild to moderate obese/very obese, BMI was calculated and then a new variable of obesity derived for further analysis.

Example 15.xiv

In a study of over-the-counter analgesic use, the survey collected information on different types of analgesics and compound products that may have been used by subjects in the previous month. In discussion with a clinical pharmacologist, distinct groups of subjects were derived for further analysis based on a priori views of which categories may be important.

15.11 **Linkage by subject of data from multiple sources and subject identification**

Issues of confidentiality and data protection, often the subject of legislation, provide an obligation on the researcher to preserve the anonymity of participants in a research project. With longitudinal studies and those that require linkage between data sets, this is not without challenges as the aim is to ensure that the records from these different sources can be combined to achieve a whole subject record. It is therefore necessary to have a study identifier that can be used throughout that preserves confidentiality. At the same time, in studies where repeated contacts are required there will be the need to link back to individual identifiers so that subjects can be contacted. Indeed, some studies may require the subject to be reminded of a previous answer to check whether there has been any change. It may be useful to use an independent item (e.g. date of birth) collected on each contact which can then be checked for consistency.

The unique study identifier can also be used to collect information that may be helpful in interpreting future results.

Example 15.xv

In a survey involving several different interviewers, each interviewer was given a separate series of subject numbers (e.g. interviewer no. 1: 0–999, interviewer no. 2: 1000–1599, and so on). Each interviewer may only have planned to survey 150 subjects, but this numbering system prevented duplication errors as well as permitting easier post hoc identification of particular interviewers for any subgroup analysis.

15.12 **Storage of data and data set**

The final aspect of data preparation to be considered is a simple, but frequently overlooked issue; that is, the establishment of an archive so that either the same investigator or others in the future can refer to the data set to undertake repeat or different analyses. Many research funders now insist on maximal data sharing, while protecting the intellectual contribution of the researcher. This is good scientific practice, in practical terms: if the principal person involved in the study, or particularly if the individuals responsible for the data set were no longer available, would the data be in a sufficiently acceptable state for another investigator to work on? In the future, it may be desirable to repeat the initial analyses as a protection against scientific fraud. Similarly, the data could usefully be combined with other similar data sets in meta-analysis or other types of pooled studies.

Chapter 16

Introductory data analysis

Descriptive epidemiology

16.1 **Introduction**

The purpose of this chapter is to outline the approaches used in reporting the study results. It is not intended to replace statistical textbooks, but will provide an introduction to the information required for measures of disease occurrence (or death) and their calculation. When computer packages are readily available to carry out such calculations, one may ask why it is necessary to be aware of such detail? In fact, their availability as something of a 'black-box' makes understanding of the basic methods used even more important: readers are encouraged to work through the examples shown using a calculator. The ability to conduct simple calculations will permit the reader, for example, to check their work or further explore data published by others. The authors have seen many examples of results presented which, on making some simple calculations, were shown to be wrong.

It is assumed that the reader has a basic knowledge of statistics and is aware of the use of summary measures including means and proportions, simple measures of variability including variance and standard deviation, and understands the conceptual basis for (i) making inferences about populations from studying samples and (ii) is familiar with the assessment of standard errors and confidence intervals (see 'Further reading').

16.2 **Reporting study results**

EQUATOR (Enhancing the QUAlity and Transparency Of health Research) network brought together reporting guidelines for many study types, for example, the guidelines for observational studies are based on STROBE (Strengthening the Reporting of Observational Studies in Epidemiology) statement (see 'Further reading'). Specifically, these guidelines stress the importance of reporting the numbers of participants at each stage of the study such as baseline and follow up, duration of follow up for cohort studies, participation rate, and number of participants with missing data. Researchers should describe characteristics of study participants (e.g. demographic or clinical), provide information on exposures and potential confounders, and report numbers of outcome events or summary measures.

Example 16.i

Table 16.1 shows an example of the description of study participants in a case–control study of rheumatoid arthritis as it could appear in a research paper. Several summary measures such as proportion, mean, and median are presented. Measures of variability include standard deviation and interquartile range. Note that the number of participants with missing data is also reported.

Table 16.1 Description of cases and controls in a hypothetical case–control study of rheumatoid arthritis

Characteristic	Cases (N = 150)	Controls (N = 300)
Participation rate (%)	82.1	67.5
Age (years), Mean (SD*)	61 (10)	63 (9)
Gender, N (%)		
Male	50 (33.3)	90 (30.0)
Female	100 (66.7)	210 (70.0)
Smoking (pack-years), Median (IQR**)	7 (1, 19)	5 (0, 12)
*BMI ***, Median (IQR)	27 (22, 30)	23 (18, 29)
Ever worked in cold environment, N (%)	35 (23.8)	51 (17.3)
Missing information, N	3	5

* Standard deviation; ** Interquartile range; *** Body Mass Index

16.3 **Incidence rate**

Chapter 2 (Section 2.1) defined incidence and described the formula for calculating an incidence rate. To recap, the calculation of an incidence rate requires (i) the number of new (incident) events and (ii) the total person-years at risk. The formula is:

$$\text{Incidence Rate}(IR) = x / npyr,$$

where x is number of incident events; $npyr$ is the number of person-years at risk.

Example 16.ii

Researchers wish to calculate incidence rate in a study of 621 individuals followed up for a total of 1,480 person-years, of whom 40 developed the disease. Following the aforementioned formula,

$$
\begin{aligned}
IR &= \quad 40 / 1,480 \\
&= \quad 0.02703 \\
&= \quad 27.03 / 1,000 \text{ person-years at risk.}
\end{aligned}
$$

In the aforementioned example, the rate was expressed as rate per 1,000 person-years to give a number that is convenient to handle. The exact denominator chosen will depend on the rarity of the event.

Example 16.iii

Figure 16.1 shows an example of the report on incidence and mortality per 100,000 for selected cancer sites.

When reporting study results, it is good practice to present confidence intervals around the effect measure (in this case the Incidence Ratio, IR). Confidence interval provides an estimation of the most likely values for the true IR in the population. Usually confidence intervals are reported at the 95% level.

The Poisson distribution can be used to calculate confidence limits around an incidence rate. This is based on the assumption that cases occur randomly in time in relation to each other. The

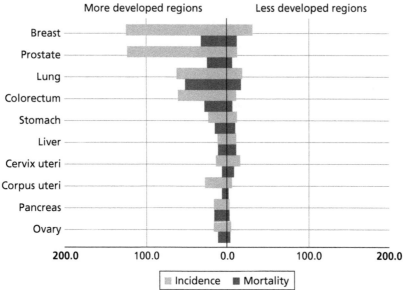

Figure 16.1 Example of incidence per 100,000 for selected cancer sites.

Source: data from IARC (Globocan software) and World Health Organization.

95% confidence interval using the Poisson distribution is obtained by looking up the values in standard statistical tables. Table 16.2 gives an abridged example from Geigy's scientific tables (see 'Further reading').

If the incidence estimate is based on more than approximately 75 cases, the normal approximation to the Poisson distribution provides a simple formula for obtaining the confidence interval. If

Table 16.2 Exact confidence intervals for number of incident events based on Poisson distribution

Number of observed events	Lower 95% limit	Upper 95% limit
0	0	3.69
1	0.03	5.57
5	1.62	11.67
10	4.80	18.39
15	8.40	24.74
20	12.22	30.89
30	20.24	42.83
40	28.58	54.47
50	37.11	65.92
75	58.99	94.01
100	81.36	121.63

x_u is the upper 95% confidence limit for the number of events and x_l is the lower 95% confidence limit for the number of events, then

$$x_u = x + 1.96\sqrt{x}$$
$$x_l = x - 1.96\sqrt{x}$$

Example 16.iv

Calculation of 95% confidence interval around the IR for data from Example 16.ii:

(a) *Using Poisson distribution:*

From Table 16.2 for x =40,

lower 95% limit = 28.58;

upper 95% limit = 54.74.

Therefore 95% confidence limits are:

28.58/1480 and 54.74/1480

= 0.0193 and 0.0370

= 19.3–37.0/1,000 person-years at risk.

(b) *Using normal approximation to Poisson distribution:*

For x = 40,

$$
\begin{aligned}
x_u \quad &= \quad 40 + 1.96\sqrt{40} \\
&= \quad 40 + 1.96 \times 6.32 \\
&= \quad 40 + 12.40 \\
&= \quad 52.40.
\end{aligned}
$$

$$
\begin{aligned}
x_l \quad &= \quad 40 - 1.96\sqrt{40} \\
&= \quad 40 - 1.96 \times 6.32 \\
&= \quad 40 - 12.40 \\
&= \quad 27.61
\end{aligned}
$$

Therefore, 95% confidence limits are:

27.61/1,480 and 52.40/1,480

= 0.0187 and 0.0354

= 18.7–35.4/1,000 person-years at risk.

The points to note in the previous example are, first, that even for 40 cases the two methods give very similar answers, and, secondly, both methods calculate the confidence interval for the number of events, which then must be divided by the person-years in the denominator to derive the actual rates.

16.4 **Prevalence**

Chapter 2 (Section 2.2) defined prevalence and described ways to measure it. Prevalence is estimated as a proportion of the relevant population and is calculated as $p = x/n$, where n = number in population; x = number with disease; p = proportion with disease.

All calculations in this section also apply to cumulative incidence, which is also expressed as a proportion.

Example 16.v

In a cross-sectional study, 621 individuals were clinically examined, of whom 40 had disease. The prevalence of disease is

p = 40/621,

  = 0.0644

  = 64.4 per 1,000 persons.

Example 16.vi

Figure 16.2 shows an example of report of prevalence over time

As with incidence rates, there are two approaches to calculating confidence intervals around a proportion (whether applied to prevalence or cumulative incidence). The first, for use with small samples, where the denominator is (say) less than 100, relies on using published tables that provide the confidence interval for every possible observed proportion of events for each denominator up to 100.

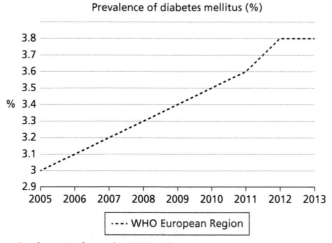

Figure 16.2 Example of report of prevalence over time.

Source: data from IARC (Globocan software) and World Health Organization.

Example 16.vii

This example shows calculation of confidence interval around prevalence proportion or cumulative incidence when the sample size is small (n < 100). Assuming a study involved 50 participants, of whom 23 had disease, then prevalence was p = 0.46. Statistical tables for exact confidence limits for a binomial proportion can be used. Table 16.3 shows a small part of the statistical table for the denominator of 50. From this table, for n = 50 and x = 23, the confidence interval for the proportion of individuals with disease is 0.318–0.607.

For a larger sample size (n > 75), the normal approximation can be used.
If p_u is the upper 95% confidence limit and p_l is the lower 95% confidence limit, then

$$p_l = p - 1.96\sqrt{\frac{p(1-p)}{n}}$$

$$p_u = p + 1.96\sqrt{\frac{p(1-p)}{n}}.$$

Example 16.viii

Using data from Example 16.v:

$$p_l = 0.0644 - 1.96\sqrt{\frac{0.0644 \times 0.9356}{621}}$$
$$= 0.0644 - 1.96\sqrt{0.000097}$$
$$= 0.0644 - 1.96 \times 0.00985$$
$$= 0.0644 - 0.0193$$
$$= 0.0451$$

$$p_u = 0.0644 + 1.96\sqrt{\frac{0.0644 \times 0.9356}{621}}$$
$$= 0.0644 + 1.96\sqrt{0.000097}$$
$$= 0.0644 + 1.96 \times 0.00985$$
$$= 0.0644 + 0.0193$$
$$= 0.0837.$$

95% confidence interval for the proportion of individuals with disease is (0.0451—0.0837) or (45.1–83.7 per 1,000 persons).

Table 16.3 Exact confidence intervals for number of incident events based on Poisson distribution

n	x	95% Confidence limits	
		Lower	Upper
50	22	0.300	0.588
	23	0.318	0.607
	24	0.337	0.262

16.5 **Crude, age-specific, and standardized rates**

The previous sections have demonstrated the calculation of rates overall in a defined population. These are known as crude rates (see Examples 16.iii and 16.vi). The same principle applies to calculating rates in population subgroups, for example, different age groups as shown previously in Example 3.i. Incidence rate in age group i can be calculated as $r_i = x_i / npyr_i$, while all-ages (crude)

incidence rate is $R = \dfrac{\sum_i x_i}{\sum_i npyr_i}$.

Example 16.ix

Table 16.4 shows an example of age-specific and all-ages incidence rates calculated using the aforementioned formula. In this example it can be seen that the incidence rate of the disease of interest increases with older age.

A frequent scenario in epidemiological investigations involves the comparison of rates of disease (whether prevalence, incidence, or mortality) between populations or indeed within a population at different points in time (see Examples 16.iii and 16.vi, respectively). Using crude rates can lead to erroneous conclusions.

Example 16.x

Let's assume that Town A has a mortality rate of 5 per 100,000 person-years at risk (pyr) and Town B a mortality rate of 10 per 100,000 pyr. Does that mean a person in Town B has double the risk of dying compared to a person in Town A? Overall the answer is yes, but the difference in mortality rate in the two towns may be explained, for example, by the fact that the residents of Town B are older.

Example 16.xi

As can be seen from Table 16.5 although Lowtown has increased incidence overall (i.e. crude rate) in comparison to Hightown, the incidence rate in every age group is, in fact, lower than in Hightown. The excess crude incidence rate in Lowtown is due entirely to a much higher proportion of its residents being in the oldest age group.

Therefore, in comparing rates between populations, it is imperative to take account of such factors which may differ between towns and have an important influence on the outcome of interest (see Chapter 18 for a fuller discussion of such confounding factors). With respect to population data, such information is often restricted to age and gender.

Table 16.4 Age-specific incidence rates

Index (*i*)	Age group (years)	Number of incident events (*x$_i$*)	Person-years at risk (*npyr$_i$*)	Incidence rate (per 10,000 person-years) (*r$_i$*)
1	0–15	2	4,432	4.51
2	16–34	6	3,978	15.08
3	35–64	13	5,396	24.09
4	65+	12	2,159	55.58
	All ages	33	15,965	20.67

Table 16.5 Comparing rates

Age group (years)	Hightown			Lowtown		
	No. of incident events	Person-years at risk	Incidence rate per 10,000	No. of incident events	Person-years at risk	Incidence rate per 10,000
0–15	10	9,415	10.6	3	4,103	7.3
16–34	18	8,346	21.6	6	3,765	15.9
35–64	20	6,215	32.2	12	4,192	28.6
65+	22	2,196	100.2	73	7,426	98.3
All ages	70	26,172	26.7	94	19,486	48.2

Consequently, it is important to examine stratum-specific rates in comparing populations with different age structures. In addition, there are methods for producing a summary measure taking account of age differences (i.e. an age-standardized rate) (see Chapter 3 (Section 3.2)). However, particularly in relation to populations with very different age structures, it should be emphasized that such measures should be calculated in addition to examining age-specific rates rather than as an alternative. The two methods of standardization are direct and indirect standardization (see Chapter 3, Sections 3.2.1 and 3.2.2, respectively).

16.6 **Direct and indirect standardization**

16.6.1 **Direct standardization**

A directly age-standardized rate is the theoretical rate which would have been observed in the population under study if the age structure of the population was that of a defined reference population. This reference population may be real or hypothetical. For example, if comparing rates between several countries, the age structure of one of the populations may be designated as the reference. Alternatively, there are reference population age structures which have been proposed for different parts of the world. As already mentioned in Chapter 3, Section 3.2.1, the World Standard Population is often used.

Example 16.xii

Figure 16.3 shows the age-standardized lung cancer mortality rates by calendar year where the World Standard Population was used for standardization.

The calculations involved in direct age standardization are as following:

Directly age-standardized rate $DASR = \sum_i \dfrac{r_i \times pyr_i}{PYR}$

Where r_i is the incidence rate in age group i in the study population, pyr_i is person-years at risk in age group i in the standard population, and PYR is the total person-years at risk in the standard population.

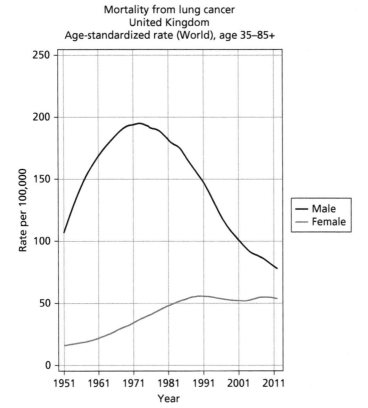

Figure 16.3 Example of age-standardized rates (World Standard Population) lung cancer mortality rate by calendar year.

Source: data from IARC (Globocan software) and World Health Organization.

Example 16.xiii

Using data from Example 16.xi, let us denote Hightown as the 'standard' population and Lowtown as the 'study' population.

$$DASR = 7.3 \times 0.36 + 15.9 \times 0.32 + 28.6 \times 0.24 + 98.3 \times 0.08 \ per \ 10,000$$

$$= 2.628 + 5.088 + 6.864 + 7.864 \ per \ 10,000$$

$$= 22.4 \ per \ 10,000.$$

Thus, the DASR in Lowtown is lower than the incidence rate in Hightown (the standard population). Therefore, the higher crude incidence rate of disease X in Lowtown is explained by the different age structures of the two towns. If Lowtown had the same age structure, then its crude rate of disease would be lower than that in Hightown.

16.6.2 **Indirect standardization**

The second method to compare rates between different populations, allowing for differences in age structure, is referred to as indirect standardization. It involves applying a set of age-specific rates from the 'standard' population to the age structure of the second population under study, to determine the 'expected' number of cases if such rates had applied in that population. This 'expected' number of cases is then compared with the actual number of cases 'observed' in the population under study. The ratio of observed/expected number of cases (often multiplied by 100) is called, when considering incidence rates, the Standardized Incidence Ratio (SIR)—with corresponding terms for Mortality and Prevalence:

$$SIR = \frac{\sum_i c_i}{\sum_i r_i \times pyr_r} \times 100$$

$$= \frac{\sum_i c_i}{\sum_i ec_i} \times 100.$$

Where r_i is the incidence rate in age group i in the standard population, c_i is the number of incident events in age group i in the study population, pyr_i is the person-years at risk in age group i in the standard population.

Expected cases $ec_i = r_i \times pyr_i$

Example 16.xiv

Using again the data from Example 16.xi, let us denote Hightown as the 'standard' population and Lowtown as the 'study' population (Table 16.7).

By definition, the SIR of a population defined as the 'standard population' will be 100. In Example 16.ix Lowtown has an SIR of 93.7 in comparison to an SIR of 100 in Hightown (the 'standard population'). Thus, the number of incident cases in Lowtown was only 93.7% of that expected if the age-specific rates of Hightown had applied.

It is important to note that if making several comparisons using indirect standardization, each time applying age-specific incidence rates from a 'standard' population (say Town A) to other populations (say Town B and Town C), then the weights used in the standardization procedure are those of the population being compared to the standard. In such circumstances each population under study can only be compared to the standard and not directly to each other (i.e. the SIRs compare Town B vs. Town A and Town C vs. Town A, but cannot be used directly to compare Town B vs. Town C). A common usage of standard ratios is in comparing rates among different population subgroups (e.g. occupational groups).

16.7 **Statistical software**

Statistical packages such as R, Stata, and SAS software perform standardization (see 'Further reading').

Example 16.xv

Boxes 16.1 *and* 16.2 *show results of direct and indirect standardization from Stata for Tables* 16.6 *and* 16.7, *respectively.*

Table 16.6 Direct age standardization

Age group		Hightown (Standard population)		Lowtown (Study population)	
Index (i)	Years	Person-years at risk (pyr_i)	Proportion (pyr_i /PYR)	Incidence rate (per 10,000) ($r_i \times 10,000$)	Weighted rate (per 10,000) ($r_i \times 10,000 \times pyr_i$ / PYR)
1	0–15	9,415	0.36	7.3	2.628
2	16–34	8,346	0.32	15.9	5.088
3	35–64	6,215	0.24	28.6	6.864
4	65+	2,196	0.08	98.3	7.864
Total		26,172	1		22.444

Table 16.7 Indirect age standardization

Age group		Standard population (Hightown)	Study population (Lowtown)		
Index (i)	Years	Incidence rate (per 10 000) ($r_i \times 10,000$)	Person-years at risk (pyr_i)	Number of incident events (c_i)	'Expected cases' (ec_i)
1	0–15	10.6	4,103	3	4.3
2	16–34	21.6	3,765	6	8.1
3	35–64	32.2	4,192	12	13.5
4	65+	100.2	7,426	73	74.4
Total				94	100.3

$$SIR = \frac{(3+6+12+73)}{(4.3+8.1+13.5+74.4)} \times 100$$

$$= \frac{94}{103.3} \times 100 = 93.7.$$

Box 16.1 Direct age standardization: Results from Stata output (data from Table 16.6)

-----Unadjusted---- Std.

Stratum	Pop.	Cases	Pop. Dist.	Stratum Rate[s]	Pop. Dst[P]	s*P
0-15	4103	3	0.211	0.0007	0.360	0.0003
16-34	3765	6	0.193	0.0016	0.319	0.0005
35-64	4192	12	0.215	0.0029	0.237	0.0007
65+	7426	73	0.381	0.0098	0.084	0.0008
Totals:	19486	94				

Adjusted Cases:		44.3
Crude Rate:		0.0048
Adjusted Rate:		0.0023
95% Conf. Interval: [0.0016, 0.0029]		

Summary of study Populations:

town	N	Crude	Adj_Rate	Confidence	Interval
2	19486	0.004824	0.002276	[0.001615,	0.002937]

Box 16.2 Indirect age standardization: Results from Stata output (data from Table 16.7)

Indirect Standardization

Stratum	Standard Population Rate	Observed Population	Cases Expected
0-15	0.0011	4,103	4.36
16-34	0.0022	3,765	8.12
35-64	0.0032	4,192	13.49
65+	0.0100	7,426	74.40
Totals:		19486	100.36

Observed Cases:	94
SMR (Obs/Exp):	0.94
SMR exact 95% Conf. Interval: [0.7569,	1.1462
Crude Rate:	0.0048
Adjusted Rate:	0.0025
95% Conf. Interval: [0.0020,	0.0031

Summary of Study Populations (Rates):

Cases Observed	Crude	Adj_Rate	Confidence	Interval
94	0.004824	0.002505	[0.002024,	0.003066]

Summary of Study Populations (SMR):

Cases Observed	Cases Expected	SMR	Exact Confidence Interval	
94	100.36	0.937	[0.756867,	1.146159]

Further reading and resources

Bland M (2015). *An Introduction to Medical Statistics*, 4th edition. Oxford University Press, Oxford, UK.

Epi Info™ https://www.cdc.gov/epiinfo [Accessed October 2017].

EQUATOR Network http://www.equator-network.org/reporting-guidelines/ [Accessed October 2017].

Lentner C (1981). *Geigy Scientific Tables: Introduction to statistics, statistical tables, mathematical formulae,* v.2. Ciba-Geigy, West Caldwell, NJ.

Package 'epitools' Version 0.5–9 for R (2017). https://cran.r-project.org/web/packages/epitools/epitools.pdf [Accessed October 2017].

StataCorp (2017). *Stata Statistical Software: Release 15*. StataCorp LLC, College Station, TX.

SAS software (SAS Institute, Cary NC) SAS/STAT(R) 12.1 STDIZE and STDRATE Procedures https://support.sas.com/en/support-home.html [Accessed October 2017].

Chapter 17

Introductory data analysis
Analytical epidemiology

17.1 Introduction

The purpose of this chapter is to outline the major analytical approaches to answering epidemiological questions with the use of data generated by the study designs described in Chapter 6. Traditionally, analysis is first undertaken to examine the main effect of the factors under study. This is followed by consideration of whether any observed major effects can be explained by their association with other variables. This issue of confounding is dealt with in Chapter 18.

Many easy-to-use statistical programs exist that permit a rapid and accurate approach to statistical analysis. In this chapter, however, formulae are presented for the main measures of effect together with worked examples. Indeed, when data are available in tabulated form, as opposed to raw data files, it is frequently an easy task to calculate the important measures 'by hand'. The formulae presented will permit the reader, for example, to check or further explore data published by others.

It is not the aim of this chapter to review all available statistical tests, and the reader is advised to refer to more comprehensive statistical textbooks (see 'Further reading'). In addition, it is assumed that the reader has a basic knowledge of statistics and is aware of the use of summary measures including means and proportions, simple measures of variability including variance and standard deviation, and understands the conceptual basis for (i) making inferences about populations from studying samples and is familiar with the assessment of standard errors and confidence intervals, and (ii) making comparisons between samples by using significance testing.

This chapter focuses primarily on the analysis of case–control (Section 6.2) and cohort studies (Section 6.3), and other study designs described in the Chapter 6 are considered briefly.

17.1.1 Statistical software

There are several statistical packages available for epidemiological analysis, which permit data entry, import from other programs such as Excel, checking and modification directly within the program. Some packages are designed specifically for the epidemiologists, such as Epi Info™, while others, such as SPSS, Stata, R, and SAS Software, have wider applications in research generally (see 'Further reading'). Most of the programs now incorporate excellent graphical features to plot and print results in publishable form. All major analytical software is regularly being upgraded and most are available in a user-friendly format. The choice of statistical package is often dictated by its availability within a workplace or educational institution. For the novice, it makes sense to work with a program for which there are experienced individuals available locally who can rapidly help to sort out any problems. Many packages have user groups and online discussion forums where help is readily available.

17.2 **Effect measurement, interval assessment, and significance testing**

Chapter 7 discussed effect measures including prevalence ratio, risk ratio, rate ratio, and odds ratio and the choice of effect measure depending on study type. Statistical analysis of any study can reveal three items of potential value: an estimate of the major effect, the precision of that estimate, and its statistical significance.

Example 17.i

In a case–control study examining the influences of working in the dyeing industry for the development of bladder carcinoma, the following results were obtained: odds ratio for ever working with dyes, odds ratio (OR) = 3.2; 95% confidence interval 1.2–8.4; p = 0.04.

The results give us different pieces of information. The odds ratio provides the best single estimate of the effect, assuming an unbiased study. The 95% confidence interval gives a range for the precision of that estimate and shows, in this example, that the data are consistent with a true effect that might only be marginal (20% increased) or indeed very large (over eightfold). The p value suggests that there is 4% probability of observing by chance the odds ratio of 3.2, when the truth is that there is no increased risk (null hypothesis H_0: true odds ratio = 1). Hence the conclusion is that working in this industry is associated with increased risk.

The p value is perhaps the least valuable of all the analytical outcomes because most epidemiological questions do not require a yes/no answer, but are concerned with magnitude. In practice, many will quote the fact that a lower 95% confidence limit greater than unity indicates a true effect, in the belief that this will increase the likelihood of publication. Indeed, studies where the confidence intervals span unity are viewed as problematic by virtue of being of insufficient size. This is unfortunate because a study that yields a 95% confidence interval for an odds ratio of 0.8–1.3 gives as much information as one that yields a 95% confidence interval of 1.1–17.4. The first result implies that if there is an increased risk, it is likely to be small. The second result implies that an increased risk is likely, but its magnitude cannot be accurately estimated.

In all examples given next, for simplicity only, 95% confidence intervals are calculated. These are the most frequently presented and accepted in practice. To obtain 90% or 99% intervals it is necessary to substitute the standard normal deviates of 1.58 and 2.64, respectively, for the figure of 1.96 in all the formulae presented.

17.3 **Analysis of cross-sectional studies**

When a cross-sectional study (Section 6.1) is measuring the relative risk (risk ratio) of disease associated with an exposure then methods for cohort studies can be used (Sections 17.5.4 and 17.5.8). Alternatively, if the cross-sectional study is being used as a method for identifying diseased and non-diseased individuals (with further data collection thereafter on exposures) then the relationship between disease and exposure can be analysed using methods for the case–control studies described next.

17.4 **Analysis of case–control studies**

In a case–control study (Section 6.2) the aim is to measure the association between a risk factor and a disease by using the odds ratio (strictly, the ratio of odds of exposure in diseased persons to the odds of exposure in the non-diseased) (Section 7.4).

This odds ratio, generally, provides a good estimate of the relative risk. However, it may not when the initial risk (e.g. the prevalence of the disease under study) is high. Around 10% has been proposed

Table 17.1 Table for calculation of odds ratio for dichotomous exposure

Exposure	Disease		Total
	Case	Control	
Present	a	b	a + b
Absent	c	d	c + d
Total	a + c	b + d	N

as a 'rule-of-thumb'. The odds ratio will be smaller than the relative risk for odds ratios of less than one, and larger than the relative risk for odds ratios of greater than one, and the discrepancy will be larger when the association is stronger (positive or negative). Nevertheless, there is no issue with using the OR, whatever the disease prevalence, provided it is interpreted as such (i.e. a ratio of odds).

Where the exposure is dichotomous, a two-by-two table can be drawn up (Table 17.1) and the OR calculated easily as the ratio of the 'cross-products':

$$\text{Odds ratio} \quad OR = (a:c)/(b:d)$$
$$= ad / bc$$

Example 17.ii

In a case–control study of 42 cases, of which 18 cases were exposed and 61 controls, of which 17 were exposed. Following Table 17.1 and the formula given here, the odds ratio can be calculated as

$$OR = 18 \times 44 / 17 \times 24 = 1.94.$$

An odds ratio of 1 implies that the odds of exposure are the same among cases and controls (i.e. there is no relationship between exposure and disease). Odds ratios greater than 1 imply that the odds of cases being exposed is greater than controls (i.e. the exposure is a potential risk factor). While odds ratios less than 1 imply that the odds of cases being exposed is less than controls (i.e. a potential protective factor).

Where the exposure is continuous, for example, blood pressure, it is often preferable to express the risk in terms of an increase or disease in risk per unit increase in exposure, for example, each 1 or 10 mmHg increase in blood pressure. Such a calculation requires the procedure of logistic regression, which is readily available in most statistical software packages.

17.4.1 Calculation of confidence interval for an odds ratio

There are two methods in common use, the 'test'-based method and Woolf's method. They normally give very similar results, and problems only arise when the numbers are small. Most computer programs specify which method is used; some present both. The 'test' method is based on the Chi-square (χ^2) statistic, which will be familiar to many readers as the standard statistical technique for comparing proportions from a contingency table.

Using notation from Table 17.1, a confidence interval around the odds ratio using 'test'-based method can be calculated as follows:

$$\chi2 = \sum \frac{(O-E)^2}{E}$$

For a: Observed, O = a;

'Expected' number is the number predicted in each cell if under the assumption of no association:

Expected, $E = (a + b)(a + c)/N$.

For b: $O = b$;

$E = (a + b)(b + d)/N$.

For c: $O = c$;

$E = (a + c)(c + d)/N$.

For d: $O = d$;

$E = (c + d)(b + d)/N$

Note that a short-cut formula can be used:

$$\chi2 = \frac{(ad - bc)^2 N}{(a+c)(a+b)(b+d)(c+d)}$$

95% confidence limits = $\text{OR}^{(1 \pm 1.96/\chi)}$

Example 17.iii

Using data from Example 17.ii and the formula shown earlier:

a: $O = 18$ $E = 35 \times 42 / 103 = 14.27$ $(O\text{-}E)^2/E = 0.97$

b: $O = 17$ $E = 35 \times 61 / 103 = 20.73$ $(O\text{-}E)^2/E = 0.67$

c: $O = 24$ $E = 42 \times 68 / 103 = 27.73$ $(O\text{-}E)^2/E = 0.50$

d: $O = 44$ $E = 61 \times 68 / 103 = 40.27$ $(O\text{-}E)^2/E = 0.35$

$\chi2 = 0.97 + 0.67 + 0.50 + 0.35 = 2.49$.

Using an alternative short-cut formula:

$$\chi2 = \frac{(18\times44 - 17\times24)^2 \times (18+17+24+44)}{(18+24)(18+17)(17+44)(24+44)} = 2.49.$$

$$\chi = \sqrt{2.49} = 1.58$$

Lower 95% confidence limit = $1.94^{(1-1.96/1.58)}$,

$= 1.94^{-0.24}$,

$= 0.85$.

Upper 95% confidence limit = $1.94^{(1+1.96/1.58)}$,

$= 1.94^{2.24}$,

$= 4.41$.

Therefore, the 95% confidence limits for OR of 1.94 are 0.85–4.41.

The formula for calculation of confidence interval around an odds ratio using Woolf's method is

$$95\% \text{ Confidence limits} = \exp\left(\log_e OR \pm 1.96\sqrt{\frac{1}{a} + \frac{1}{b} + \frac{1}{c} + \frac{1}{d}}\right)$$

(Note: *exp* is the inverse of the natural logarithm function. This function is available on most calculators.)

Example 17.iv

Using data from the Example 17.ii and using Woolf's method as just shown:
OR = 1.94;
$Log_eOR = 0.663$.

$$Lower\ 95\%\ confidence\ limit = \exp(0.663 - 1.96\sqrt{\frac{1}{18} + \frac{1}{17} + \frac{1}{24} + \frac{1}{44}})$$

$$= \exp(0.663 - 1.96\sqrt{0.179})$$

$$= \exp(0.663 - 1.96 \times 0.423)$$

$$= \exp(0.663 - 0.829)$$

$$= \exp(-0.166)$$

$$= 0.85$$

$$Upper\ 95\%\ confidence\ limit = \exp(0.663 + 1.96\sqrt{\frac{1}{18} + \frac{1}{17} + \frac{1}{24} + \frac{1}{44}})$$

$$= \exp(0.663 + 1.96\sqrt{0.179})$$

$$= \exp(0.663 + 1.96 \times 0.423)$$

$$= \exp(0.663 + 0.829)$$

$$= \exp(1.492)$$

$$= 4.45$$

Therefore the 95% confidence limits for OR of 1.94 are 0.85–4.45.

The previous examples illustrate that both methods give very similar results. Note that the odds ratio (1.94) does not lie mathematically in the centre between the two limits (around 1.8 for the aforementioned confidence interval), reflecting its logarithmic properties. The consequence of this is that displaying confidence intervals graphically should be done on a logarithmic scale, which would then reflect the equal proportional distances from the observed odds ratio.

17.4.2 Logistic regression

In practice, logistic regression is normally used to estimate odds ratios and confidence intervals. This type of regression models the probability of an outcome, for example, probability of disease Y. Because this probability could take values from 0 to 1, the natural logarithm of odds, Y/(1–Y), is used instead, making it more suitable for a regression:

$$log_e[Y/(1-Y)] = a + bX,\ where\ X\ is\ a\ predictor\ (e.g.\ smoking\ status).$$

The exponential of the coefficient *b* results in the odds ratio.

The advantage of logistic regression is that it can analyse the effect of not just one predictor, but several risk factors on the outcome simultaneously (Chapter 18) (multiple logistic regression).

Example 17.v

For data in Example 17.ii, the output from logistic regression is shown on Box 17.1. It can be seen that the OR = 1.94 as in the Example 17.ii, and the 95% confidence interval is (0.85–4.45), is similar to Example 17.iv.

It is important to note that, for logistic regression, some statistical packages require the outcome to be coded as 1 (e.g. cancer) or 0 (no cancer). Coding the outcome as 2 (instead of 0) can potentially lead to an incorrect (inverse) estimate of the odds ratio. Therefore, particular attention should be paid when defining the outcome categories within statistical packages.

Box 17.1 Example of computer outputs in calculation of odds ratio using logistic regression

	Disease		
Exposure	Control	Case	Total
No	44	24	68
Yes	17	18	35
Total	61	42	103

Logistic regression	Number of obs	=	103
	LR chi2 (1)	=	2.47
	Prob > chi2	=	0.1158
Log likelihood=–68.394752	Pseudo R2	=	0.0178

Disease	Odds Ratio	Std. Err.	z	P>|z|	[95% Conf.	Interval]
Exposure	1.941176	.8207597	1.57	0.117	.8475469	4.445968
_cons	.5454545	.1384143	-2.39	0.017	.3317096	.8969312

Note:_cons estimates baseline odds.

17.4.3 Calculation of odds ratios with multiple levels of exposure

Frequently, the exposure can be considered after categorizing into several different levels. Indeed, dichotomizing exposures into an arbitrary yes/no does not use all the data, whereas demonstration of a trend of increasing risk with increasing exposure is valuable evidence of a real effect (dose–response effect).

The major analytical principle is to relate the risk in each exposure stratum to that of one reference stratum, normally that presumed to be at lowest risk, or absence of exposure. This stratum, by definition, will have an odds ratio of 1.

The choice of the number of strata to be used is dependent on the numbers available and the biological sense of splitting up the exposure. The best statistical use is made when the strata have equal numbers and thus, in the absence of powerful biological or clinical arguments, the entire cohort is divided up by tertiles, quartiles, or quintiles (see Section 7.8). There is no further gain in demonstrating a dose response in going beyond five categories. For other exposures, unequal categorization may be more appropriate, for example, for smoking: never smoked, ex-smoker, currently less than 5 cigarettes per day, 5–20 per day, and more than 20 per day (Table 7.1).

Table 17.2 shows how to calculate odds ratios with multiple levels of exposure.

Example 17.vi

Table 17.3 details the calculation of odds ratios with multiple levels of exposure, in this example the level of obesity measured as body mass index (BMI). Note a trend of increasing odds (risk) of disease with increasing levels of obesity.

Table 17.2 Calculation of odds ratio with multiple levels of exposure

Exposure level	Cases	Controls	Odds ratio
1	a_1	b_1	$\dfrac{a_1 b_1}{a_1 b_1} = 1$
2	a_2	b_2	$\dfrac{a_2 b_1}{a_1 b_2}$
3	a_3	b_3	$\dfrac{a_3 b_1}{a_1 b_3}$
...	...	...	...
i	a_i	b_i	$\dfrac{a_i b_1}{a_1 b_i}$

Table 17.3 Example of calculation of odds ratio with multiple levels of exposure

BMI stratum	Cases	Controls	Odds ratio
1 (Low)	21	30	$\dfrac{21 \times 30}{21 \times 30} = 1$
2	31	26	$\dfrac{31 \times 30}{21 \times 26} = 1.70$
3	24	11	$\dfrac{24 \times 30}{21 \times 11} = 3.12$
4 (High)	17	4	$\dfrac{17 \times 30}{21 \times 4} = 6.07$

17.4.4 Estimation of linear trend

In Example 17.vi, the data suggest that there is a trend of increasing risk with increasing levels of obesity. This can be formally tested for statistical significance by using the χ^2 test for trend. Table 17.4a shows the data layout for determination of the presence of linear trend with increasing exposure. Notation is as following:

x_i is the arbitrary score given to exposure stratum i;
n_i is the number of cases and controls in stratum i;
d_i is the number of cases in stratum i;
N is the total number of cases and controls.

χ^2 test for trend is calculates as following:

$$\chi^2_{trend\ 1df} = \frac{N\left[N(\Sigma d_i x_i) - \Sigma d_i (n_i x_i)\right]^2}{\Sigma d_i (N - \Sigma d_i)\left[N(\Sigma n_i x_i)^2 - (\Sigma n_i x_i)^2\right]}$$

The resultant value for χ^2 has one degree of freedom. From statistical tables (see 'Further reading') for $p = 0.05$, $\chi^2_{1df} = 3.84$. Thus, values in excess of 3.84 are said to describe a significant trend, although in practice inspection of the data will yield the same conclusion.

Table 17.4a Table for data layout to determine presence of linear trend with increasing exposure

Exposure level	Cases	Controls	x_i	n_i	d_i	$n_i x_i$	$d_i x_i$	$n_i x_i^2$
1	a_1	b_1	1	a_1+b_1	a_1	$1(a_1+b_1)$	$1(a_1)$	$1^2(a_1+b_1)$
2	a_2	b_2	2	a_2+b_2	a_2	$2(a_2+b_2)$	$2(a_2)$	$2^2(a_2+b_2)$
3	a_3	b_3	3	a_3+b_3	a_3	$3(a_3+b_3)$	$3(a_3)$	$3^2(a_3+b_3)$
...	...	...	...	...	...	...	...	...
i	a_i	b_i	i	a_i+b_i	a_i	$i(a_i+b_i)$	$i(a_i)$	$i^2(a_i+b_i)$
Total				N	Σd_i	$\Sigma n_i x_i$	$\Sigma d_i x_i$	$\Sigma n_i x_i^2$

Example 17.vii

Table 17.4b shows the data layout based on the information from Table 17.4a and the corresponding Example 17.vi. Following the previous formula for χ^2 test for trend:

$$\chi^2_{trend\ 1df} = \frac{164 \times [164 \times 223 - 93 \times 354]^2}{93 \times (164-93) \times [164 \times 930 - (354)^2]}$$

$$= \frac{164 \times [36572 - 32922]^2}{93 \times 71 \times [152520 - 125316]}$$

$$= \frac{164 \times (3650)^2}{93 \times 71 \times 27204}$$

$$= 12.16$$

From statistical tables (see 'Further reading') for $\chi^2 = 12.16$ with one degree of freedom $p = 0.0005$ which suggests a significant trend, as is confirmed by examining the values of the odds ratios by BMI stratum in Table 17.3.

Inspection of the data will also permit observation of trends that are not linear, including the so-called J-shaped curve, where low dose exposure is associated with a higher risk than an intermediate dose, but subsequent increases in exposure are associated with an increase in risk.

Table 17.4b Example of data to determine presence of linear trend with increasing exposure

Exposure level	x_i	n_i	d_i	$n_i x_i$	$d_i x_i$	$n_i x_i^2$
1	1	51	21	51	21	51
2	2	57	31	114	62	228
3	3	35	24	105	72	315
4	4	21	17	84	68	336
Total		164	93	354	223	930

Example 17.viii

Figure 17.1 shows a hypothetical example of a J-curve which indicates that patients with very low blood pressure or high blood pressure are at increased risk of stroke, compared to patients with diastolic blood pressure of 80–89 mmHg, whose odds ratio is set to 1. Note that the odds ratios (and 95% confidence intervals) are plotted on a vertical logarithmic scale.

While categorization of continuous exposures has advantages such as relative ease of understanding, calculation, and interpretation, it is important to be aware of numerous disadvantages. There is no single method of categorization; for example, should quartiles of the distribution of cases or controls, or cases and controls combined, be used in a case–control study? Should exposure be categorized into two, three, four, or five groups, or should instead predetermined categories (such as 10-year age groups or blood pressure classified *a priori* as low, normal, or high) be used? Different choices of categories may lead to different results and potentially different conclusions. There is also no uniform agreement on the reference category; for example, whether to use an extreme (i.e. lowest or highest), 'never' or 'zero' exposure, 'normal' category, or most common group as a reference. Manipulation of categories in order to find a significant result can lead to false positive findings, and/or an exaggerated estimate of the relationship between exposure and outcome. Finally, there is potential loss of efficiency when using categorized exposure compared to a continuous variable in the regression analysis. Therefore, it is a good research practice to justify the use of categories and to predefine them at the stage of developing the analysis plan.

17.4.5 **Analysis of matched pairs**

The calculation of an odds ratio for matched pairs in matched case–control studies (see Section 6.2) is different from that for an unmatched analysis. In practice, a study that is designed as matched may frequently be analysed as though it were unmatched because, as a consequence of dropouts and withdrawals, there are incomplete pairs. Therefore, where an unmatched analysis will include all the subjects seen, a matched analysis will include only complete matched sets. For the simplest form of 1:1 matching, the calculation of the odds ratio can be rapidly achieved. It is important to note that the unit included in each cell of the table is a pair rather than an individual. The odds ratio is calculated as the ratio of the discordant pairs. Thus, in simple terms the odds ratio will be greater than unity if there are more pairs with the case exposed and the control not exposed than the reverse.

Table 17.5a shows the data arrangement and formula to calculate odds ratio for matched pairs.

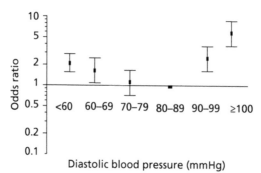

Figure 17.1 Example of J-shaped relationship between exposure and disease.

Table 17.5a Calculation of odds ratio for matched pairs

Control	Case	
	Exposure present	**Exposure absent**
Exposure present	p	q
Exposure absent	r	s

OR = r/q

Example 17.ix

In a study of 78 matched case–control pairs, in 11 pairs both smoked, in 17 pairs neither smoked, in 36 pairs the case smoked and the control did not smoke, whereas in the remaining 14 pairs the converse was the case. Following Table 17.5a and producing Table 17.5b, the OR = 36/14 = 2.57.

It is clear that it is the exposure-discordant pairs that are informative. In studies where there are multiple controls per case or, as is often the case in practice, the study ends up with a variable number of controls per case, the calculations become rather complex.

The conditional logistic regression procedure available in statistical software packages can undertake this kind of analysis as well as examining exposure, either at multiple levels or as a continuous variable similar to the way that the unconditional logistic regression (Section 17.4.2) does for unmatched case–control studies.

17.4.6 Calculation of confidence interval around odds ratio derived from a matched-pair analysis

As with the calculation of a confidence interval around an unmatched derived odds ratio, a test-based calculation can be used such as McNemar's test for matched pairs.

Following notation in Table 17.5a, the formula for calculation of a confidence interval around an odds ratio derived from a matched-pair analysis is as follows:

$$95\% \text{ confidence interval} = OR^{\left(1-\frac{1.96}{\chi}\right)}, \text{ where } \chi^2 = \frac{\left[(r-q)-1\right]^2}{r+q}$$

Example 17.x

Using data and results from Example 17.ix and Table 17.5b,

$$\chi^2 = \frac{\left[(36-14)-1\right]^2}{36+14} = 8.82; \; \chi = \sqrt{8.82} = 2.97$$

$$\text{Lower 95\% confidence limit} = 2.57^{\left(1-\frac{1.96}{2.97}\right)} = 2.57^{(0.34)} = 1.38$$

$$\text{Upper 95\% confidence limit} = 2.57^{\left(1+\frac{1.96}{2.97}\right)} = 2.57^{(1.66)} = 4.79$$

Therefore 95% confidence interval for OR 2.57 is (1.38–4.79).

Table 17.5b Example of data from a matched case–control study

Control	Case	
	Smoker	**Non-smoker**
Smoker	11	14
Non-smoker	36	17

Table 17.6a Calculation of rate ratio (RtR) estimate from incidence (density) rates

Exposure	Person-years at risk	Number with outcome	Incidence rate
Present	$npyr_e$	x_e	$x_e/npyr_e$
Absent	$npyr_0$	x_0	$x_0/npyr_0$

$RtR = (x_e/npyr_e) / (x_0/npyr_0)$

17.5 **Analysis of cohort studies**

17.5.1 **Calculation of rate ratio from incidence data**

A ratio of incidence rates between two exposure groups provides an estimate of the rate ratio, with the incidence rates being calculated as shown in Table 17.6a.

Example 17.xi

A follow-up study comparing the incidence of melanoma stratified at baseline according to the presence of a significant number of benign lesions; the results obtained are shown in Table 17.6b. Following the formula in Table 17.6a, the RtR = 15.70/4.82 = 3.26.

17.5.2 **Calculation of population attributable risk**

The rate difference is also of importance, being the incidence in the exposed minus that in the non-exposed, and gives the absolute (rather than the relative) change in incidence associated with exposure. If data are available on the proportion of individuals in the population who are exposed, it is also possible to calculate the proportion of the total number of cases arising within the population that are due to the exposure.

Assuming that I_e is the incidence in the exposed and I_0 is the incidence in the non-exposed population, then (I_e-I_0) is the incidence in exposed due to exposure.

The proportion of incidence in the exposed population due to exposure can be calculated as $\dfrac{I_e - I_0}{I_e}$.

Table 17.6b Example of data from follow-up study comparing the incidence of melanoma

Exposure	Person-years at risk	Number of melanoma cases	Incidence rate
High lesion count	12,100	19	15.70/10,000
Low lesion count	41,500	20	4.82/10,000

Given that the rate ratio is calculated as RtR = I_e/I_0, then $\dfrac{I_e - I_0}{I_e} = \dfrac{RtR - 1}{RtR}$.

If the proportion of the population exposed is p_e, the proportion of all cases in a population due to exposure (known as the population attributable risk) is $\dfrac{(I_e - I_0)p_e}{I_e p_e + I_0(1 - p_e)} = \dfrac{p_e(RtR - 1)}{1 + p_e(RtR - 1)}$.

Example 17.xii

In a prospective study of oral contraceptives use and stroke, a RtR of 3.1 was found for ever users. The proportion of everyday users of oral contraceptives in the population studied was 0.6.

Proportion of risk in oral contraceptive users due to oral contraceptive use $= \dfrac{3.1 - 1}{3.1} = 0.68.$

Proportion of cases in female population due to oral contraceptive use $= \dfrac{0.6(3.1 - 1)}{1 + 0.6(3.1 - 1)} = 0.56.$

Thus, in this example, 68% of the stroke risk in oral contraceptive users is due to their use of oral contraceptives, and the remainder is due to their background (population) risk. Further, given the frequency of oral contraceptive use in the female population, it can be estimated that 56% of all the cases that arise can be explained by their use. Alternatively, if these data were true, eliminating oral contraceptive use might have the potential for reducing the number of cases of stroke in a female population by over half.

17.5.3 Calculation of confidence interval around incidence rate ratio

As with the calculation of the confidence interval around an incidence rate, the crucial factor is the number of cases; the number of person-years at risk does not influence the calculation.

To calculate the confidence interval around an incidence rate ratio, an approximation may be found from the following formulae (using notation from Table 17.6a):

$$95\% \text{ confidence interval} = \exp\left(\log_e RtR \pm 1.96 \sqrt{\dfrac{1}{x_0} + \dfrac{1}{x_e}} \right)$$

(Note: *exp* is the inverse of the natural logarithm function. This function is available on most calculators.)

As with the confidence interval around an odds ratio (see Section 17.4.1), the distribution is logarithmic.

Table 17.7a Table for calculation of risk ratio estimate from prevalence or cumulative incidence data

Exposure	Disease		Total
	Case	Not case	
Exposed	a	b	a + b
Not exposed	c	d	c + d

Example 17.xiii

Using data from Example 17.xi and Table 17.6a,

$$\text{Lower 95\% confidence limit} = \exp\left(\log_e 3.26 - 1.96\sqrt{\frac{1}{19} + \frac{1}{20}}\right)$$

$$= \exp\left(1.18 - 1.96\sqrt{\frac{1}{19} + \frac{1}{20}}\right)$$

$$= \exp\left(1.18 - 1.96\sqrt{0.1026}\right)$$

$$= \exp\left(1.18 - 0.63\right)$$

$$= \exp\left(0.55\right)$$

$$= 1.73.$$

$$\text{Upper 95\% confidence limit} = \exp\left(1.18 + 0.63\right) = \exp\left(1.81\right)$$

$$= 6.11.$$

17.5.4 Calculation of risk ratio estimate from prevalence or cumulative incidence data

This, as discussed in Section 17.3, is relevant to a comparison of prevalence proportions or cumulative incidence. The risk ratio is simply the ratio of the two proportions (see notation in Table 17.7a).

Risk in exposed = $a/(a + b)$
Risk in not exposed = $c/(c + d)$
RiR = $[a/(a + b)]/[c/(c + d)]$

Example 17.xiv

In a cohort study, 221 infants, of whom 49 weighed under 2,000 g at birth, were followed up to age 6 years; 18 of the low birth-weight group, and 29 of the normal birth-weight group, had learning difficulties. Table 17.7b follows data format from Table 17.7a.

Risk of learning difficulty in low birth-weight group = 18/49; risk of learning difficulty in normal birth-weight group = 29/172. Therefore, RiR = (18/49)/(29/172) = 2.18.

17.5.5 Calculation of a confidence interval around a risk ratio

As with other confidence-interval calculations, there is the possibility of using either a 'test'-based approach or a logarithmic transformation: both give very similar results.

Table 17.7b Example of data for calculation of risk ratio estimate

Birth weight	Learning difficulties		Total
	Yes	No	
Low (< 2,000 g)	18	31	49
Normal (≥ 2,000 g)	29	143	172

Confidence interval for risk ratio using a test-based method:

95% confidence interval $= RiR^{\left(1 \pm 1.96/\chi\right)}$, where χ^2 can be calculated using the short-cut formula from Section 17.4.1.

Example 17.xv

For data in Example 17.xiv and Table 17.7b, $\chi^2 = 9.00$ and therefore $\chi = 3$.

Lower 95% confidence limit $= 2.18^{\left(1-1.96/3\right)} = 2.18^{(0.347)} = 1.31$

Upper 95% confidence limit $= 2.18^{\left(1+1.96/3\right)} = 2.18^{(1.653)} = 3.63$

Therefore RiR = 2.18 95% CI (1.31–3.63).

17.5.6 Life-table method for incidence data

One problem with comparing incidence rates, as in Section 17.5.1, is that such a comparison takes no account of the time to an event. A simple example will suffice to clarify the point. The ultimate cumulative incidence of death in any group of individuals is always 100%; the point of interest is the time course of the deaths. Thus, it is frequently the rate ratio of an event at a particular point in time that is of interest: this is often referred to as the *hazard ratio*. The life-table approach permits a calculation of the probability of an event at a particular time since the start of observation. The probability at the end of the second year (say) for developing an event is equivalent to the probability of developing the event during the first year multiplied by the probability of developing the event in the second year, if free from the event at the start of the second year.

Table 17.8a illustrates the use of life-table methods for analysis of incidence data.

Example 17.xvi

One hundred smokers, after receiving intensive health education, gave up smoking. At the end of each of the subsequent five years, 5, 10, 8, 7, and 6 subjects, respectively, had restarted the habit. Table 17.8b shows the use of a life table for these data.

It can be noted that in this example the cumulative probability of remaining a non-smoker at the end of the five years could have been calculated much more easily by noting that at the end of the fifth year there were 64 of the original 100 subjects who had not relapsed.

Table 17.8a Use of life-table methods for analysis of incidence data

Time interval (*i*)	Number entering interval (*n_i*)	Number developing event (*x_i*)	Probability of event within interval (*x_i/n_i*)	Probability of no event within interval (*p_i*)	Cumulative probability of no event
1	n_1	x_1	x_1/n_1	$1-x_1/n_1 = p_1$	p_1
2	$n_1 - x_1 = n_2$	x_2	x_2/n_2	$1-x_2/n_2 = p_2$	p_1p_2
...	...	...	...	...	...
i	$n_{i-1} - x_{i-1} = n_i$	x_i	x_i/n_i	$1-x_i/n_i = p_i$	$p_1p_2 \ldots p_i$

Table 17.8b Example of life-table data

Time interval (years) (*i*)	Number entering interval (*n$_i$*)	Number restarting smoking (*x$_i$*)	Probability of restarting smoking (in given year) (*x$_i$ /n$_i$*)	Probability of remaining non-smoker (in given year) (*p$_i$*)	Cumulative success (*p$_1$p$_2$ ... p$_i$*)
1	100	5	0.05	0.95	0.95
2	95	10	0.105	0.895	0.85
3	85	8	0.094	0.906	0.77
4	77	7	0.091	0.909	0.70
5	70	6	0.086	0.914	0.64

However, in practice, it is exceedingly unlikely that all subjects entered at time '0' will have exactly five years of follow-up. Some will die; others will be lost to follow-up for a variety of other reasons. More importantly, few studies recruit all individuals at a single point in time. Thus, in considering the disease risk following an occupational exposure, the duration of follow-up will vary, being the interval since a particular subject was first employed to the date that the follow-up of that individual was completed: the censorship date. Some individuals may therefore have had 10 years of follow-up, whereas others, depending on the study design, had perhaps less than one year. Thus, there is frequently incomplete information, a phenomenon known as right censorship (i.e. incidence data are missing to the 'right' of the conceptual data line). If the assumption is made that the risk of disease is unrelated to the chances of being 'censored', each individual can be included up until the time they are censored. When this analysis is not undertaken by computer, the approach is to assume that the individual was censored midway through an interval and hence contributed half a person–time of follow-up for that interval.

Example 17.xvii

Taking the same data as in Example 17.xvi and adding information on the losses or end of follow-up during each interval produces the result as shown in Table 17.8c. Clearly, the cumulative success for remaining a non-smoker is actually lower than that seen in Table 17.8b, owing to the censored observations.

Data from these calculations can be used to plot 'survival' (i.e. event-free survival) curves from which the event-free survival can be read off at a particular time of interest. It is easier to

Table 17.8c Use of life-table methods (with losses)

Time interval (years) (*I*)	Number entering interval (*m$_i$*)	Number 'lost' during interval (*l$_i$*)	Number at risk, (*n$_i$*)	Number restarting smoking, (*x$_i$*)	Probability of restarting smoking, (*x$_i$ /n$_i$*)	Probability of remaining non-smoker (*p$_i$*)	Cumulative success (*p$_1$p$_2$ ... p$_i$*)
1	100	4	98	5	0.051	0.949	0.949
2	91	3	89.5	10	0.112	0.888	0.842
3	78	2	77	8	0.104	0.896	0.755
4	68	5	65.5	7	0.107	0.893	0.674
5	56	4	54	6	0.111	0.889	0.599

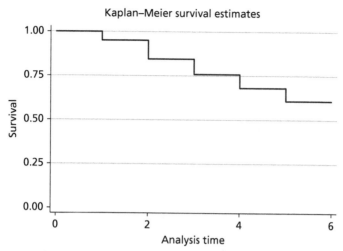

Figure 17.2 Example of survival curve for data in Table 17.8c.

undertake this analysis by computer, which uses the actual date of each event to generate a more accurate curve than can be obtained by the interval approach used just now; however, the principle is the same. The curves generated are often known as Kaplan–Meier curves and the survival estimate at a particular point in time is known as the Kaplan–Meier estimate. It is also possible to calculate the confidence interval around the estimates at each time point.

Example 17.xviii

Figure 17.2 shows an example of a survival curve drawn using the data from Example 17.xvi

17.5.7 **Comparison of survival curves**

A comparison of the curves for disease-free survival (say) between two exposure groups can give an estimate of the effect of the exposure. Survival curves can be compared for statistical significance by using the logrank test, which can be done easily using a calculator; a suitable layout is shown in Table 17.9a.

If the numbers of events in both groups were distributed randomly, related only to the number at risk in each group, then, in any given time interval i:

Table 17.9a Data layout for logrank test

Time interval	Group A		Group B		Combined	
	At risk	Number of observed events	At risk	Number of observed events	At risk	Number of observed events
1	n_{1A}	o_{1A}	n_{1B}	o_{1B}	$n_{1A} + n_{1B}$	$o_{1A} + o_{1B}$
...	...	...	...	...	...	...
i	n_{iA}	o_{iA}	n_{iB}	o_{iB}	$n_{iA} + n_{iB}$	$o_{iA} + o_{iB}$

Expected number of events in Group A, $e_{iA} = \dfrac{n_{iA}}{n_{iA} + n_{iB}}(o_{iA} + o_{iB})$;

Expected number of events in Group B, $e_{iB} = \dfrac{n_{iB}}{n_{iA} + n_{iB}}(o_{iA} + o_{iB})$;

Then for all time intervals considered from 1 to i:

Total number of observed events in Group A $= \sum\limits_{1}^{i} o_{iA}$

Total number of observed events in Group B $= \sum\limits_{1}^{i} o_{iB}$

Total number of expected events in Group A $= \sum\limits_{1}^{i} e_{iA}$

Total number of expected events in Group B $= \sum\limits_{1}^{i} e_{iB}$

logrank test gives the value for χ_{1df}^2 as

$$\frac{\left(\sum o_{iA} - \sum e_{iA}\right)^2}{\sum e_{iA}} + \frac{\left(\sum o_{iB} - \sum e_{iB}\right)^2}{\sum e_{iB}}.$$

Example 17.xix

Using data from Example 17.xvii and Table 17.8c for Group A and adding data for Group B (Table 17.9b),

$$\chi_{1df}^2 = \frac{(36 - 30.21)^2}{30.21} + \frac{(27 - 32.79)^2}{32.79} = 1.11 + 1.02 = 2.13.$$

As in Section 17.4.3, from statistical tables (see further reading) for $p = 0.05$, $\chi_{1df}^2 = 3.84$. Thus we conclude that the curves from two groups are unlikely to represent different responses.

Table 17.9b Example of logrank test

Time interval	At risk		Observed events		Expected events	
	Group A, n_{iA}	Group B, n_{iB}	Group A, o_{iA}	Group B, o_{iB}	Group A, e_{iA}	Group B, e_{iB}
1	98	97	5	4	4.52 [a]	4.48
2	89.5	91	10	6	7.93	8.07
3	77	82	8	5	6.30	6.70
4	65.5	74.5	7	5	5.61	6.39
5	54	66	6	7	5.85	7.15
Total			36	27	30.21	32.79

Note: a $e_{1A} = \dfrac{98}{97 + 98} \times (4 + 5)$

17.5.8 **Cox regression**

Whereas the Kaplan–Meier method and logrank test are useful for comparing survival curves, Cox regression (or proportional hazards regression) allows analysis of the effect of several risk factors on survival (Chapter 18). The probability of the outcome of interest (such as death or disease recurrence) is called the hazard, H(t) at time t. The baseline hazard function $H_0(t)$ at time t is the hazard when not exposed to factors under study. The ratio $H(t)/H_0(t)$ is the hazard ratio. The hazard is modelled as $log_e(H(t)/H_0(t)) = b_1X_1 + b_2X_2 + \ldots + b_iX_i$, where $X_1 \ldots X_i$ are predictors (such as level of physical activity, smoking, and so on).

For a dichotomous predictor, $exp(b_i)$ can be interpreted as the instantaneous relative risk of an event, at any time, for an individual with the risk factor present compared to an individual with the risk factor absent (e.g. current smokers vs. current non-smokers).

One of the assumptions of Cox regression is proportional hazard assumption, which means that the survival curves for two strata must have hazard functions that are proportional over time (i.e. constant relative hazard).

Example 17.xx

For comparison of survival in two groups (plotted in Figure 17.3) the output from Cox regression is shown on Box 17.2. It can be seen that the curves look very similar which is confirmed by the hazard ratio close to one, HR = 0.99 and 95% confidence interval 0.92–1.07 leading to conclusion that there is no statistically significant difference between the two treatment groups.

Cox proportional hazards model can be adapted for the estimation of prevalence ratios in cross-sectional studies by imposing a condition of constant follow-up time (e.g. time $t = 1$) for all study participants (see 'Further reading').

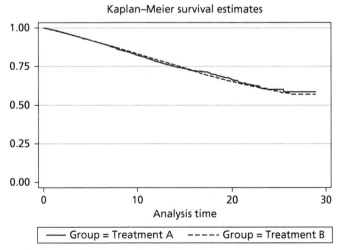

Figure 17.3 Example of survival curves for two treatment groups.

Box 17.2 Example of computer output from Cox regression

stcox group

failure_d: outcome

analysis time_t: time

id: patid

Interation 0:   log likelihood=−260668.63

Interation 1:   log likelihood=−260668.58

Interation 2:   log likelihood=−260668.58

Refining estimates:

Interation 0:   log likelihood=−260668.58

Cox regression -- Breslow method for ties

No. of subjects =	117,126		Number of obs =	117,126
No. of failures =	23,414			
Time at risk =	−1212079.734			
			LR chi2(1) =	0.10
Log likelihood =	−260668.58		Prob > chi2 =	0.7522

_t	Haz. Ratio	Std. Err.	z	P>|z|	[95% Conf.	Interval]
group	.9877399	.0385185	−0.32	0.752	.915058	1.066195

17.6 Analysis of other types of observational studies

17.6.1 Analysis of case-crossover studies

A case-crossover study (see Section 6.4.1 and 'Further reading') can be analysed as a stratified cohort study (see Section 6.3 and Chapter 18), in which case the incidence rate ratio can be estimated using the Mantel–Haenszel method (see Section 18.4.2). Each participant represents a strata. The person–time data are the number of episodes that each participant is exposed and the number of episodes that each participant is not exposed. Strata with no outcome event of interest do not contribute to the estimate of relative risk.

Using notation from Table 17.10, the Mantel–Haenszel estimate of relative risk can be calculated as follows:

$$RR_{MH} = \frac{\sum_i a_i N_{0i} / T_i}{\sum_i b_i N_{1i} / T_i}$$

Table 17.10 Notation for participant i in case-crossover Mantel–Haenszel analysis

	Disease		Total
Case	a_i	b_i	M_{1i}
Person–time	N_{1i}	N_{0i}	T_i

There are several methods to estimate confidence interval, but this is beyond the scope of this book (see 'Further reading').

Example 17.xxi

A case-crossover study was conducted to investigate the relationship between coffee consumption and subsequent myocardial infarction (MI). Coffee exposure within the hour before MI onset is of interest. The hypothetical data are presented in Table 17.11. Note that only two patients consumed coffee less than one hour before MI.

$$\text{Mantel–Haenszel estimate of relative risk } RR_{M-H} = \frac{(8,401+5,116+0+0+0+0+0)}{(0+0+730+36+1,820+24+365)}$$

$$= \frac{13,517}{2,975} = 4.54$$

A case-crossover study can be also analysed as a matched case–control study (see Section 17.4.5). In this situation each case episode and its matched control episodes(s) form a stratum. Conditional logistic regression can also be used for analysis of such data.

17.6.2 Analysis of case–cohort studies

Methods for cohort studies described in Section 17.5 can also be used for analysis of case–cohort studies, for example, Cox regression. To tackle the issue of oversampling mentioned in Section 6.4, weighted Cox proportional hazards regression model is used (see 'Further reading').

17.6.3 Analysis of migrant studies

Migrant studies (see 'Further reading') are often descriptive in nature, and therefore methods discussed in Chapter 16 can be applied. Usually incidence or mortality in the migrant group in the new host country are compared to the population in the home country, indigenous population of the host country, or other migrant groups in the host country. Comparison between the first-generation migrants and their descendants in the host country can also be useful. Further analysis within the migrant group in the host country can be performed by duration of residence in the host country or age at migration. If data on risk factors are available at an individual level, the methods described in Sections 17.4 and 17.5 can also be used, including multivariate analysis (see Chapter 18).

17.6.4 Analysis of Mendelian randomization studies

The aim of statistical analysis of Mendelian randomization studies (Section 6.4.4) is to determine the magnitude of the causal association between a modifiable exposure of interest and an outcome. The important assumptions that underpin the Mendelian randomization approach are

Table 17.11 Notation for participant i in case-crossover Mantel–Haenszel analysis

i	Last time coffee consumed prior to onset of myocardial infarction (MI)	Exposure < 1 hour before MI?	α_i	b_i	Usual frequency of coffee consumption during past year	Exposure during the past year (hours) N_{1i}	Non-exposure during the past year (hours) (assuming there were 365.25 ×24 = 8,766 hours in a year) N_{0i}
1	30 min	yes	1	0	Once per day	1 × 365 (in a year) = 365	8,766 – 365 = 8,401
2	45 min	Yes	1	0	10/day	10 × 365 = 3,650	8,766 – 3650 = 5,116
3	7 hours	No	0	1	Twice a day	2 hours × 365 days = 730	8,766 – 730 = 8,036
4	3 hours	No	0	1	3/month	3 × 12 months = 36	8,766 – 36 = 8,730
5	24 hours	No	0	1	5/day	5 × 365 = 1,820	8,466 – 1,820 = 6,946
6	8 hours	No	0	1	Twice a month	2 × 12 months = 24	8,766 – 24 = 8,442
7	2 days	No	0	1	Once per day	1 × 365 = 365	8,766 – 365 = 8,401

that the genotype is associated with the modifiable (non-genetic) exposure of interest; that the genotype is not associated with confounding factors that bias conventional epidemiological associations between modifiable risk factors and outcomes; and that the genotype is related to the outcome only via its association with the modifiable exposure.

One method of analysis is known as triangulation. Using genetic information, a genetic risk score can be constructed.

Example 17.xxii

Researchers identified from published literature 11 single nucleotide polymorphisms (SNPs) related to the exposure of interest, and derived a combined genetic risk score for each participant from analysis of collected blood samples.

The association between the exposure and the genetic risk score can then be determined using linear regression. Association between the exposure and the outcome can be estimated using methods described in Sections 17.4 or 17.5, for example, using odds ratio estimated from logistic regression. In addition, the relationship between genetic score and outcome can also be determined and then compared to combination of two previous associations.

Another, more complex method is called instrumental variable (IV) analysis (see 'Further reading') which is based on statistical models-derived variables that represent an intermediate between a cause and the outcome. However, such analysis requires advanced statistical knowledge.

17.6.5 **Analysis of ecologic studies**

Section 6.4.5 explained that ecological studies consider groups, rather than individuals, as units of analysis. Pearson correlation or Spearman rank correlation and regression analysis predicting disease rate from average exposure is often used for statistical analysis. Weighted regression can be used to allow for variation in the size of groups, for example, size of schools, population size of cities or countries. It is important to note however that regression coefficients cannot be interpreted as the change in disease rate with the unit of change in exposure. In studies where both individual level data (on patients) and group level data (e.g. on medical practices) are available, analysis called multilevel modelling, hierarchical regression, or a mixed effects model can be used. However, such advanced techniques are beyond the scope of this book (see 'Further reading').

17.7 **Analysis of randomized controlled studies**

Analysis of randomized controlled trials (see Section 6.5) usually involves survival analysis described in Section 17.5, such as Kaplan–Meier and Cox regression. Such trials should usually be analysed following the 'intention to treat' principle when all study participants are included in the analysis according to the original treatment group allocation, irrespective of whether they actually received the treatment to which they were randomized. An alternative approach is a 'per protocol' analysis where participants are analysed according to the treatment they actually received. It is also important to describe baseline characteristics of each group, similar to Table 16.1 in Chapter 16. These characteristics usually include demographic data such as age, gender, ethnicity, or social class, and baseline severity of illness measures and other variables known to be to be related to the primary outcome of the study. Such analysis is useful in describing the study participants and assessing the similarities of the treatment groups. However, performing statistical tests of significance to evaluate whether the observed baseline differences could have occurred by chance is not recommended, because in a correctly randomized study any such observed significant difference will be due to chance. There are many other issues to consider when analysing data collected from randomized controlled studies which are covered in more specialized textbooks (see 'Further reading').

17.8 **Conclusion**

The exciting point in any epidemiological study comes when the raw data collected are analysed to reveal the answer to the main question posed, be it an incidence rate, an odds ratio, or other measure. In practice, the calculations are most often performed by computer, but the investigator needs to be aware of how the results were arrived at. For all studies it is necessary to calculate not only an estimate of the main effect, but also a confidence interval around that result.

Further reading

Textbooks

Bland M (2015). *An Introduction to Medical Statistics*, 4th edition. Oxford University Press, Oxford, UK.

Clayton D, Hills M (2013). *Statistical Models in Epidemiology*. Oxford University Press, Oxford, UK.

Lindley DV, Scott WF (1995). *New Cambridge Elementary Statistical Tables*. Cambridge University Press, Cambridge.

Rothman KJ (1986). *Modern Epidemiology*. Little, Brown and Company, Boston/Toronto.

Cross-sectional studies

Barros, Aluísio JD, Hirakata VN (2003). Alternatives for logistic regression in cross-sectional studies: an empirical comparison of models that directly estimate the prevalence ratio. *BMC Med Res Methodol*, **3**, 21.

Case–control studies

Davies HT, Crombie IK, Tavakoli M (1998). When can odds ratios mislead? *BMJ*, **316**(7136), 989–91.

Hosmer Jr. DW, Lemeshow S, Sturdivant RX (2013). *Applied Logistic Regression*, 3rd edition. John Wiley & Sons, Hoboken, NJ.

Turner EL, Dobson JE, Pocock SJ (2010). Categorisation of continuous risk factors in epidemiological publications: a survey of current practice. *Epidemiol Perspect Innov*, **7**, 9.

Cohort studies

Cox DR (1972). Regression models and life-tables (with discussion). *Journal of the Royal Statistical Society Series B*, **34**, 187–220.

Case-crossover studies

Marshall RJ, Jackson RT (1993). Analysis of case-crossover designs. *Statist Med*, **12**, 2333–41.

Case–cohort studies

Sharp SJ, Poulaliou M, Thompson SG, White IR, Wood AM (2014). A review of published analyses of case-cohort studies and recommendations for future reporting. *PLoS One*, **9**, e101176.

Migrant studies

Kolonel LN, Wilkens LR (2006). Migrant studies. In: Schottenfeld D, Fraumeni JF (eds) *Cancer Epidemiology and Prevention*, 3rd edition. Oxford University Press, New York, NY.

Parkin DM, Khlat M (1996). Studies of cancer in migrants: rationale and methodology. *Eur J Cancer*, **32A**(5), 761–71.

Mendelian randomization studies

De Silva NM, Freathy RM, Palmer TM, *et al.* (2011). Mendelian randomization studies do not support a role for raised circulating triglyceride levels influencing type 2 diabetes, glucose levels, or insulin resistance. *Diabetes,* **60**(3), 1008–18.

Lawlor DA, Harbord RM, Sterne JAC, Timpson N, Davey Smith DS (2008). Mendelian randomization: using genes as instruments for making causal inferences in epidemiology. *Statist Med,* **27**, 1133–63

Ecologic studies

Goldstein H (2003). *Multilevel Statistical Models.* Arnold, London, UK.

Randomized controlled studies

Peduzzi P, Henderson W, Hartigan P, Lavori P (2002). Analysis of randomized controlled trials. *Epidemiol Rev,* **24**(1), 26–38.

Statistical software

Epi Info™ https://www.cdc.gov/epiinfo [Accessed October 2017].

IBM SPSS Statistics for Windows, Version 22.0. IBM Corp, Armonk, New York, NY https://www.ibm.com/analytics/us/en/technology/spss/ [Accessed October 2017].

SAS software. SAS Institute Inc., Cary, NC, USA. https://www.sas.com [Accessed October 2017].

STATA data analysis and statistical software https://www.stata.com/ [Accessed October 2017].

The R Project for Statistical Computing https://www.r-project.org/ [Accessed October 2017].

Chapter 18

Confounding

18.1 **Introduction**

The concept of confounding is best introduced by way of a simple example:

Example 18.i

In a prospective cohort study, coal miners who worked at the coalface were found to have twice the incidence of carcinoma of the lung as miners who worked on the surface. It was questioned whether this represented a real increase in risk associated with face work or whether the increased risk could be explained by face workers smoking more than surface workers.

In this example the question is raised as to whether the apparent relationship between the disease and the risk factor is explained (*confounded*) by their joint association with the 'true' risk factor of smoking. Unlike the discussion of bias in Chapter 19, the issue here is not one of impaired validity; if the study had been carefully conducted then the relationship observed was correct. The problem of confounding is therefore one of interpretation. (Some textbooks of epidemiology refer to 'confounding bias', a conjunction that is misleading and unhelpful.)

Further evaluation of this simple example reveals some key points about confounding.

i) Confounding can only be proved after appropriate analysis; in Example 18.i, confounding due to cigarette smoking is *suspected* but remains to be demonstrated *in this study*. Consequently, the observation that a particular variable is (or is not) a confounder in another similar study does not answer the question as to whether it is acting similarly in the current investigation.

ii) Confounding as an explanation of an association is not (or is only extremely rarely) an all-or-nothing phenomenon. The effect of confounding will be, more usually, to alter the strength of an apparent relationship between two variables (e.g. risk factor and disease). The effect of the confounder may make the apparent relationship disappear. An accurate estimate of the strength of any observed association requires consideration of the effects of all likely important confounders.

Occasionally, however, *adjusting* for a confounder can strengthen the observed association, as in the example given next (negative confounding).

Example 18.ii

A prospective study comparing pregnancy outcome in smokers and non-smokers suggested that the former resulted in babies of lower birth weight. It was known that smoking varies with maternal age and that the latter also affects birth weight (lower maternal age is associated with low birth weight). Adjusting for maternal age increased the strength of the association. This would be explained by older pregnant women being more likely to be smokers.

The demonstration that adjustment for possible confounding allows a judgement of where the real effect lies: care must be taken before inferring a cause-and-effect relationship. Although common sense and previous experience are helpful, it may be impossible to reach a clear conclusion, as the following example shows.

Example 18.iii

A study was undertaken in a particular migrant population sample living in London, to determine whether blood pressure was related to the duration of living in the United Kingdom. A strong association was found which disappeared after adjusting for the possible confounding effect of age. As most of the migrant population had migrated to the United Kingdom at broadly the same age, it was impossible to distinguish between the two alternative hypotheses: (i) that duration in the United Kingdom explained an observed hypertensive effect of age, or (ii) that age explained an observed hypertensive effect of duration in the United Kingdom.

Confounding should also be distinguished from one variable acting *on the path* in explaining an association (i.e. an intermediate variable that exists as a consequence of the exposure and therefore should not be adjusted for).

Example 18.iv

The demonstration that individuals who have a high energy (calorie) intake have an increased risk of developing maturity onset (type II) diabetes is probably mediated via obesity. It would thus be nonsensical to adjust for body weight because this would eliminate the relationship, and the real risk from overeating would be masked. (This relationship is illustrated in Fig. 18.1)

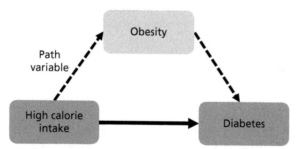

Figure 18.1 Relationship between the risk of developing diabetes and obesity.

Example 18.v

A study investigated whether loss of a close family member was associated with an increased heart disease risk. The study had data on both a depression and a physical activity score assessed one year after the bereavement. There was a strong association between the bereavement and disease risk which almost disappeared after adjusting for depression and activity. This result should be interpreted that bereavement is most likely not associated, but that there is an association which is mediated by the consequences of depression and lower physical activity.

One of the major advances in the application of epidemiological methods in the past decade has been brought about by the widespread availability of statistical software for personal computers that enables the simultaneous adjustment of an association for multiple potential confounders. Indeed, in the same analysis it is now relatively easy to examine the strength of association, not only of the main variable under study, *the main effect*, but also of a variety of potentially important confounders. In practice, therefore, it is possible to examine several variables simultaneously for their *independent* effects and it is not necessary to specify which effect is the main one of interest. This is discussed in detail in Section 18.4.4. Thus, the conclusion is that although it is easy to adjust for confounders with many epidemiological analysis packages, it is vital to have a sensible and biologically/clinically coherent model of how the different variables are expected to be connected to each other and the main effect.

Example 18.vi

A research study aimed to look at the association between height, weight, sports activity, cigarette smoking, and chronic back pain. All these predictors were mutually associated. In considering the scope for confounding the researchers had a clear model informed by biological and other evidence that, for example:

Weight predicted height and not the other way around

Weight and smoking were correlated but that the former was more likely to be associated with back pain than the latter: thus, adjusting the obesity relationship for smoking habit would not make sense

It was more likely that those who smoked would do less physical activity than those that didn't smoke

However, it is clear that confounding can be a problem and hinders appropriate interpretations; it is important that it should be minimized where possible and evaluated for its impact where not.

18.2 Minimizing confounding in study design

The first step is to think about the potential confounders in a proposed study. A list can be drawn up from the results of previous studies and from consensus opinion.

The consequence of drawing up such a list is that it is incumbent on the investigator to attempt to collect these data from the study's subjects, if at all possible. The list should, however, be of manageable size. It is useful for the investigator to adopt the role of a potential reviewer or other critical reader who might ask whether an association revealed could be explained by a confounder that the investigator had not considered.

18.2.1 Selection of study subjects

Matching

One approach to minimize the risk of confounding is to make the groups being compared as similar as possible in respect of potential confounders by using either individual or frequency matching, as discussed in Chapter 8. The problems with this strategy as outlined are first, that the effects of the matched variables cannot be examined and, secondly, that the matching process is inefficient in time, may be difficult in respect of a large number of potential confounders and can seriously reduce the numbers available for study.

The unknown confounders

In comparative studies there is often the concern that any difference observed between the groups under study may result from confounding, though the exact nature of the confounding variable(s) remains obscure, preventing their ascertainment. This is a particular problem in case–control studies where cases are not selected from a true population base. These unknown confounders can therefore be controlled by attempting to recruit controls from a similar base. Two examples illustrate the point.

Example 18.vii

A case–control study of a rare disease recruited cases from the register of a specialist unit in a major academic centre. The investigator was unsure what factors, such as socioeconomic, educational, and so on, determined whether a patient with that disease would be referred to such a unit. The anxiety was that these very factors might confound any observed association between the exposures studied and the disease. To minimize this, it was felt that an appropriate comparison group would be cases with a broad range of other diseases referred to the same unit, but for which there was no evidence that the exposure under investigation was linked.

Example 18.viii

In a case–control study of an even rarer disease, after a nationwide campaign on social media an investigator was able to identify 80 cases nationwide. The population base for these cases was unknown and the investigator was concerned that any association uncovered might be explained by unknown confounders relating to the use of Facebook. It was decided to use Facebook to recruit friends of the cases (without the disease!) as a control group in an attempt to minimize any unknown confounders associated with use of Facebook.

18.3 **Conduct of study**

There is little that can be done during the data collection phase to reduce confounding. In studies with sequential recruitment over a long period of time, it might be appropriate to monitor the subjects to ensure a reasonable balance between the major potential confounders such as age and sex. This is of particular relevance in studies where the target number to be recruited is small. Although far from ideal, it may sometimes be necessary to add in collection of data on a potential confounder that was not thought through at the start of the study.

Example 18.ix

A prospective cohort study investigated the frequency of shoulder, neck pain and headache in office workers in relation to the number of weekly hours spent in front of a computer monitor. Early in the data collection phase of the study, the investigators became aware that those who were high users also worked longer hours and were often working under greater pressure. Initially they had not thought to collect data on the latter variables, but the study had to be amended to allow such information to be obtained. Thus, at the analysis stage a subgroup analysis would be planned to include those with this extra information.

In the example just given there was missing data on possible key confounders because of change in the study protocol. In 'real life' there is often missing data on potential confounders for a variety of reasons. This is particularly true when using routine data sources. Thus, the analysis of subgroups, with and without these data items, can be attempted.

18.4 **Analysis**

There are four approaches to examining how relevant confounding may be in a completed study. The details of the analytical methods involved are beyond the scope of this volume, and adjusting for possible confounders is a major topic in its own right. In the following discussion, the aim is to present the major uses of the different strategies with illustrations and to provide appropriate cautions about their use.

18.4.1 **Baseline comparison of potential confounders**

The first stage is to draw up a table comparing the frequency distributions of the potential confounders (or their summary statistics such as means, medians, and so on) to determine whether a serious problem is likely. Thus, in Table 18.1 data are presented from a case–control study comparing the distribution of some potential confounding variables. The differences are relatively small, but the controls are slightly older, more likely to be female, to be current smokers, and to have spent more years in full-time education. None of these differences seem large and they are intuitively unlikely to affect the results to any major extent.

This reasoning has the disadvantage of being 'ecological' in so far as the two groups may have similar overall age distributions and overall sex distributions but (for example) in one group the

Table 18.1 Comparison of potential confounding variables between study groups

	Case, $N = 80$	Controls, $N = 94$
Age: mean (standard deviation)	41.4 (6.2)	42.3 (7.1)
Female (%)	31 (38.8)	40 (42.6)
Current smokers (%)	19 (23.8)	25 (26.6)
Years full-time education: mean (standard deviation)	9.8 (2.1)	10.3 (2.0)

males might be much older than the females, and vice versa. If the effect of the main variable under study is itself altered by this interaction this could be a problem. None the less, this 'baseline' comparison is an important first step, and it might provide some reassurance.

18.4.2 **Stratification**

Inspection of raw data may suggest that there are important differences between the groups being compared in relation to the distribution of a potential confounder, to the extent that these differences might explain the observed result. In those instances where it is possible (given the available numbers) and biologically sensible to divide up the subjects into different categories (strata) of the possible confounders, a stratified analysis is an appropriate first step. Consider the data provided in Table 18.2. The same data will be used to illustrate the approach to be adopted if the study is (i) a cohort study with the end point being a risk ratio of the cumulative incidences, or (ii) a case–control study with the end point being an odds ratio.

In this example the risk of disease in the exposed population appears to be twice that in the unexposed after crude analysis. However, the same study's data revealed (Table 18.2b) that, overall, males have an approximately threefold increased risk compared with females and thus it is pertinent to enquire whether the difference between exposed and non-exposed in Table 18.2a could be explained by differences in the sex distribution between the exposure groups. The relevant data are given in Table 18.2c, which indeed show that the males are heavily weighted towards being exposed. As a consequence, analysis by sex-specific strata shows that within strata there is probably no increased risk due to exposure. The original observed relationship between exposure and disease was therefore confounded by sex.

It is possible to calculate relatively easily, with a hand calculator, an adjusted relative risk or odds ratio by using the data from stratified two-by-two tables (Table 18.3). The principle is to calculate an 'average' or weighted effect estimate across the strata examined. The calculations for an odds ratio are shown in Table 18.3a and for a risk ratio in Table 18.3b. The upper box in both tables shows the calculation for the first stratum and the second box gives the calculation for the 'ith' stratum. The summary estimate is then obtained by summation across the i strata analysed. The application of this formula to the data in Table 18.2 is given and shows how adjusting for sex virtually abolishes any effect of exposure. The results are summarized in Table 18.4.

The weighted odds ratio is referred to as the Mantel–Haenszel estimate after the authors who first described the procedure. It is also necessary to calculate confidence intervals around these estimates, and formulae are readily available. Indeed, many simple statistical packages calculate these relatively easily. Table 18.4 gives the confidence interval results from the data in Table 18.2.

There are some limitations to the use of this method. First, it may not be appropriate to consider a confounder in a categorical state when its effect may be continuous. Secondly, small numbers in some strata preclude a valid application of the method. Thirdly, for practical reasons, it is often

Table 18.2 Investigation of possible confounding by stratification

a) Crude analysis

Exposure status (number)	Disease		Cumulative incidence (%)	Risk ratio	Odds ratio
	Yes	No			
Exposed (500)	15	485	3	2.0	2.0
Non-exposed (2,500)	38	2,462	1.5		

b) Relationship to possible confounder of sex

Sex stratum(number)		Cumulative incidence (%)	Risk ratio	Odds ratio
	Yes	No			
Male (1,000)	31	969	3.1	2.8	2.9
Female (2,000)	22	1,978	1.1		

c) Analysis stratified by sex

Sex stratum	Exposure status (number)	Yes	No	Cumulative incidence (%)	Risk ratio	Odds ratio
Male	Exposed (400)	14	386	3.5	1.2	1.2
	Non-exposed (600)	17	583	2.8		
Female	Exposed (100)	1	99	1.0	0.9	0.9
	Non-exposed (1,900)	21	1,879	1.1		

impossible to stratify by more than one variable simultaneously, for example, age and sex, whereas such adjustment is normally considered desirable. Fourthly, a summary measure is not appropriate when there is evidence of heterogeneity across strata (i.e. the association between exposure and disease is substantially different between strata). Thus, such an analysis is rarely performed given the more powerful software packages available to adjust for multiple potential confounders. However, the exercise can be a useful first step if a stratification issue is suspected.

18.4.3 Standardization

An alternative, but related, approach to stratification is standardization. The principle of this has been outlined in Sections 3.2 and 16.4. It permits comparison of two or more groups, by forcing a similar distribution for a potential confounder. Age is the most typical variable used for standardization. Consider the data in Table 18.5, the crude data being the same as in Table 18.2. When stratified by age (Table 18.5b), it is clearly seen that incidence rises with increasing age. Thus, a difference in age distribution between the exposed and unexposed groups should be considered to determine whether this might explain their observed difference in incidence. As the data are revealed (Table 18.5c), the differences between the exposure groups within each age band are less striking than the overall difference. A comparison of the age distributions (Table 18.5d) shows that the exposed individuals are weighted towards being older (44% aged over 65 compared with 31% of the non-exposed). Standardization is therefore the process of applying a single or standard set of weights (in this case age-specific proportions) to both groups. In Table 18.5e, the weights that are applied are those from the non-exposed group. When these weights are applied to the age-specific incidence figures in the exposed group, this results in an age-standardized incidence in

Table 18.3a Calculation of Mantel–Haenszel summary

a) Odds ratio (OR)

i) First stratum of confounder

Exposure	Disease	
	+ve	-ve
+ve	a_1	b_1
-ve	c_1	d_1

ii) ith stratum of confounder

Exposure	Disease	
	+ve	-ve
+ve	a_i	b_i
-ve	c_i	d_i

Summary OR $= \sum_1^i \dfrac{a_i d_i}{n_i} \Big/ \sum_1^i \dfrac{b_i c_i}{n_i}$

Using data from Table 18.2, summary odds ratio

$$= \left\{ \left(\frac{14 \times 583}{1,000} \right) + \left(\frac{1 \times 1,879}{2,000} \right) \right\} \Big/ \left\{ \left(\frac{386 \times 17}{1,000} \right) + \left(\frac{21 \times 99}{2,000} \right) \right\}$$

$= (8.16 + 0.94)/(6.56 + 1.04)$

$= 9.10/7.60$

$= 1.2$

Table 18.3b Calculation of Mantel–Haenszel summary

a) Risk ratio (RR)

i) First stratum of confounder

Exposure	Disease	
	+ve	-ve
+ve	a_1	b_1
-ve	c_1	d_1

ii) ith stratum of confounder

Exposure	Disease	
	+ve	-ve
+ve	a_i	b_i
-ve	c_i	d_i

Summary RR $= \sum_1^i \dfrac{a_i(c_i + d_i)}{n_i} \Big/ \sum_1^i \dfrac{c_i(a_i + b_i)}{n_i}$

Using data from Table 18.2, summary risk ratio

$$= \left\{ \left(\frac{14 \times 600}{1,000} \right) + \left(\frac{1 \times 1,900}{2,000} \right) \right\} \Big/ \left\{ \left(\frac{17 \times 400}{1,000} \right) + \left(\frac{21 \times 100}{2,000} \right) \right\}$$

$= (8.40 + 0.95) / (6.80 + 1.05)$

$= 9.35/7.85$

$= 1.2$

Table 18.4 Calculation of confidence limits from the data in Table 18.2

Crude odds ratio for all strata	2.00
Mantel–Haenszel weighted OR	1.20
95% confidence limits	0.58, 2.44
Crude risk ratio for all strata	2.00
Mantel–Haenszel weighted OR	1.20
95% confidence limits	0.62, 2.30

the exposed group of 2.5%, slightly less than the observed incidence of 3%. This incidence is not a 'real' figure in any way, but describes the incidence that would have been obtained in the exposed population if their age distribution had been that of the non-exposed. The consequence of this is to lower the apparent risk ratio from 2 to 1.65, suggesting that exposure is still associated with an increased disease risk, but not as large as suggested by the crude data.

The standardization can be done 'the other way round' (i.e. applying the weights from the exposed to the non-exposed). When this is done using the exposed weights from Table 18.5d, an age-standardized rate of 1.8 is obtained for the unexposed group. The result of this is to lower the risk ratio from 2 to 1.65 (3/1.8): an identical result. This process can be repeated for other potential confounding variables. Standardization simultaneously across two or more variables is also possible, for example, applying weights specific to age and sex. As with stratification, the limiting factor is the numbers in each level, and standardization is not normally practicable unless the data sets are very large.

18.4.4 **Multivariate techniques**

By far the most commonly used approach to assessing the size and direction of confounders is to use one of the established statistical packages for epidemiological data analysis such as 'STATA', 'SPSS', and 'SAS' (see 'Further reading' in Chapter 17). These and other packages permit the adjustment of associations simultaneously for several potential confounders in order to obtain an accurate estimate of their independent effects. Thus, in one routine the effects of (say) age, sex, and socioeconomic status as well as the main exposure under investigation can be quantified. All software programs will generate standard error values and/or confidence intervals around the estimates obtained. In addition, it is possible to look for interactions between a confounder and a main effect; for example, is the risk from an exposure which is different in different age groups? Similarly, it also possible to examine interactions between confounders, for example, is the relationship between young males and the main effect different to that in older males or younger females?

Logistic regression is the most commonly used method for examining associations in case–control studies where the outcome is dichotomous (i.e. predicting whether a subject is a case or a control). The output is expressed in terms of coefficients, which are interpreted as giving the change in the logarithm[1] of the odds of being a case per unit change in the risk factor considered. In a case–control study of diabetes the coefficient resulting from a logistic regression for age was +0.1225. This was calculated as being equivalent to an increased disease risk of $\exp^2(0.1225) = 1.13$ for each increase in age of one year (within the age range studied; see Section 17.4.2).

Table 18.5 Investigation of possible confounding by standardization

a) Crude analysis

Exposure status (number)	Disease		Incidence (%)	RR
	Yes	No		
Exposed (500)	15	485	3	2.0
Non-exposed (2,500)	38	2,462	1.5	

b) Relationship to possible confounder of age

Age stratum(number)	Disease		Incidence (%)
	Yes	No	
25–44 (1,000)	6	994	0.6
45–64 (1,000)	14	986	1.4
65+ (1,000)	33	967	3.3

c) Analysis stratified by age

Age stratum	Exposed				Non—Exposed			
	Disease		Incidence (%)		Disease		Incidence (%)	RR
	Yes	No			Yes	No		
25–44	1	99	1.0		5	895	0.5	2.0
45–64	4	176	2.2		10	810	1.2	1.8
65+	10	210	4.5		23	757	2.9	1.6

d) Age distribution of exposed/non-exposed

Age	Exposed		Non-exposed	
	Number	Proportion	Number	Proportion
25–44	100	0.20	900	0.36
45–64	180	0.36	820	0.33
65+	220	0.44	780	0.31
Total	500	1.00	2,500	1.00

e) Apply non-exposed age weighting to incidence rates of exposure

Age	Exposed incidence I (%)	Non-exposed weight W	Weighted incidence IW (%)
25–44	1.0	0.36	0.36
45–64	2.2	0.33	0.73
65+	4.5	0.31	1.40
All	3.0		2.5 (ΣIW)

f) Summary of analysis

Ratio of crude incidence = 3/1.5 = 2

Ratio of age-adjusted incidence = 2.5/1.5 = 1.65

Logistic regression is only one multivariate method of adjustment. Among several other methods used, particularly in cohort studies, are Poisson regression and Cox's (proportional hazards) regression (see Section 17.5.8 for further information on Cox's regression). The former is used in studies where the outcome is the development of a rare incident event, and the latter is used in survival analyses when the time to the development of an event is the outcome of interest. The details and constraints of all these approaches are outside the scope of this volume, and expert statistical help will probably be required. One problem is that the availability of statistical software means that these analyses can be done with only one line of programming. The danger is that incorrect inferences will be made. Many would argue that it would have been better if these sophisticated statistical techniques were not so accessible to the novice!

One final point about confounding is that it is only possible to adjust for the variables that have been considered. In all observational (non-randomized) studies the concern is about unmeasured confounders. Often therefore in writing up the discussion part of an epidemiological study, the author will write something along the lines of 'we attempted to adjust for all the major confounders we were aware of, but the possibility remains that unmeasured confounders relating (say) to the method of recruitment, might explain some of the association we observed'!

Notes

1. In base e
2. Anti-logarithm

Chapter 19

Bias

19.1 Introduction

Bias is the largest source of anxiety for those undertaking an epidemiological study. It can be usefully defined as a systematic deviation from the truth (i.e. the study produces an incorrect conclusion), either about the existence of an association or about its strength. In studies comparing two populations, such as case–control or cohort studies, the results of bias can be in either direction, it may:

◆ falsely show the presence of an association which in truth was not present; *or*

◆ falsely show the absence of an association which in truth was present.

Clearly, bias is not an 'all or nothing' phenomenon and the aggregated impact of the different sources of bias will therefore typically falsely express the magnitude of an effect in either direction as opposed to changing the answer to the 'yes/no' question.

Bias can also exist in cross-sectional prevalence surveys, in which case bias results in a false estimate of the true occurrence of the disease.

Bias results from problems in the design or conduct/progress of the study. The importance of this is that such problems cannot be overcome by analysis, in contrast to those due to confounding (see Chapter 18). The examples next illustrate bias resulting from issues with study design (Example 19.i) and with issues in the way the study progressed, resulting in a non-response bias that had not been predicted (Example 19.ii).

Example 19.i

In a cohort study of coal miners, it was discovered that the coalface workers had twice the incidence of chronic bronchitis as the surface workers, based on sickness absence records. It was questioned whether part of the higher incidence was due to bias in so far as coalface workers with respiratory symptoms might be more likely to have work absences. This possibility could not be assessed from the available data.

Example 19.ii

A prevalence survey of diabetes required those in the target population to attend for a blood test, there was a 60% response rate. The investigators were concerned about non-response bias and indeed on telephoning a sample of non-responders they found that those who attended for a blood test were much more likely to have a family history of diabetes.

The message is that biases have to be considered at the design stage and during conduct of the study and not at the end of the study, although it is incumbent on investigators to consider the action of potential biases in explaining the study results.

19.1.1 Direction of bias

The direction of any potential bias should always be considered and, indeed, may be 'helpful'. Consider the following example:

Example 19.iii

In a case–control study, where the exposure of interest was alcohol intake, an investigator took, as the source of controls, friends of the cases. At the end of the study, which showed that the cases had an increased exposure to alcohol, criticism was levelled on the basis of the possibility that the source of controls represents a potential bias (i.e. friends may be selectively more similar to their matched case in relation to alcohol consumption). The investigator pointed out that if this were true, it would have acted in a direction to make it more difficult to find a real effect. Thus, if this bias had not been present then the real difference would have been larger.

Such a situation is not uncommon, and the point is a valid one: the design of the study made it harder for the researcher to reveal a true increase in the cases. This is not necessarily a useful strategy to adopt in designing a study. This study was at risk of missing a real effect. However, for those reading and reviewing such a study, it would be inappropriate to reject the findings of a positive result based on that source of bias. It emphasizes a point often overlooked by students. It is not enough to identify that a study may be affected by bias, but instead it is more useful to think of the likely direction and magnitude of any bias.

19.1.2 **Non-directional misclassification**

Another frequent situation relates to a study involving a comparison, where the same level of error occurs in both groups under study.

Example 19.iv

In a case–control study of osteoarthritis of the knee, one of the exposure variables under study was subject-recalled weight at age 25. The study suggested that those with arthritis had a higher average weight at this age, but the study was criticized about the likely errors in recalling weight many years previously. The investigators accepted this, but argued that despite being an inaccurate method of assessing weight, the errors would be similar in both groups. Hence the errors should act in the direction of making it more difficult to detect a real difference, and thus the fact that this study found a difference is likely to represent a real effect. In this case, the investigators were making the assumption that the level of inaccuracy was similar in both groups.

A word of caution is required. The aforementioned two comments seem to suggest that study designs that are clearly imperfect are acceptable if they come to the 'right' answer. This is not ideal for three reasons:

i) In both instances the investigator was lucky not to have missed a real association!

ii) Studies, such as those in Examples 19.ii and 19.iii, should aim not only at assessing whether there is an association, but also to estimate its magnitude. An underestimate of the true effect is not an ideal solution.

iii) Such studies are *inefficient*, in so far as to observe an effect it is necessary to study more subjects at greater cost.

Example 19.v

A study showed that older people were more likely to fall if they had problems with their vision. The size of the effect was modest and the costs of introducing a system to screen and correct for visual problems was thought not to be cost-effective in terms of the number of falls saved. However, the study design was associated with several random errors in measurement, both in assessing vision and gathering falls data. It is possible that a more robust study design would have generated a more positive result and thus provide stronger evidence for public health intervention.

Clearly it is preferable, if the choice has to be made, to slant the study design to bias against the hypothesis under test, but there are, as stated, important negative consequences.

19.2 **Major sources of bias**

It is useful to separate biases into two groups: those that result from the subjects studied and those that result from errors in information gathering. Biases that result from the sample of subjects studied mean that assumptions about randomness and representativeness cannot be assumed and the conclusions to be drawn are strictly limited. Biases in information gathering will have effects that depend on whether the data were gathered for the purposes of ascertainment of cases or of exposure. Each of the major sources of bias will be discussed, examples given, and strategies suggested for their reduction.

19.2.1 **Internal and external validity**

Bias affects the validity of a study. It is important however to differentiate *internal validity* from *external validity*. Internal validity refers to whether the results obtained (e.g. in measuring prevalence or studying associations) reflect the 'truth' in the study population. The internal validity of the study can be compromised by selection bias (Section 19.3), information bias (Section 19.4) and confounding (Chapter 18). External validity refers to the extent to which the study results can be generalized to populations other than that included in the study. To a certain extent this is a matter of judgement taking into account relevant factors. A common misconception is that in order to generalize to a wider population, the study population must be 'representative' of that wider population (see further reading).

Example 19.vi

The classic observations of a relationship between smoking and lung cancer came from studying British doctors. Could such observations be generalized outside this population group? It seemed unlikely that the carcinogenic effects of smoking would be altered either by one's occupation or nationality—therefore it seemed reasonable to extrapolate this result more generally—and subsequent studies worldwide have supported this initial observation.

19.3 **Selection bias**

The first possibility for selection bias comes from the selection of subjects for *participation*.

Example 19.vii

In a case–control study of psoriasis and smoking, an investigator selected the cases from patients attending the clinic of a specialist dermatologist. Clearly, such patients are not a random sample of the conceptual population of all patients with psoriasis and are likely to have more severe disease. Thus, any risk factors derived from those cases may represent risk factors for severity rather than psoriasis **susceptibility** *per se. In addition, the referral practice for that dermatologist may be determined by several sociodemographic and related variables, each of which might contribute to suggesting a spurious relationship with a putative risk factor.*

In this example, the problem is clearly laid out, which results from selecting cases of a disease from a specialist referral population. Electronic record systems in both primary and secondary care in theory should permit ascertainment of all possible cases within a target population. The researcher needs to be satisfied that the quality of the records, both in terms of completeness of ascertainment and quality of diagnosis, is sufficient across the target population.

Example 19.viii

In a study of multiple sclerosis, an investigator recruited cases from those who had attended a specialist service within a three-month period. As a consequence of this recruitment method, individuals who had severe disease and had died, or conversely those with mild disease and did not currently attend for treatment, were excluded. The better approach would have been for the recruitment of all cases who had been diagnosed during a specified period of time: an incident cohort. It might have been possible to do this retrospectively if a register had existed of all new cases attending in the period of interest.

19.3.1 **Non-response bias**

The most frequent source of concern to investigators in any epidemiological study is that of non-response bias. This applies equally to cross-sectional prevalence surveys, case–control studies, and even prospective cohort investigations where the non-response results from both failure to participate at the recruitment stage and losses to follow-up. The principal point at issue is whether those who are studied are selectively different from those who choose not to participate, in respect of the variable under study, such as disease or exposure status. In free-living populations there will always be a proportion of individuals who will decline to complete a questionnaire, be interviewed, or to attend for an examination. Although each study will have its own sources of this bias, most studies suggest that the likelihood of non-response is greater in younger males and those of lower socioeconomic status and education level. Persons who perceive a study as less relevant to them are also more likely not to take part. Interestingly these are often the same groups that do not vote in elections!

In case–control studies, cases are likely to be much more willing to take part than controls, and this probably reflects the greater perceived relevance to cases. In cross-sectional studies, those with a disease are more likely to respond than those who are completely well. However, some health surveys have found that study subjects with positive health behaviours (and consequently better health) were more likely to participate than those who did not. This emphasizes that without any information on non-participants, it may be difficult to be certain about the direction of any non-response bias.

Example 19.ix

A random population sample was mailed and invited to attend a special screening clinic for diabetes. The response rate was 42% and overrepresented those with a family history of diabetes and those who had symptoms of thirst and urinary frequency. Thus, this sample could not yield an accurate estimate of disease prevalence.

There is no 'magic' percentage response when bias can be confidently excluded. Conversely, a low response does not indicate that bias is present. Indeed, it may be easier to interpret a study with a low response rate but which included an analysis of the potential non-response bias in comparison to a study with a high response rate but without any information about non-participants.

Example 19.x

In a prospective cohort study, looking at the development of an otherwise rare disease in two occupationally exposed groups (high and low exposure) 88% were successfully followed up for 10 years. The investigator was concerned that even this relatively small loss to follow-up could be problematic if those who had developed the disease had died or had moved away to stay close to family (i.e. development of the disease was associated with an increased likelihood of loss).

Example 19.xi

In a molecular genetic study of a rare disease, an investigator invited both cases and controls to give a blood sample. The response rates were low at 35% in the cases and 27% in the controls. The investigator argued that given the lack of known phenotypic consequence of the genetic variants he was investigating, he could not conceive of a mechanism by which the likelihood of responding was related to the genetic factor under study.

Given the frequent potential for non-response bias, it is appropriate to consider strategies for its control. Clearly, the study should be designed and conducted to minimize the non-response rate, and strategies for this have been described previously (see Chapter 13). It is also important to attempt to ensure that non-response is not related to the variable under study, though this might create ethical difficulties.

Example 19.xii

A population-based screening survey for vertebral osteoporosis involved inviting a random sample of the population 60 years and over to attend for X-ray screening. Pilot studies suggested that the response rate in the target population might be low at around 55%. The investigator was concerned that those who attended might be biased towards those who perceived themselves at higher risk owing to presence of back pain as well as factors such as family history, and so on. He therefore described the study loosely in terms of a research study of 'spinal health', but an ethical committee insisted that it would be inappropriate not to reveal to participants the true aim of the study.

The strategy that normally must be used is a post hoc investigation to attempt to uncover the presence and strength of any non-response bias. The results of such an exercise must be considered when interpreting the data found. There are several possible approaches.

19.3.2 Approaches to assessing non-response bias

Demographic approach

Data are normally available from the sampling frame on the age and sex distribution of responders and non-responders. These should be evaluated in relation to the observed effects of age and sex on the main variable under study.

Example 19.xiii

A prevalence study aimed to identify the overall prevalence of depression in the entire adult population of a small town. There were marked differences in participation rates in the different age and gender groups. The researchers 'weighted back' the depression prevalences to the numbers in each age sex group in the population to estimate the overall prevalence. This process assumed that the depression prevalence within each age sex group was similar in participants and non-participants, which may not be true.

'Reluctant responders'

In most surveys, subjects who initially do not participate are invited a second or even a third time to take part. A comparison of the distribution of the main variable under study between first-time and subsequent responders may be instructive. Failure to find a difference would provide some support against response being related to the outcome measured. In contrast, a finding that the prevalence of the disease decreased with time to response would give rise to concern that the prevalence among non-participants was even more extreme.

Alternative data

Depending on the sampling frame, it might be possible to obtain data about the non-responders from an alternative source that might give either direct or indirect data on any difference between responders and non-responders.

Example 19.xiv

A prevalence study of cardiovascular risk factors was undertaken on an occupational group to assess that population's mean cardiovascular disease risk score. Around 60% of the subjects targeted for participation actually agreed to be screened. The investigator was provided with aggregated data from the pre-employment medical examinations of both responders and non-responders. She was able to discover that the non-responders to the current screening study had a higher mean body mass index (BMI) and were more likely to smoke at employment entry than the screening responders. This confirmed the suspicion of a significant likelihood of non-response bias in any report of the prevalence of cardiovascular disease risk in this population. Indeed, through modelling the study statistician was able to estimate the size of the bias to generate an estimated cardiovascular risk profile for this population.

Sample survey

One useful approach is to survey a small sample of the non-responders, possibly using a different approach; for example, a telephone interview, to try to seek out differences. It is impossible to obtain a truly random sample of non-responders in this way because there will always be a small percentage of individuals who refuse any participation. Depending on the nature of the investigation, again either direct or indirect data relating to the major variable under study may be obtained. Thus, in a screening survey to attend for blood-pressure measurement, non-responders may be willing to provide information on body weight and family history by telephone.

With respect to the aforementioned approaches to assessing non-response bias, depending on the precise data available, it may be possible to 'adjust' the results at the analysis stage for the possible effects of this bias.

It is not unreasonable to attempt to recalculate what would have been the outcome of the study under several realistic assumptions of bias, for example, if the non-responders were (say) half as likely to have the disease or symptoms as the responders. In that way, a single study can generate several estimates of the main result, each gathered under a different set of assumptions, with the reader left to consider the merits of each estimate.

19.3.3 **Other forms of selection bias**

There are many other possible ways by which selection bias may occur, but the aforementioned are the most important. There may, however, be special situations where surprising biases can arise. In many instances this can result in cases being more likely to be identified if they were exposed to the subject of interest.

Example 19.xv

In a case–control study, a general practitioner used her computerized diagnostic index to retrieve information on patients who had consulted with migraine in the previous 24 months. By comparing their records with those of an age-matched random sample, she demonstrated that the condition was linked to the use of the oral contraceptive pill (OCP). Her results, however, could have been explained by surveillance bias in that women on the OCP were reviewed every six months and were asked about their general health. Hence this surveillance was likely to result in an increased detection of migraine in OCP users compared with non- users.

Indeed media, both traditional and 'social media', can lead to spikes in concern about specific exposures and, as a consequence, individuals with health concerns and who had been exposed might be selectively likely to be ascertained.

Example 19.xvi

Following an influenza outbreak, mass immunization with a new vaccine was undertaken which led to reports of cases of narcolepsy. What was impossible to disentangle, given the rapid media attention, was whether the vaccine led to a true increase in narcolepsy, or whether concerns about the vaccine led to earlier presentation with symptoms of sleepiness in those who had been vaccinated.

Other selection biases can be more subtle.

Example 19.xvii

In a case–control study, it was found that oestrogen use was related to the risk of uterine fibroids. The possibility needed to be addressed of protopathic bias (i.e. that early unrecognized disease led to an increased chance of exposure). Thus, in this case, the possibility was considered that women with unusual uterine bleeding as a first sign of fibroids, but for whom the diagnosis was not made until a later date, had been started on hormones as a means of controlling the symptom. The cases that subsequently became known were therefore more likely to have been 'exposed'.

19.4 **Information bias**

The origin of information bias may lie either within the observer or the subject.

19.4.1 **Observer bias**

Comparative studies, involving interviews or clinical examination, rely on the impartiality of the observer. Structured interviews, using standardized wording of introductions to questions and clearly standardized examination techniques, may help. However, if the observer is aware of the disease (or exposure) status of the participant, it may be impossible to rule out a 'nudging' towards the hypothesis being tested. Ideally, the observer should be unaware (be blinded) as to the status of the subject although, particularly in case–control studies, this is frequently impossible to maintain. Strict training of interviewers helps and ensuring, for example, that there are not different interviewers for cases and controls but that the participants are, as far as possible, randomly allocated to the study team. A not uncommon source of bias occurs when there is a delay between interviewing cases and interviewing controls. Thus, the cases could (say) be interviewed in winter and the controls interviewed in the summer. These differences may be important if a seasonally affected exposure such as diet is being investigated. Alternatively, in a case–control study, subjects with a disease may have thought at some length about past relevant exposures, in comparison to controls who may have never previously considered these.

External observation and recording the interview can be a useful quality control measure. Even noting the duration of the interviews may be useful.

19.4.2 **Subject bias**

This most typically takes the form of recall bias. For example, in a case–control study subjects who have a disease may be more likely to recall exposures than those who are not disease-free. It is human nature to attempt to explain the occurrence of an unpleasant event like an illness by a simple exposure. Thus, in clinical practice, many patients invoke a stressful (life) event as the cause of their symptoms, even though the relationship in time is coincidental.

Example 19.xviii

Mothers of newborn infants with a neonatal problem (the cases) were asked about flu-like illnesses during pregnancy, and their answers compared with those from mothers with a normal infant. It is perhaps not surprising that the cases recalled more episodes of flu as the mothers themselves were concerned about what factors in pregnancy might have caused the problem in their newborn.

Attempts can be made to reduce this bias by:

i) making the subjects blind to the hypothesis under test (not always practical);

ii) using exposures that can be corroborated from other sources such as contemporary records or interviews with household contacts;

iii) minimizing the period of recall to maximize accuracy, although clearly the study may have to involve a longer period of recall;

iv) selecting a comparison group for whom the potential for recall bias is likely to be similar;

v) adopting more stringent methods for reducing differential recall.

Example 19.xix

In the case–control study earlier, recall bias may have been minimized by advising the mothers in both the case and the control group that they were going to be asked about flu symptoms during pregnancy. Giving prior notice allowed the mothers to speak to household contacts, work colleagues, and others to attempt a more complete ascertainment of previous flu.

There is no reason to believe that recall bias results in the false reporting of events, either exposure or disease, that had not occurred. The problem typically lies in more accurate recall by (say) cases rather than controls. Recall may be heightened and may be more inaccurate temporally, with an artificial collapsing of the time interval.

Example 19.xx

A case–control study of inflammatory bowel disease suggested a greater exposure to stressful life events in the six months preceding disease onset in the cases. However, a sample survey of household contacts, in both cases and controls, suggested that although there was no bias in recall of whether or not an event had occurred, the cases (but not the controls) were more likely to have errors in the dating of the event towards a closer time interval to disease onset.

Example 19.xxi

In a case–control study of adults with chronic widespread body pain, subjects were asked about events in childhood including hospitalization and operation. Analysis revealed strong associations between case status and reporting these events. However, because of concern about subject bias (in particular, differential recall between cases and controls), information on these events was also collected from the medical records of cases and controls. Using the latter data, there was however no association between the record-derived exposure and case status. To explain this a further analysis revealed that cases had a much better recall of the documented hospitalizations and operations, while controls 'forgot' about half of all such events (see further reading).

19.5 **Is an unbiased study ever possible?**

The previous comments are likely to have led to the pessimistic conclusion that it is either impossible or impracticable to perform an unbiased study. Indeed, in epidemiological classes, a favourite exercise is to take a published paper, preferably from a renowned source, and suggest many reasons why the conclusions may be invalid owing to issues in the design and conduct of the study leading to biased estimates of disease burden or associations! The message from this chapter aims to be more practical. It is possible, in both the design and the conduct of a study within the available resources, to attempt to minimize the potential for bias. However, the skill of the epidemiologist lies not in conducting the perfect study, but in documenting and assessing the likely impact of its imperfections. However, perhaps the major task at the end of the study is for the investigator to be self-critical and consider carefully what potential for bias remained and how far the data collected permit an estimate of the likely effect of any bias. Ultimately, if possible, the aim is to provide a useful commentary on how far the results observed should be interpreted given the potential sources of bias.

Further reading

Recall bias

McBeth J, Morris S, Benjamin S, Silman AJ, Macfarlane GJ (2001). Associations between adverse events in childhood and chronic widespread pain in adulthood: are they explained by differential recall? *J Rheumatol*, **28**(10), 2305–309.

Study populations

Macfarlane GJ, Beasley M, Smith BH, Jones GT, Macfarlane TV (2015). Can large surveys conducted on highly selected populations provide valid information on the epidemiology of common health conditions? An analysis of UK Biobank data on musculoskeletal pain. *Br J Pain*, **9**(4), 203–12.

Rothman KJ, Gallacher JE, Hatch EE (2013). Why representativeness should be avoided. *Int J Epidemiol*, **42**(4), 1012–14.

Chapter 20

Association or causation

20.1 **Introduction**

Much epidemiological research aims to determine and quantify the relation between a predictor, or group of predictors and an outcome. In previous chapters the methodologies and approaches that can be employed have been discussed, with the end point of studies being an estimate of the relationship between predictors and outcomes. What emerge are measures of association.

An association may be false or its strength inaccurate because of biases in the method (Chapter 19) or the failure to allow for confounding (Chapter 18). Ultimately, observational epidemiological studies aim to result in an estimate of an association that reflects a real underlying relationship. The consequence being that this would lead to an understanding of causation with the option of strategies for developing interventions or the understanding of the role of current interventions. The appropriateness of all these steps is dependent on the validity of the association.

Example 20.i

Several epidemiological studies have shown an association between salt intake and high blood pressure. Such studies have led to many mechanistic studies on why salt should lead to a consistently raised blood pressure and to assess the value of reducing salt intake either to prevent hypertension, or as a means of management in patients who are diagnosed.

In broad terms the original observed association(s) were not only real, but also *causative*, that is, high salt intake is a cause of elevated blood pressure (at least in susceptible individuals). Substitute in red meat for salt and bowel cancer for high blood pressure in Example 20.i, then it is still the case that epidemiological studies show an association. What is much less clear is whether this is causative: robust mechanisms are lacking, and it is not clear about the benefits of cutting red meat out of the diet either to prevent or impact on the severity of bowel cancer.

In theory, for both the aforementioned examples a randomized controlled trial where there is an experimental intervention can, and in the case of salt restriction, has been done. For most associations such randomized controlled trials (RCTs) are impossible and there must be a reliance on data from observational studies; together with evidence from other types of research. As will be discussed next there has not been, and could not be, a randomized controlled trial of a normal population, randomizing half to start and continue smoking and the other half never to smoke, to prove that smoking causes several common serious disorders.

This chapter thus focuses on what can be inferred from associations about causation.

20.2 **If not causative what are the possibilities?**

If an association is not causative, there are several options.

i) There were unmeasured (or poorly measured) confounders

Example 20.ii

A case–control study of inflammatory disorders was focused on determining whether risk was reduced by high consumption of vitamin C. The study demonstrated a clear association. Comparing the highest quintile of consumption with the lowest, the OR was 0.7 with a 95% confidence interval (0.6, 0.8). Such a study is subject to many unmeasured confounders particularly as diets high in vitamin C from fruit and vegetables, will be high in other vitamins and trace substances. Such diets may also be low, because of food choices, in nutrients that are harmful. It could not be concluded from this study therefore that high levels of vitamin C were causally related to a lower risk of inflammatory conditions. See 'Further reading'.

ii) The association was real, but the link was not causative

Example 20.iii

A prospective cohort study showed that young men with high levels of alcohol intake were at risk of self-harm. Whereas the alcohol may have contributed to that, it was more likely that there was an underlying problem that led to the alcohol consumption and the latter was not causally related to the self-harm. Thus, high alcohol consumption was on the path between an unknown aetiological factor and self-harm.

iii) The association was on *the path* between the real causative agent and outcome of interest

Example 20.iv

A prospective cohort study showed that children who scored highly on a depressive mood scale had high rates of substance abuse later in adolescent life. It may be that the depressed mood led to the substance abuse, or there was a common factor leading to both, for example, prior physical, sexual, or emotional abuse. Thus, substance abuse was on the path of a causative relationship between prior physical, sexual, or emotional abuse and mood disorder.

iv) The association was real, but the direction was the reverse

Example 20.v

So-called reverse causality is not uncommon in epidemiological studies. A case–control study of patients with chronic pain showed that cases were much more likely than controls to report poor quality sleep (OR 3.8, 95% CI 1.9, 7.6). What is unclear is whether poor quality sleep leads to an increased risk of pain, or whether having pain results in poorer quality sleep. (In this example though it might be possible to disentangle these effects by mounting an intervention study depriving subjects of sleep!) See 'Further reading'.

Furthermore, all the earlier examples exclude the possibility that an association was demonstrated but was actually due to random error (type I error).

The main conclusion is that epidemiological studies can show strong associations but are almost impossible on their own to demonstrate the causal chain. Indeed, even it was possible to identify all true confounders and adjust for them, although the direction and strength of the association seems to be clear, 'causation' cannot be assumed.

20.3 **When is an association likely to indicate causation?**

Over 50 years ago, Sir Austin Bradford Hill listed nine tests that can be applied to give a sense of whether an association might indicate real causation. They are still widely applied today and are listed in Table 20.1. There are no rules about how far each test must be applied and whether all need to be satisfied. There is also discussion as to how useful they are given the limitations in different situations (see 'Further reading'). The interpretation and limitations are illustrated with examples.

Table 20.1 Bradford Hill test for causation

Bradford Hill test for causation
Temporal relationship
Strength of association
Dose response
Consistency between studies
Biological plausibility
Other explanations
Possibility to alter by intervention
Specificity
Coherence of evidence

20.3.1 Temporal relationship

The underlying concept is that a risk factor cannot be considered causative unless it can be shown that it antedated the onset of the disorder. This is the only 'criterion' on the list which must be satisfied.

Example 20.vi

In studies suggesting the development of physical or behavioural disorders following immunization in infancy, the question is always raised as to whether the disorder was present prior to the immunization but just not recognized. In one recent well-publicized case there was a suggestion that a vaccine against H1N1 was associated with the development of narcolepsy. The latter is a difficult disorder to prove and awareness of symptoms, rather than their new onset, was precipitated by the vaccine.

20.3.2 Strength of association

It seems logical that the stronger the measure of association, the greater the likelihood that it is causative. A relative risk of 10 would be superficially more likely to be 'real' than one of 1.5. Certainly, weaker relationships are more likely (all other things being equal) to be explained by confounding (i.e. there would only need to be one or a small number of confounders with a weak relationship to the exposure). However, a weak relationship does not necessarily exclude a causative role. Conversely, a strong relationship could emerge from a tight relationship between a confounder and the main effector, but only the former was measured. Genetic epidemiology studies are particularly susceptible to such possible misinterpretation.

Example 20.vii

One of the first 'modern' genetic association studies showed a very strong association between HLAB27 and ankylosing spondylitis over 40 years ago. This observation has been consistently replicated and the odds ratio can be as high as 200 but it is still unknown if this is a causative relationship. By contrast, several genome wide association studies of very large numbers of cases and controls have demonstrated odds ratios for some common gene variants that are statistically significant but typically below 1.5. These variants may very well have a biological role in disease, but the odds ratios are low because of population stratification and disorder heterogeneity.

20.3.3 **Dose response relationship**

In general, the greater the 'dose' of exposure the greater would be the expected effect on risk. Conversely if there was no dose response effect, this might argue against a causative role. The problem comes when there might be a threshold, a plateau, or other effects that preclude demonstrating a true dose response. Very few exposures would show a true linear or greater than linear effect. Dose can also be derived in different ways.

> **Example 20.viii**
>
> *A dose response relationship between alcohol intake exists for many disorders but the nature of that dose response varies. In some it is years of regular drinking that is the strongest, in others it is the maximum number of units of alcohol, whereas for others it is the frequency of 'binge drinking'. Given the added complexities of variation over time in amount and frequency of alcohol consumption, within individuals, together with changing types of alcohol imbibed, it is not surprising that showing consistent trends of increasing risk for some disorders can be challenging.*

20.3.4 **Consistency between studies**

Much of the epidemiological literature is based on attempted replication of studies to show consistency between populations studied. Again, it seems logical that the less consistent the finding of an association, the less likely it is to be causative. The converse does not necessarily apply; replicate studies may consistently be subject to all the other issues discussed. Replication is particularly valuable if studies are conducted in different geographical locations and using different designs.

20.3.5 **Biological plausibility**

The discussion section of many epidemiological papers, especially those demonstrating a previously unrecognized association, attempt to enhance the relevance of their findings by attempting to find a biological basis or pathway for the link. Absence of such a link is not proof of no causation. Indeed, the demonstration of a strong association may be the spur to look for biological causes. The association between smoking and lung cancer did not emerge against a strong background of basic science, suggesting that inhaled tobacco smoke caused cancerous changes in the laboratory. Rather, the epidemiological observations led to such investigations. There is also the challenge that there are frequently several biological pathways, which might be conflicting in their effects when investigated in laboratory animals or human volunteers, and it is tempting to identify the studies that support the epidemiological claim but ignore the others that do not.

20.3.6 **Other explanations**

This is an interesting exercise but demands of the researcher that in interpreting the results, all other explanations are considered, both biases in the data and confounding but also the issues listed earlier in Section 20.2. It is not necessarily the case that such explanations are better, but listing those explicitly will help the reader reach a judgement about the likelihood of causation.

20.3.7 **Possibility to alter by intervention**

From a public health or clinical medicine perspective, an association would be shown to be causative if one could eliminate or modify in an experimental manner and show a change in disease occurrence. Of course, one could conduct such an intervention, targeting air pollution through reductions in car emissions in a city, for example, and demonstrate a reduction in respiratory disease. This would still not be conclusive evidence of causality since other factors such as reduction in cigarette smoking may explain the change. A cluster randomized controlled trial would provide stronger evidence on whether reduction in air pollution was causally related to the health outcome.

Example 20.ix

The possibility that fluoride may be protective against dental decay came from several observational (case-control and cohort) studies showing associations between fluoride intake and (absence of) dental decay. There have been, and still are, ongoing studies of the use of fluoride in toothpaste or added to the drinking water. These trials are not easy to conduct, and a recent Cochrane review concluded: 'We did not identify any evidence, meeting the review's inclusion criteria, to determine the effectiveness of water fluoridation for preventing caries in adults.' It is interesting to speculate whether, given all the circumstances, it would be possible in practice to undertake and complete a robust trial.

20.3.8 **Specificity**

The Bradford Hill 'criteria' seem to be based on single exposures and single disorder relationships. He argued that an effect which was specific for a particular risk factor/disorder relationship was more likely to be causative. This does not though reflect most circumstances of the relationship between a risk factor and a disease. Most of the relevant studies, both aetiological and clinical, examine associations between multiple exposures, and their interactions in relation to a chosen outcome. What emerges is less a list of 'causes', but more a sense of the types of populations at risk.

20.3.9 **Necessity vs. sufficiency**

a) It is very rare to have situations in which disease *always* follows exposure and exposure always leads to the disorder or disease. On extreme example might be very infectious diseases such as Ebola where single contact will always cause the disease—but one doesn't need an epidemiological study to show that Ebola virus caused the outbreak, or that exposure to the virus was both *necessary* (no cases without infections) *and sufficient* (almost all the exposed individuals became ill).

b) More frequent is the situation which requires exposure, but most individuals exposed do not develop the disease. Many other infectious diseases fall into this category. Another example is mesothelioma following asbestos exposure. In that example the exposure to asbestos is *necessary* (mesothelioma will not occur in its absence) *but not sufficient* (as most exposed individuals would not develop mesothelioma).

c) Of greater frequency is the situation where the exposure *always* leads to the disorder but most individuals with outcome do not have that exposure but develop it from other causes. As an example, exposure to significant ionizing radiation can be *sufficient* to lead to the development of some cancers *but not necessary*, as the same cancers can develop via other pathways.

d) By far the most frequent situation is when exposure only rarely leads to the disorder and also that individuals with the disorder are only rarely exposed. This does not preclude the exposure being causative but does make it challenging to identify in epidemiological investigations.

20.3.10 **Coherence**

In some ways a 'catch all' in so far as the different data from all sources adds up, as it might do in a legal case. Evidence may be circumstantial but supportive. Many examples might serve to illustrate but if a case was being made that use of airbags prevents deaths from road traffic accidents, supporting evidence might include:

- Ecological evidence, countries/populations with the lowest level of airbags fitted have the highest number of road deaths;
- Populations where there have been new laws making airbags mandatory in new cars show a change towards a reduction in deaths after the law have been introduced;
- Post-mortem and police reports of series of road traffic deaths show fewer cases in cars with airbags;
- Test laboratory experiments demonstrate substantially reduced injuries in experiments in which airbags are deployed.

None of these individual lines of evidence is robust enough to demonstrate cause and effect, but they all provide supportive evidence.

Example 20.x

Most nulliparous women will not develop breast cancer before the age of 50. Further most cases of breast cancer that are diagnosed in women under the age of 50, are in women who have had at least one pregnancy. Yet epidemiological studies show that nulliparity is a risk factor. In this instance there is no specificity between risk factor and disease.

20.4 **Causes or risk factors**

As discussed earlier in relation to specificity, most disorders do not have a single cause. Apart from single gene disorders and conditions that result from a single profound insult such as infection, toxic exposure, or injury, the overwhelming majority of disorders require the interplay of several different factors. A deep discussion about the difference between 'a cause' and 'a risk factor' is beyond the scope of this volume. Indeed, the question of what is a 'cause' becomes a philosophical one. Thus, even accepting Hill's criteria, it is difficult to operationalize when it is legitimate to refer to an association being causal. At a clinical or public health level, identification of a cause logically infers that the risk can be mitigated or potentially mitigated by an intervention. This is not true about other 'irreversible' risk factors that can be equal in their predictive strength. Thus age, gender, and ethnicity are risk factors, at least in part, for most chronic disorders. Their relationship may not be explained by any confounder, and they may satisfy most of the Hill criteria.

20.4.1 **Aetiological heterogeneity**

A continuing challenge for those conducting or interpreting the results of an epidemiological study is the possibility that the sample of cases ascertained, which might be very similar in their clinical expression, are very different in their background risk profile. What might be a major cause in some subjects, might be minor or absent in others. This variation in the risk profile can be termed 'aetiological heterogeneity'. Thus, individuals with apparently the same clinical disorder have different combinations of risk factors, be they genetic, environmental, or a combination. More detailed assessment of the cases might help separate out disease subgroups, which can be analysed separately.

Example 20.xi

Several risk factors for coronary artery disease are well known: raised cholesterol components, cigarette smoking, raised blood pressure, and so on. They may all be considered causes but are not the only cause as

normotensive, non-smokers with a low cholesterol can still develop coronary artery disease. Focusing at-
tention on that low-risk group may be useful in unravelling what are the principal causes in that latter,
low-risk group.

20.4.2 **Alternative to clinical trials**

The randomized clinical trial is considered a gold standard by which one can prove causal links, although such trials, be they for primary or secondary prevention, are difficult to conduct espe-cially if involving lifestyle changes. Compliance may be low and it may be difficult to allow for other changes in lifestyle at the same time. Furthermore, in such trials, publicity and changing attitudes might result in the non-intervention arm changing their lifestyle. Even the simplest trials are very expensive to conduct and they generally only answer a single question.

Example 20.xii

Although excess sodium (salt) intake is implicated as a risk factor for hypertension in several types of epi-demiological study and is biologically coherent, proving this as a cause can only come from a randomized trial. Whereas there are several trials of the benefits of salt restriction in patients with established (mild) hypertension, there are very few trials with a community-wide attempt to prevent the 'disease'. Furthermore, although it might seem obvious that excess salt intake is a cause of hypertension, it can be argued that this is only relevant in subjects with a genetic predisposition.

Mendelian randomization

The previous example highlights the potential that genetic investigation can 'in reverse' identify the possible role for lifestyle risk factors that are difficult to study in trials and where confounding limits the interpretation of observational epidemiological studies. *Mendelian randomization* (de-scribed in Chapter 6) is based on the use of genetic variants to study environmental factors (par-ticularly where the environmental factor–disease link is likely subject to important confounding).

Example 20.xiii

An early example of the use of Mendelian randomization was in the role of calcium in osteoporosis and the in-fluence of lactose intolerance genes, which would result in individuals having low milk and consequently cal-cium intake into their diets. Thus, studies that showed that individuals with such a genetic background were at high risk of disorders such as osteoporosis added to the evidence that low calcium intake is a risk factor. Clearly, most subjects with osteoporosis are not lactose intolerant but unless there was another biologically coherent pathway by which such a genetic background would lead to osteoporosis, a low calcium intake (or other nutrient that predominantly comes from dairy products) would provide the most logical explanation.

Propensity modelling

Another increasingly used technique in observational epidemiology to investigate causation in the absence of a randomized trial is *propensity modelling* (see 'Further reading'). The value of a ran-domized trial is that there is no bias in allocation of interventions between the groups studied, whereas in an observational study there may be other differences which cannot be allowed for. In epidemiological research it is most often used in observational clinical studies to examine outcomes to interventions that have not been randomly allocated. In general terms, the variables that could potentially influence the treatment decision are modelled to produce a propensity score equivalent to a probability of being treated based on those variables in the entire cohort. The subjects in the cohort who were given the treatment under investigation are then matched for the propensity score to those who weren't, and their outcomes compared. This is best explained by a simplified example.

Example 20.xiv

A study aimed to determine if the use of a new biologically active drug in patients with rheumatoid arthritis was associated with an increased risk of specific long-term hazards such as malignancy. It was not possible, obviously, to examine this question in a randomized controlled trial. The researchers had two large prospective cohorts: one which had been treated with the new drug and the other with other more conventional therapies. The treatment decision had not been random and there may well have been underlying differences, for example, in the severity of the arthritis that both influenced the decision to use the new drug and also affect the likelihood of cancer. They postulated several such variables such as age, gender, disease severity, smoking, and derived a predictive equation based on such variables in their cohort that would yield a probability, or propensity score, of any individual being treated with the new drug. In the model that was developed, for example, a male, aged 48, non-smoker with a high level of disease activity, would have a propensity score of 0.75 of having the new drug. Within their large cohorts there were subjects with a propensity score of around that level, in both the group treated and not treated with the biologically active drug.

The researchers then matched each of their subjects who were treated with an untreated subject, but who had similar propensity scores. Thus, the resulting two groups based on the potential confounders had equal likelihoods of being treated with the new drug, but in reality only half had been. The researchers argued that the reasons for the difference in the treatment they had were related to factors such as patient or physician preference, which would not of themselves be of relevance to the outcome. This analysis was a useful surrogate for a randomized clinical trial. Thus, any differences in outcome between the two treatment groups was unlikely to be explained by bias in allocation.

This method is increasingly used in pharmaco-epidemiology studies and is superior to adjusting for confounders in the standard way. Its use is widespread in situations where only observational studies can be carried out. The method is not without problems and is challenging when the timing of giving specific treatments is also relevant to take on board. In such instances, other methods such as the use of *marginal structural models* may be preferred.

Further reading

Mendelian randomization

Davey Smith G, Ebrahim S (2005). What can mendelian randomisation tell us about modifiable behavioural and environmental exposures? *BMJ*, **330**(7499), 1076–9.

Propensity modelling

Austin PC (2011). An introduction to propensity score methods for reducing the effects of confounding in observational studies. *Multivariate Behav Res*, **46**(3), 399–424.

Tests for causation

Fedak KM, Bernal A, Capshaw ZA, Gross S (2015). Applying the Bradford Hill criteria in the 21st century: how data integration has changed causal inference in molecular epidemiology. *Emerg Themes Epidemiol*, **12**, 14.

Hill AB (1965). The environment and disease: association or causation? *Proc R Soc Med*, **58**, 295–300.

When association is not causative

Ness AR (2001). Commentary: beyond beta-carotene-antioxidants and cardiovascular disease. *Int J Epidemiol*, **30**(1), 143–44.

Sabia S, Dugravot A, Dartigues JF, *et al.* (2017). Physical activity, cognitive decline, and risk of dementia: 28 year follow-up of Whitehall II cohort study. *BMJ*, **357**, j2709.

Part G

Coherence of evidence across studies

Chapter 21

Reviews of evidence

21.1 Introduction

This chapter reviews the ways of summarizing and evaluating evidence from epidemiological studies. Summary of evidence is needed in every day clinical practice and for public health. We live in a time of information overload, and it is impossible to read all the available scientific journals, even on a narrow scientific topic. Simply using search terms such as 'cancer' will result in millions of results in Google Scholar or PubMed (a service of the US National Library of Medicine®) database. Given the ever-increasing volume of medical literature and time constraints, summary of evidence plays a big role in decision-making.

The World Health Organization established the Evidence-Informed Policy Network (EVIPNet) to promote the systematic use of research evidence in health policymaking in 'order to strengthen health systems and get the right programs, services and drugs to those who need them'. Summary of evidence plays an important role in establishing clinical and cost-effectiveness of interventions, and is crucial, for example, to the UK's National Institute for Health and Care Excellence (NICE) health technology assessment process. Technology appraisals involve recommendations on the use of new and existing treatments within the National Health Service (NHS) in the United Kingdom. Evidence synthesis is important when several studies are conducted trying to answer the same research questions, but the results are conflicting. It can help to guide recommendations for managing clinical conditions; identifying future research priorities; can be used in justifying applications for research funding; and is increasingly becoming part of student dissertations.

Example 21.i

While browsing the internet, a researcher stumbles on a web site that claims that coffee causes back pain. Searching using the phrase 'does coffee cause back pain' using a general search engine results in more popular articles. How can the scientific evidence for such a claim be assessed? It is tempting to use a general search engine to look for this information, however such searches will, most likely, result in anecdotal evidence, personal stories, and discussion fora.

21.2 What is evidence?

The *Oxford English Dictionary* defines evidence as 'the available body of facts or information indicating whether a belief or proposition is true or valid'. Current best evidence is up-to-date information from relevant, valid research studies. Evidence can be related to the effects of different medications and other forms of healthcare, the potential for harm from exposure to particular agents, the accuracy of diagnostic tests, or the predictive power of prognostic factors. Professor David Sackett defined evidence-based medicine as 'the conscientious, explicit, judicious use of current best evidence in making decisions about the care of individual patients' (Sackett *et al.*, 1996).

But where does evidence come from? Evidence is often summarized in a literature review, which is a state-of-the-art synthesis of current evidence on a given research question. Reviews have been a part of the healthcare literature for a long time: they may be called literature reviews, narrative reviews, critical reviews, or commentaries on a given topic. They were usually written by experts in the field: for example, earlier reviews have habitually only one author. Such reviews are often qualitative in nature, and mostly verbally describe results of previous studies. Usually, they involve informal and subjective methods of collecting information. Often, there is no explanation why some studies are chosen over the others, or how the studies were found.

Example 21.ii

Searching PubMed with a word 'review' it is possible to find references to reviews published as early as 1840s. One interesting example was published in 1853 by the Association Medical Journal (now called the British Medical Journal (BMJ)) under the category 'periscopic review'. This section contains short evaluations of evidence on various topics. The article describes evidence 'founded on upon the works referred to, and upon information gleaned from other sources', related to therapeutic uses of the common ash tree (Fraxinus excelsior). This brief review summarized patient cases and treatment experiences of physicians from different countries. It concluded that 'additional information is obviously required regarding the medicinal properties of the bark and leaves of the common ash'. The author(s) then ask if any of the journal readers could contribute 'towards supplying the deficiency'.

A future research agenda is also proposed: 'We believe that an investigation of the medicinal properties of ash leaves would, if properly conducted, yield some useful results.'

21.2.1 **Levels of evidence**

Chapter 6 considered various study designs used in epidemiology. The Oxford Centre for Evidence-Based Medicine (CEBM) summarizes a hierarchy of levels of evidence depending on the research question and study design (see 'Further reading'). Generally, systematic reviews, randomized trials, and inception cohort studies represent the highest level of evidence dependent on the study design. However, it is strongly advised that the summary table should be read together with the accompanying Introductory Document and Background Document, both available from CEBM website (see 'Further reading').

21.3 **What is a systematic review?**

A systematic review is a review in which there is a comprehensive search for relevant studies on a specific topic, and those identified then appraised and condensed according to a predetermined and explicit method. Systematic reviews are increasingly replacing traditional narrative reviews and expert commentaries as a way of summarizing research evidence. They are a result of an attempt to bring the same level of accuracy to reviewing research evidence as should be used in generating the evidence. They should be based on peer-reviewed protocols so that they can be replicated if necessary.

The number of published systematic reviews and meta-analyses have increased dramatically in the past 30 years.

Example 21.iii

A search in the PubMed database for meta-analyses or systematic reviews (using exact words) among publications on pain resulted in only two publications in 1985 and 1,541 in 2015, representing an increase from 0.04% to 4%.

21.3.1 **Advantages of systematic reviews**

Systematic reviews have advantages over traditional reviews because they are more objective and less prone to bias. The literature search involved in the production of such a review is comprehensive and repeatable, with a clear description of the methods used. They contain explicit criteria for choosing studies and also include assessment and discussion of the quality of the primary studies. Provided the studies contain quantitative data then a meta-analysis can be conducted, which will be discussed in Chapter 22. Readers should be able to replicate or verify any systematic review.

21.4 **How to conduct a systematic review**

Box 21.1 lists the steps involved in the process of conducting a systematic review. Because systematic reviews involve substantial time and resources, numerous tools were devised to automate steps in the process of conducting a systematic review (see 'Further reading').

21.4.1 **Defining the research question**

The acronym PICO, where P stands for **P**articipants (or patients/population), I is for **I**ntervention (or Exposure or Prognostic Factor), C is for **C**omparisons (or controls) and O is for **O**utcomes helps to remember the structure of the review question.

Example 21.v

When evaluating evidence on the link between coffee consumption and back pain, there are several PICO options depending on research question, for example, 'Do adult patients with back pain, compared to persons without back pain, have higher coffee consumption?' or 'In adults, does high coffee consumption, compared to low consumption, increase the incidence rate of back pain?' or 'In patients with a history of back pain, does low coffee consumption, compared to high consumption, reduce the recurrence rate?'.

Box 21.1 **Steps involved in the process of conducting a systematic review.**

Steps in conducting systematic review

1. Defining a research question
2. Identifying reasons for a systematic review and checking if it has been done already
3. Planning and resourcing
4. Review registration
5. Searching for evidence
6. Selecting studies for inclusion
7. Data extraction and management
8. Critical appraisal of studies (quality assessment)
9. Data synthesis
10. Publication
11. Archiving and updating

21.4.2 **Why is the review required?**

Several reasons were described at the beginning of the chapter as to why evidence needs to be evaluated. It is also important to establish that it has not been done already or there may be similar ongoing systematic reviews, in which case starting a new review would be a waste of resources. However, it may be that an existing systematic review is out of date and several new relevant studies have been conducted, in which case an update is justified.

21.4.3 **Planning and resourcing**

It is important to appreciate that a properly conducted systematic review is a major undertaking which needs time and resources. It requires a multidisciplinary team of researchers (the responsibility of each collaborator involved in the review should be decided in advance), substantial staff and computer resources, access to library and to appropriate online databases. Many papers may require payment in order to access them and this has to be factored into costings.

Some research funding bodies have specific calls for evaluation of evidence, and so it may be possible to apply for a research grant.

> **Example 21.vii**
>
> *If a systematic review on the relationship between coffee and back pain was being undertaken then a suitable multidisciplinary team might involve: an epidemiologist, clinical pain specialist, biochemist, nutritionist, and statistician.*

21.4.4 **Review registration**

Once the research question has been decided and the review team is assembled, it is advisable that the review is registered to avoid replicating what is already underway. There are examples of systematic reviews published at the same time and answering similar research questions, which obviously represents a wasteful duplication of effort and resources.

It is possible to register a systematic review with various relevant organizations. When registering such a review, a protocol is usually required. There are guidelines for writing them, and they can be published (see 'Further reading').

21.4.5 **Searching for evidence**

Some ways of finding evidence include reading textbooks, attending conferences, or asking colleagues (or journal readers such as in Example 21.ii). Other sources include specialist web sites, clinical guidelines, research interest groups, and reviews.

However, to search systematically and reproducibly there are online databases such as MEDLINE, CENTRAL, PubMed, Embase, CINAHL, and Google scholar. This activity has its own methodology, and it is a good idea to obtain some training on literature search by attending a dedicated training course, learning using online tutorials and training materials, or asking for help from a librarian or review methodologist with experience in conducting literature search.

A good starting point is a recent systematic review on similar topic which can give some idea of type of databases and other sites that can be searched but also useful keywords and search strategies. The principle is similar: use 'OR' where either word is acceptable in search results, for example, cancer OR neoplasms. Searching for cancer AND smoking will retrieve results containing articles which have information on both. Search can usually be limited to articles published in English language or studies in humans only. Databases can be on different platforms and therefore the search commands can be different. Some databases have some saved expert searches which can be used by others (see 'Further reading').

Example 21.viii

Box 21.2 *shows an example of a MEDLINE search for publications related to Example 21.i. The search uses medical subject headings (MeSH) as well as free text words.*

To validate their search strategy, review authors often perform hand searching in a small sample of journals known to be important in the area of research and where relevant articles are likely to be published. It can be done by either looking through a sample of journals for preset dates or looking online at the list of contents. Another step is to search references of selected articles to minimize the risk of relevant older studies being missed.

Citations found can then be exported from databases into specific reference management software. Duplicates will then need to be identified and removed—otherwise there can be considerable time wasted from screening and reviewing the same article many times. Software is available to help undertake this task (see 'Further reading').

Box 21.2 An example of a MEDLINE Ovid search for publications on relationship between coffee and back pain

Back pain	1. dorsalgia.ti,ab.
	2. exp Back Pain/
	3. (backache or back-ache).ti,ab.
	4. exp Back Pain/
	5. ((back or lumb$) adj3 pain).ti,ab.
	6. coccyx.ti,ab.
	7. coccydynia.ti,ab.
	8. sciatica.ti,ab.
	9. exp sciatic neuropathy/
	10. spondylosis.ti,ab.
	11. lumbago.ti,ab.
	12. back disorder$.ti,ab.
	13. or/1-12
Coffee	14. Coffee/
	15. Caffeine/
	16. (coffee or caffeine or caffeinated or decaffeinated).tw.
	17. or/14-16
Combining back pain and coffee	18. 13 and 17
Limiting to humans	19. (animals not (humans and animals)).sh.
	20. 18 not 19

21.4.6 **Selecting studies for inclusion**

The next step is to scan the titles and abstracts of all studies identified by the electronic searches for relevant publications. This is usually done by two reviewers, independently, and disagreements resolved by discussion. Following that, full texts of articles are obtained for further assessment.

Many research papers are published in 'open access' which means they are available free of charge on the public internet, allowing anyone to download, print copy, or distribute the paper to others for research purpose. It is important to check the licence agreement when downloading a paper. However, in some cases the full text is only available for an additional fee. Academic institutions are often able to obtain full text papers under certain conditions. It is also possible to write to the authors explaining the purpose of the project and asking for a copy. Full text pre-publication copies are also often available on the authors' institutional websites in specially designed databases and sites such as social networking site for researchers (e.g. ResearchGate).

Reasons for exclusion should be reported, and therefore it is useful to create eligibility assessment form which can be used either in paper or electronic form. The results should be illustrated on a PRISMA Flow Diagram. Such a diagram is a graphical representation of the flow of citations reviewed during a systematic review and shows the number of selected publications at each stage of identification, screening, eligibility, and final inclusion. It is possible to download a PRISMA Flow Diagram template from the PRISMA website (see 'Further reading').

Example 21.ix: Flow diagram

The authors of a systematic review found 685 papers while searching in MEDLINE, Embase, and CINAHL databases and 3 papers from other sources. After removing duplicates, abstracts of 121 titles were screened. Of those, 32 potential studies remained to be evaluated for inclusion using full texts. At this point papers had to be discarded for not meeting the eligibility criteria: 11 were removed because they did not investigate the relevant outcome and 8 studies did not investigate the exposure under study. Furthermore 5 studies were excluded for not reporting a relationship between exposure and outcome. A further study had to be discarded because the diagnosis among study subjects was not made by a clinician, as required by the protocol. Of the 7 remaining papers, 6 studies reported sufficient data for meta-analysis.

Figure 21.1 shows hypothetical data was generated using PRISMA Flow Diagram Generator. Reasons for exclusion can also be stated in the chart (see 'Further reading').

21.4.7 **Data extraction and management**

Once the eligible studies are identified, data extraction needs to be performed by two members of the research team, independently (to minimize extraction errors), using a specially designed data extraction form. As in Section 21.4.6, any disagreements can be resolved by discussion and by checking the original paper.

Such a form can include the researcher performing data extraction, date of data extraction, type of publication (e.g. journal article, conference abstract), publication year, the country in which the study was conducted, characteristics of the study participants (e.g. age, gender, ethnicity), details of how exposure and outcomes were measured, sample size/power calculation, number of participants, participation rate, and source of funding. This form can be on paper or electronic. It is useful to pilot the form in advance to make sure all the necessary information is extracted. Box 21.3 shows an example of the data extraction form.

Sometimes the required data are not reported in published manuscripts. For example, particularly in older papers, the authors may not provide the number of participants in each group or report p values only. A study may report several exposures combined (e.g. several medications under one broad category such as non-steroidal anti-inflammatory drugs) while the review

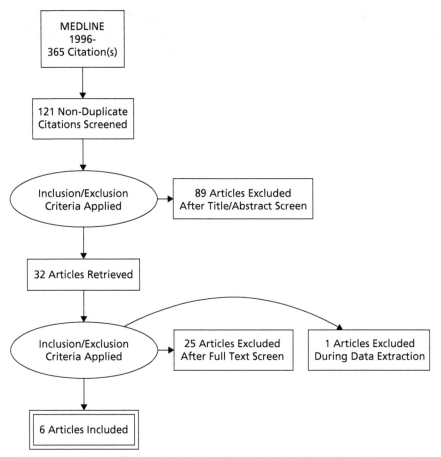

Figure 21.1 PRISMA diagram for hypothetical data (obtained using PRISMA Flow Diagram Generator).

focuses on one specific exposure (or a particular medication, such as aspirin). In such situations it can be a good idea to contact manuscript authors. Full text papers have an address for correspondence which usually includes an email address. However, in older publications the address may be no longer valid because the author has moved to another institution or retired.

Example 21.x

In a systematic review, the researchers needed to contact an author to ascertain further details of exposure measurement to determine whether the study was eligible for inclusion in their review. However, the email in the address for correspondence was no longer valid. Some detective work was required. This included looking at more recent publications by the same author, and conducting a search on social media platforms.

Ideally, if available, researchers can provide data that are missing in the published manuscript in an aggregated form suitable for meta-analysis. However, often due to limited resources, the authors might offer the full (anonymized) original data set. In such a case, the authors of the systematic review may need to conduct the analysis which require additional resources and statistical expertise. A legal agreement may be required to transfer data, creating a further delay. For these reasons review authors often decide to use published data only.

Box 21.4 shows an example of an email to the authors of the original study with request for additional information.

Box 21.3 An example of a data extraction form

Systematic review title

Reviewer: ....

Study name/ID .... First author ....

Year of publication .... Country ....

Funding:

Pharmaceutical industry ☐

Other   ☐   Please specify ....

Study desion:

Case control ☐   RCT ☐

Cohort   ☐

Participants:

Population source ....   Total N ....

Participation rate ....

Inclusion/exclusion criteria ....

....

Age ....   Gender ....

Exposure:

....

....

Comparison:

Group1 ....

Group2 ....

Group3 ....

Definition of outcome...

21.4.8 Assessing study quality and risk of bias

Quality is a complex concept which can be difficult to measure. Critical appraisal is the use of explicit, transparent methods to assess the data in published research. However, the reporting in published studies is often inadequate or incomplete (due to space restrictions), which can increase the difficulty of assessing the quality. Most of the quality assessment tools used in systematic

---

Box 21.4 Example of an email to the authors with request for additional information

Dear [author title and name],

We are working on a systematic review investigating the relationship between coffee intake and back pain (PROSPERO registration [number]). In your study [reference], you report results for caffeinated and decaffeinated coffee intake combined. We appreciate that this study was conducted a long time ago, but wonder if you still have access to the original data? We would be very grateful if you could provide us with the data similar to data reported in Table 2 of the paper, but separately for caffeinated and decaffeinated coffee intake. Alternatively, we are happy to conduct this additional analysis ourselves provided that you are able to share the original data with us.

Please let us know if this is possible.

Thank you very much in advance.

Yours sincerely,

[reviewer title and name] (on behalf of the review team)

---

reviews involve some measure of the methodological strength, or bias (please refer to Chapter 19 of the book). Differences in risks of bias can help explain differences in the results of the studies included in a systematic review (heterogeneity).

Some examples of scales to assess study quality are given in 'Further reading'. It is a good idea to design a quality/risk of bias assessment form, similar to the data extraction form shown in Box 21.3.

21.4.9 **Data synthesis**

Once all the necessary information from each individual study is extracted, this information needs to be summarized (see Chapter 22).

21.4.10 **Publication**

On completion of the review, the results can be submitted for publication. It is important to check journal author guidelines carefully, as most journals have a manuscript size limit. Systematic reviews are usually lengthy, and therefore it may require shortening the text. Select only essential tables and figures to be published in the journal and present additional, lengthy tables, and other items such as search strategy in an online supplement. Online-only journals have usually less restriction on manuscript size.

There are specific publication guidelines for systematic reviews and meta-analyses (see 'Further reading').

21.4.11 **Post-publication issues**

Keeping the systematic review data in such a way that is easily assessed or modified is important, and tools exist to facilitate archiving of reviews.

Systematic reviews are most useful when they are regularly updated. New evidence can accumulate rapidly, and users should check for more recent studies to see whether new evidence has altered the findings. It is possible to set up regular automatic notifications from relevant databases using the original search strategy for when a new study is published.

The quality of published systematic reviews is highly variable, and there are tools for assessing their methodological quality (see 'Further reading').

Systematic review of systematic reviews is a logical next step forward, bringing together a summary of reviews in one place and allowing the findings of separate reviews to be compared (see 'Further reading').

Further reading

This chapter can only provide an outline of how to conduct a systematic review of epidemiological evidence. There is a considerable body of material available which provides more detailed information on how to conduct this activity.

Levels of evidence

Howick J, Chalmers I, Glasziou P, *et al.* (2016). *The 2011 Oxford CEBM Levels of Evidence (Introductory Document)*. Oxford Centre for Evidence-Based Medicine, Oxford, UK. http://www.cebm.net/index. aspx?o=5653 [Accessed August 2018].

Howick J, Chalmers I, Glasziou P, *et al.* (2016). *Explanation of the 2011 Oxford Centre for Evidence-Based Medicine (OCEBM) Levels of Evidence (Background Document)*. Oxford Centre for Evidence-Based Medicine, Oxford, UK. http://www.cebm.net/index.aspx?o=5653 [Accessed August 2018].

OCEBM Levels of Evidence Working Group (2016). *The Oxford Levels of Evidence 2*. Oxford Centre for Evidence-Based Medicine, Oxford, UK. http://www.cebm.net/index.aspx?o=5653 [Accessed August 2018].

Systematic review

Higgins JPT, Green S (eds) (2011). *Cochrane Handbook for Systematic Reviews of Interventions* Version 5.1.0 [updated March 2011]. The Cochrane Collaboration. Available at: http://handbook.cochrane.org [Accessed August 2018].

Schünemann H, Brożek J, Guyatt G, Oxman A (eds) (2013). *Handbook for Grading the Quality of Evidence and the Strength of Recommendations using the GRADE Approach* [Updated October 2013]. https://gdt. gradepro.org/app/handbook/handbook.html#h.w6r7mtvq3mjz [Accessed August 2018].

Systematic review registration

Campbell Collaboration. So you want to write a Campbell systematic review? https://www. campbellcollaboration.org/research-resources/writing-a-campbell-systematic-review.html [Accessed August 2018].

International prospective register of systematic reviews PROSPERO https://www.crd.york.ac.uk/ PROSPERO/ [Accessed August 2018].

Proposing and registering new Cochrane reviews http://community.cochrane.org/review-production/ production-resources/proposing-and-registering-new-cochrane-reviews [Accessed August 2018].

Registered systematic reviews, Joanna Briggs Institute http://joannabriggs.org/research/registered_titles. aspx [Accessed August 2018].

Protocols for systematic reviews

Moher D, Shamseer L, Clarke M, *et al.* (2015). Preferred reporting items for systematic review and meta-analysis protocols (PRISMA-P) 2015 statement. *Syst Rev*, **4**(1), 1.

Searching for evidence

Campbell Collaboration https://campbellcollaboration.org/ [Accessed July 2018].

Centre for Reviews and Dissemination (CRD) at the University of York databases DARE (Database of Abstracts of Reviews of Effects), NHS EED (NHS Economic Evaluation Database) and HTA (Health Technology Assessment) https://www.crd.york.ac.uk/CRDWeb/ [Accessed July 2018].

ClinicalTrials.gov https://www.clinicaltrials.gov/ [Accessed July 2018].

Cochrane Central Register of Controlled Trials (CENTRAL) http://www.cochranelibrary.com/about/central-landing-page.html [Accessed July 2018].

Cochrane Library http://www.cochranelibrary.com/ [Accessed August 2018].

European Medicines Agency (EMA) http://www.ema.europa.eu/ema/ [Accessed July 2018].

Google Scholar https://scholar.google.co.uk/ [Accessed August 2018].

International Agency for Research on Cancer (IARC). Monographs on the evaluation of carcinogenic risks to humans http://monographs.iarc.fr/index.php [Accessed July 2018].

Joanna Briggs Institute http://joannabriggs.org/ [Accessed August 2018].

PubMed https://www.ncbi.nlm.nih.gov/pubmed [Accessed August 2018].

Research Gate https://www.researchgate.net/ [Accessed August 2018].

Scottish Intercollegiate Guidelines Network (SIGN) http://sign.ac.uk/ [Accessed August 2018].

The National Institute for Health and Care Excellence (NICE) https://www.nice.org.uk/ [Accessed August 2018].

US Food and Drug Administration (FDA) https://www.fda.gov/ [Accessed July 2018].

WHO International Clinical Trials Registry Platform (ICTRP) http://www.who.int/ictrp/en/ [Accessed July 2018].

Citation management

EndNote http://endnote.com/ [Accessed July 2018].

Mendeley https://www.mendeley.com/ [Accessed July 2018].

Zotero https://www.zotero.org/ [Accessed July 2018].

De-duplication

Rathbone J, Carter M, Hoffmann T, Glasziou P (2015). Better duplicate detection for systematic reviewers: evaluation of systematic review assistant-deduplication module. *Syst Rev*, **4**, 6.

Data extraction and management

Review Manager 5 (RevMan 5) http://community.cochrane.org/tools/review-production-tools/revman-5 [Accessed August 2018].

RevMan Web http://community.cochrane.org/tools/review-production-tools/revman-web [Accessed August 2018].

Quality assessment tools

Effective Public Health Practice Project Quality Assessment Tool (EPHPP) for quantitative studies https://merst.ca/ephpp/ [Accessed April 2018].

Higgins JPT, Altman DG, Gøtzsche PC, *et al.* (2011). The Cochrane Collaboration's tool for assessing risk of bias in randomised trials. *BMJ*, **343**, d5928.

Jadad AR, Moore RA, Carroll D, *et al.* (1996). Assessing the quality of reports of randomized clinical trials: is blinding necessary? *Control Clin Trials*, **17**, 1–12.

Scottish Intercollegiate Guidelines Network (SIGN). Critical appraisal notes and checklists http://www.sign.ac.uk/checklists-and-notes.html [Accessed August 2018].

Wells GA, Shea B, O'Connell D, *et al.* The Newcastle-Ottawa Scale (NOS) for assessing the quality of nonrandomised studies in meta-analyses. Available at: http://www.ohri.ca/programs/clinical_epidemiology/oxford.asp [Accessed August 2018].

Publication

Stroup DF, Berlin JA, Morton SC, *et al.* (2000). Meta-analysis of observational studies in epidemiology: a proposal for reporting. Meta-analysis Of Observational Studies in Epidemiology (MOOSE) group. *JAMA*, **283**(15), 2008–12.

The Preferred Reporting Items for Systematic Reviews and Meta-Analyses (PRISMA) statement http://prisma-statement.org/ [Accessed August 2018].

Automation

Al-Zubidy A, Carver JC. Review of systematic literature review tools http://carver.cs.ua.edu/Papers/TechnicalReports/2014/SERG-2014-03.pdf [Accessed August 2018].

The Systematic Review Toolbox http://systematicreviewtools.com/ [Accessed July 2018].

Tsafnat G, Glasziou P, Choong MK, *et al.* (2014). Systematic review automation technologies. *Syst Rev*, **3**, 74.

Archiving

Review Manager 5 (RevMan 5) http://community.cochrane.org/tools/review-production-tools/revman-5 [Accessed August 2018].

RevMan **Web** http://community.cochrane.org/tools/review-production-tools/revman-web [Accessed August 2018].

The Systematic Review Data Repository (SRDR) https://srdr.training.ahrq.gov/ [Accessed August 2018].

Quality of systematic reviews

Assessing methodological quality of systematic reviews (AMSTAR) http://amstar.ca/ [Accessed August 2018].

Systematic review of systematic reviews

Smith V, Devane D, Begley CM, Clarke M (2011). Methodology in conducting a systematic review of systematic reviews of healthcare interventions. *BMC Med Res Methodol*, **11**, 15.

Chapter 22

Meta-analysis

22.1 **Introduction**

While Chapter 21 discussed how to find and evaluate evidence, this chapter will consider how to summarize the identified evidence in a meaningful way.

The idea of combining data from several studies is relatively old. Karl Pearson, British biostatistician known for the Chi-square test, in his report on 'Certain enteric fever inoculation statistics' in 1904 noted that 'Many of the groups ... are far too small to allow of any definite opinion being formed at all, having regard to the size of the probable error involved. Accordingly, it was needful to group them into larger series'. However, the relevant methodology has been developed relatively recently, as was illustrated in Example 21.iii.

Meta-analysis refers to the statistical analysis of results from individual studies for the purpose of integrating the findings. It includes approaches to control for chance and potential bias.

There are other terms related to meta-analysis such as quantitative review, combined analysis, pooled analysis, or quantitative synthesis. Some of them use different methods, for example, meta-analysis of published data considers each study as a unit of analysis while individual patient data (IPD) analysis (also sometimes called pooled analysis) includes the original data from each study on a participant level. Prospective planned IPD analysis involves several centres following the same study protocol to facilitate bringing data together and to ensure comparability.

By combining individual studies, a meta-analysis increases the power to study a particular research question.

22.2 **Whether to conduct a meta-analysis**

Meta-analysis usually follows on from a systematic review once the eligible studies are identified. However, it is important to point out that the term *meta-analysis* should not be used interchangeably with the term *systematic review* as it may be not possible or appropriate to combine the primary data described in the review.

Meta-analysis requires sufficiently uniform information from each study, and not all studies may provide the data in the required form. There may also be an issue of heterogeneity, for example, studies of different design, recruiting different clinical populations, measuring outcomes in different ways and at different time points (see Section 22.8 for further information).

Therefore, the first decision will be whether there are enough studies which are sufficiently similar and provide similar type of data to numerically combine them.

Example 22.i

A systematic review was conducted examining whether, among persons with asthma, aspects of diet were related to severity of reported symptoms. A total of five studies were identified. However, the populations were very different (some were based on self-reported diagnosis and others at specialist respiratory centres), and diet had been collected (24-hour recall, 7 day weighed food intake) and analysed in very different ways (one study used food groups, another used individual nutrient intake). It was decided therefore that it was not possible to combine the data from these studies.

Example 22.ii

A systematic review reported 20 studies examining the relationship between physical activity and breast cancer. Of these, 13 were cohort studies. Although they had measured physical activity in different ways, each allowed identification of one or more groups with a level of physical activity below recommended levels. Each of the included studies had required pathologically confirmed cases of breast cancer in order to be included. Further, they each reported rate ratios for the association under study. The researchers concluded that the studies were sufficiently similar and could be considered for a meta-analysis.

This chapter describes the steps involved in the process of meta-analysis. It is assumed that a systematic review was conducted, and a final set of studies for inclusion has been identified.

22.3 Extraction and assembling of information

Section 21.4.7 describes the procedure for data extraction and management in systematic reviews. This is an important step which should be conducted with care and independently by at least two reviewers to minimize data extraction errors.

Data in published manuscripts are often incomplete. Section 21.4.7 and Example 21.x discussed the approach to obtaining information from the authors of primary studies that is clearly available.

Example 22.iii

In a systematic review of maternal obesity and birth defects in the offspring, the researchers decided to measure obesity using body mass index (BMI). However, several studies only reported mean and standard deviation (SD) for weight and height. The researchers contacted the authors to obtain information for BMI, which is a function of weight and height.

Example 22.iv

While conducting a systematic review of association between sedentary time with cardiometabolic risk in teenagers, researchers noted that one study reported only mean time, without any measure of variability such as SD or confidence interval. Researchers contacted the authors of the original manuscript who were happy to provide the missing information.

However, if the authors of the studies are either not willing or unable to provide the necessary data, various methods can be used to estimate it (see 'Further reading') so that excluding relevant studies with missing information can be avoided.

22.4 Data entry and homogenization

Once data extraction is performed, data need to be entered into relevant software for the purpose of statistical analysis. At this stage, it is essential that the extracted data are comparable and measured on the same scale.

Example 22.v

While conducting a systematic review of the association between obesity and migraine in women, researchers noted that studies reported weight either in kilograms or pounds, height in metres, centimetres, or inches, or pain levels often reported on either 10 cm or 100 mm visual analogues scale, and therefore conversion was necessary.

Occasionally, studies report only proportions or the actual numbers in each group, and therefore additional calculations to determine the effect size are required.

When different studies use different effect measures, they must be converted into some common measure. Mean or median and interquartile range, standard deviation, variance, standard error, or confidence intervals are often reported for continuous outcomes. For binary outcomes, odds ratios, relative risks, or incidence rate ratios (adjusted for confounding factors or crude) and confidence intervals are usually shown. When some studies use continuous data, others use binary data, and others use correlational data, formulae can be applied to convert effect sizes (see 'Further reading').

When types of outcomes differ between studies, a separate meta-analysis of each type of outcome can be conducted but may result in several meta-analyses with less studies included in each meta-analysis because it is unlikely that all studies report all types of outcome. However, if studies and their reporting are very different, careful consideration should be given when deciding if it makes sense to include such disparate studies in a meta-analysis, as previously discussed.

Example 22.vi

A systematic review of the relationship between blood pressure and cardiovascular risk included studies that measure home blood pressure monitoring (HBPM) readings, ambulatory blood pressure monitoring (ABPM), 24-hour blood pressure monitoring, or an average of two single measurements obtained during visits to family physician. These are potentially different measures that may be used in defining hypertension.

22.5 Description of the included studies

A first step in summarizing the evidence is the description of individual studies. Tables giving descriptive information for each included study may contain the following information (typically obtained using a data extraction form as described in Section 21.4.7): name of the first author; year of publication; name of journal where study is published; geographical location of study; study design; population source; data collection procedures; inclusion and exclusion criteria; duration of follow-up (months); sample size; and participation rate. Statistical methods and adjustment for confounding factors in observational studies is often described. Cochrane reviews usually also contain a brief description of each individual study separately. In addition, a table describing excluded studies and reason for exclusions is typically provided (see 'Further reading').

22.6 Description of individual studies' results

Results from each study can be summarized in a table. For each outcome of interest, such a table usually includes name of the first author or study name, year of publication, number of participants in each group, value of effect measure, and confidence interval.

22.7 **Forest plot**

A forest plot is helpful in showing the information from the individual studies in a single figure. (Historically, the origin of the name 'forest' seems unclear but it is most likely refers to a 'forest of lines'.) The plot illustrates point estimates from individual studies as a symbol (usually square) of a size proportional to the study weight. A horizontal line across the square shows the confidence interval. The overall estimate from the meta-analysis and its confidence interval appear at the bottom of the plot, represented by a diamond. The centre of the diamond represents the overall estimate, and its horizontal points represent the confidence interval bounds.

Example 22.vii

Figure 22.1 shows a forest plot for a hypothetical meta-analysis of nine case–control studies. It can be seen that the results of the studies differ. Four studies (B, E, G, H) show an increase in risk while other four studies (A, C, D, I) show a decrease in risk. One study (F) have effect estimate (OR) close to one. The highest OR was noted in Study H and the lowest in Study A.

22.8 Investigating heterogeneity

Heterogeneity in meta-analysis refers to the variation in outcomes between studies. Some variation (random) is acceptable, whereas other variation seems to be outside random expectations (i.e. suggesting bias). The first step in investigating heterogeneity is to visually examine the forest plot. Are there any studies that can be considered outliers? If so, it is useful at this point to double-check that the data extracted from the original publications are correct and no mistakes were made when converting between different measurement units (please refer to Section 22.2.2), study results, or during the data entry.

Example 22.viii

After examination of the forest plot presented on Figure 22.1, researchers checked their data entry again. They realized that the data for cases and controls in study H were entered the wrong way around. After correcting the information on Study H, they produced a new forest plot (illustrated on Figure 22.2) which shows less variation between studies.

22.8.1 Galbraith plot

A Galbraith plot can be seen as either an alternative or supplement to forest plot. It is a scatter plot in which the horizontal axis shows inverse of the standard error, while the vertical axis shows the

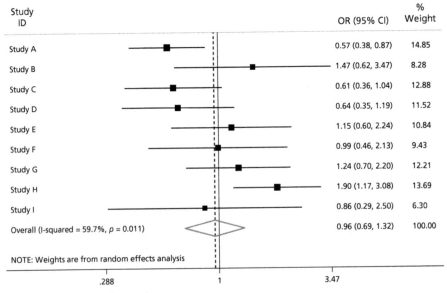

Figure 22.1 Example of a forest plot.

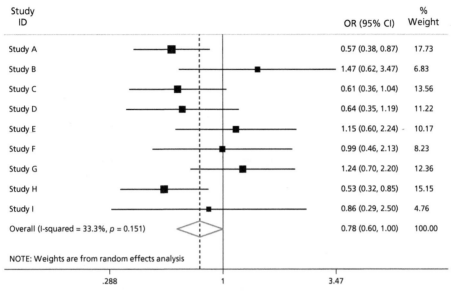

Figure 22.2 Example of forest plot after correcting data for Study H.

effect divided by the standard error, and each study is represented by a point. A line can be plotted with slope representing the combined effect, together with two further lines representing upper and lower limits of an approximate 95% confidence region. It is expected that on average 95% of points will be between these limits if there is no heterogeneity. This plot is useful because studies outside the limits are easily identified and may be considered outliers. Subsets of studies can also be differentiated through the use of different symbols, which may help to identify possible sources of heterogeneity. Systematic investigation of between-study heterogeneity, as a function of differences in design features, types of analyses, and population characteristics, can help to explain inconsistency between study results.

Example 22.ix

A Galbraith plot on Figure 22.3 used the same data as forest plot on Figure 22.1. It can be seen that Study H and Study A are outside the approximate 95% confidence region and therefore should be investigated further. Example 22.vii also noted that these studies are possibly different from the rest of the studies included in the meta-analysis.

22.8.2 **Considering sources of heterogeneity**

There are several possible biases in meta-analyses. For example, study inclusion criteria could potentially be defined in such a way as to exclude any potentially contradicting studies. Bias in provision of data can occur when researchers are not able or willing to provide further information or share data, or when the data has been irretrievably lost (see Section 21.4.7).

Citation bias occurs when reference lists of manuscripts include studies that are strongly supportive of the published results. Database and language bias relates to dominance of research reports from developed countries and publications in English language. Multiple publication bias occurs when multiple manuscripts from the same study published with different results or on different subsets of data. Not all journals are indexed in major databases and there is an issue of elapsed time before publication, including publication and indexing gaps.

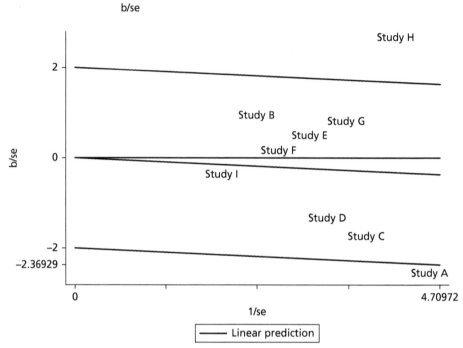

Figure 22.3 Example of Galbraith plot.

Example 22.x

While working on a systematic review, researchers discovered that investigators of one study kept publishing an update every couple of years, sometimes with different first author. In this case the publication which most closely meets the objectives of the review should be used. For example, the publication which has follow-up reported at the required time or with the eligible outcome measures. All other things being equal one would normally take the publication reporting the largest numbers, which is likely to be the most recent.

Publication bias is the term for what occurs whenever the research that appears in the published literature is systematically unrepresentative of the population of completed studies. Therefore, meta-analysis can potentially lead to wrong conclusions. Much conducted research is never published, and positive results are more likely to be published than null results; or there may be a combination of both authors not writing up and submitting manuscripts with null results, and editors being less likely to accept them.

22.8.3 Funnel plot

A funnel plot is a graph designed to investigate publication bias. It is a scatter plot of the effect estimates versus some measure of their precision, such as standard error, variance, inverse of variance, or sample size. In the absence of bias, the plot looks like a symmetrical inverted funnel (Figure 22.4). If there is bias, for example, because smaller studies showing no statistically significant effects remain unpublished, then such publication bias will lead to an asymmetrical appearance of the funnel plot (Figure 22.5). It should be noted however that funnel plot asymmetry may also reflect other types of bias.

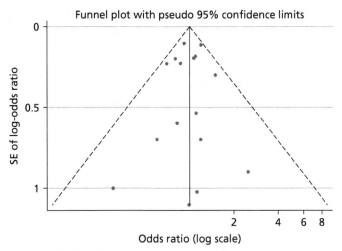

Figure 22.4 An example of a funnel plot.

Example 22.xi

Researchers conducted a meta-analysis examining the relationship, in prospective studies, between working as a teacher (in comparison to other occupations) and mental health. They were concerned that only 'positive' studies had been reported, since if researchers did not find a relationship they would not attempt to publish these 'null' results. They therefore constructed a funnel plot, which demonstrated that mainly significant results had been published, as evidenced by part of the plot being sparse.

Visual evaluation of funnel plots may be subjective, and therefore more formal statistical methods to investigate publication bias were proposed such as Beggs's test and Eggar's test. These tests explore whether the study estimates are related to the size of the study (see 'Further reading').

'Trim and fill' is a non-parametric method developed for estimating the number of missing studies that might exist in a meta-analysis, and the effect that these studies might have had on the overall estimate. It is also possible to model the selection process that determines which results are

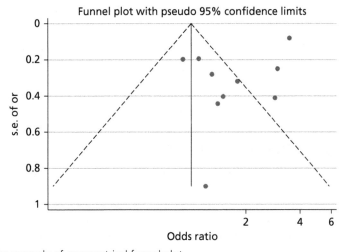

Figure 22.5 An example of asymmetrical funnel plot.

published, based on the assumption that the study p value affects its probability of publication (selection models). It is important to point out that these methods require a large number of studies and they are not sufficiently powerful in most meta-analyses.

22.8.4 Measuring heterogeneity

Statistical heterogeneity can be identified by testing the null hypothesis that the studies all have the same effect. The Cochran's Q test for heterogeneity looks at the differences between observed effects for the studies and the pooled effect estimate. Q is distributed as a chi-square statistic with degrees of freedom calculated as the number of studies minus one.

Non-significant results of this test cannot be interpreted as evidence of homogeneity. Test for heterogeneity has low power as the number of studies in meta-analysis is usually low, and it may fail to detect heterogeneity as statistically significant when it exists. To compensate for the low power of the test, sometimes a higher significance level is used, for example, $p < 0.1$.

If heterogeneity is found, it suggests that differences between studies exist and it may be invalid to pool the results and generate a single summary estimate. The Chi-square test described here provides a test of significance for heterogeneity, but it does not measure it. An index of heterogeneity can be defined as I^2, which is interpreted as the percentage of variability due to heterogeneity rather than chance, and is calculated as following:

$$I^2 = (Q - \text{degrees of freedom}) / Q \times 100\%.$$

The value which Q is expected to have if there is no heterogeneity is equal to its degrees of freedom. If I^2 is negative, it can be set to zero. Hence I^2 is the percentage of the Chi-squared statistic which is not explained by the variation within the studies. It represents the percentage of the total variation, which is due to variation between studies. Interpretation of the value of I^2 is arbitrary. Higgins *et al.* (2003) (see 'Further reading') suggests interpreting the value of I^2 of 0% as no heterogeneity, 25% as low heterogeneity, 50% as moderate heterogeneity, and 75% as high heterogeneity.

Example 22.xii

Figure 22.1 shows the value of I^2 = 59.7%, while after correcting the error for Study H on Figure 22.2, the value changed to I^2 = 33.3%.

What can be done about heterogeneity? If it is present, it is important to describe the variation, investigate sources of it, explain, remove it, or account for it. There are several options if statistical heterogeneity is identified among a group of studies that would otherwise be considered suitable for a meta-analysis: use subgroup analyses; use sensitivity analyses; or use a random effects model. Alternatively, authors may decide not to perform a meta-analysis.

22.9 Calculating the overall effect

Use of an arithmetic average is not an appropriate way of computing the overall effect because studies of different sample sizes have different statistical power. Therefore, a weighted average of the results should be used, in which the larger studies have more influence on the overall estimate. The two statistical techniques used in meta-analysis are fixed effect models and random effect models. The choice between them depends on the way the variability of the results between the studies is treated.

Fixed effect models are based on the assumption that a single (or 'fixed') effect is common to every study, while a random effects meta-analysis estimates the mean of a distribution of effects. The term 'random' reflects the fact that the studies included in the analysis are assumed to be a random sample of all possible studies that meet the inclusion criteria for a systematic review.

The consequence of using a random rather than a fixed effect model is that the confidence intervals for the summary estimate are usually wider. Also, a random effects model is therefore considered to be more conservative than a fixed effects model. Estimates from random effects models tend to be more sensitive to publication bias than fixed effect estimates, because smaller studies have larger relative weights. How can one decide whether to undertake a fixed effect or random effect analysis? It is usually decided a priori that the studies are sufficiently different to dictate a random effect model.

Example 22.xiii

A group of researchers selected 10 similar hospitals in a defined geographical area and conducted a randomized clinical trial within each hospital involving a randomly selected group of patients of the same age and sex, using the same study protocol. It can be assumed that all studies are based on the same population. The fixed effect model can be used to combine results from each individual hospital.

Example 22.xiv

After conducting a systematic review, researchers located several published studies that were conducted by different research groups in different countries at different times. While the studies investigated seemingly comparable interventions, it can be argued that the true impact of the exposure varies from study to study. It is likely that the patient population (sex, age, comorbid diseases) differed between studies, and that the intervention was therefore more effective in some populations than in others. It's also possible that the intervention itself (the precise dosage, type of medication and length of follow-up) differed from one study to the next and that this could have an impact on the effect size. The random effects model would fit such data.

The scenario described in the Example 22.xiii, where all studies are assumed to be sampled from the same population, is relatively rare. In most meta-analyses, the data are similar to that presented in Example 22.xiv.

Example 22.xv

For data described in Figure 22.2, fixed effect estimate is 0.74 (0.61, 0.91) and random effect is 0.78 (0.60, 1.00). It can be seen that the confidence interval for the summary effect is wider under the random effects model than under the fixed effect model. When studies are collected from published literature, the random effects model is generally more appropriate. It is important to point out that the strategy of using a fixed effect model first and then, if the test for heterogeneity (refer to Section 22.8.4) is significant, switching to a random effects model should not be used. This is because the test for heterogeneity cannot be interpreted as evidence of homogeneity and because it usually has low statistical power. The decision to use the random effects model should be based on understanding of whether or not all studies share a common effect size, and not on the outcome of a statistical test.

22.10 **Subgroup analysis**

Subgroup analysis involves splitting studies into subgroups by specific features such as participant characteristic (sex, age, clinical diagnoses, or geographical region) or study design characteristic (type of intervention, length of follow-up, type of outcome measure used). Subsets should be specified a priori at the protocol stage. The more subgroup analyses are performed, the more likely a false positive result is found simply due to chance. Subgroup analysis should be considered as a hypotheses-generating exercise for testing in the future and should have a scientific rationale. In addition to investigating heterogeneity, subgroup analyses can be used to answer specific questions about particular groups of participants, types of exposure, or types of study.

Example 22.xvi

A meta-analysis was conducted to quantify how effective were weight intervention programmes for reducing the weight of participants. Before the meta-analysis was conducted, it was specified that subgroup analyses would be conducted on three groups according to whether they were overweight, obese, or morbidly obese.

22.11 **Meta-regression**

Meta-regression is a tool used in meta-analysis to examine the impact of study characteristics (e.g. age, proportion of females, intended dose of drug or baseline risk) on effect size using regression techniques.

Example 22.xvii

A hypothetical example of meta-regression is shown on Figure 22.6. The figure illustrates log odds ratio of cardiovascular death in 14 trials of thiazide diuretics versus placebo in patients with hypertension, according to reduction in blood pressure, together with a summary random effects meta-regression. The area of each circle is inversely proportional to the variance of the log relative risk estimate.

However, when there is a small number of studies and multiple study characteristics, there is high risk of obtaining a spurious result.

22.12 **Sensitivity analysis**

A sensitivity analysis investigates robustness of the findings to the decisions made in the process of obtaining them. It involves the removal of studies that meet certain criteria (e.g. poor quality, pharmaceutical sponsorship, publication as a conference abstract) to determine their effect on the overall result. For example, a poorly designed large study might be overrepresented in the analysis compared with a small but well-conducted study. A sensitivity analysis could be performed in which the large poorly designed study is removed and the meta-analysis is repeated with the

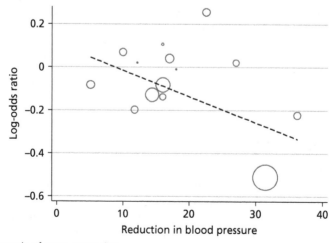

Figure 22.6 Example of meta-regression.

remaining studies to assess if the overall effect estimate remains the same. Like subgroup analysis, sensitivity analysis should be determined *a priori*, if possible. Reporting of effects of sensitivity analyses usually done narratively.

Example 22.xviii

A meta-analysis was conducted of trials of a drug to reduce inflammation in the lining of the gut. It was planned a priori *to commencing the study to conduct two subgroup analyses (a) by different classes of drug, and (b) according to whether the study was funded by a pharmaceutical company or not.*

Example 22.xix

A meta-analysis aimed to examine the effects of acupuncture (compared to conventional care) for stress and identified randomized controlled trials which had a specific measure collected. The trial wished to examine how long any effects lasted. However, trials collected data at different time points. Therefore, the outcomes were grouped into < 6 months, 6–12 months (inclusive), and > 12 months. Separate meta-analyses were conducted for each time point. It is possible however (and more efficient) to analyse multiple outcomes using multivariate methods (see 'Further reading').

22.13 Meta-analysis using individual patient data (pooled analysis)

Individual patient data meta-analysis (pooled analysis) considers primary study data obtained from authors of the papers rather than published estimates. Relative to published data, individual-level data usually provide greater flexibility to address issues of control for confounding and exploration of effect modification or subgroup effects. However, heterogeneity between studies would still exist. A major impediment to this type of meta-analysis is the effort of obtaining the original data.

In the past decades, a phenomenon of several research centres, often international, getting together, creating large research consortia, and combining the individual patient data to study a particular disease has become common.

Example 22.xx

The International Head and Neck Cancer Epidemiology (INHANCE) Consortium was established in 2004, based on the collaboration of research groups leading large molecular epidemiology studies of head and neck cancer that are either ongoing or have been recently completed. Questionnaire data on over 26,000 cases and 34,000 controls, and biological samples from a majority of the study population are available. These studies have been conducted in various regions of the world.

22.14 Meta-analysis of studies conducted using identical protocol (prospective meta-analysis)

The prospectively planned IPD meta-analyses includes pooling data as part of the protocol to standardize data collection procedures. Joint planning of the data collection and analysis increases the homogeneity of the included data set. However, heterogeneity between the study centres may still exist due to differences in populations and in the relevant confounding variables, and in differences in obtaining controls (e.g. hospital-based controls in some centres and population-based in others). Furthermore, the costs for this meta-analysis are high and the planning, which is substantial, may be not easy.

Example 22.xxi

The International Agency for Research on Cancer (IARC) initiated the Alcohol-Related Cancers And Genetic susceptibility in Europe (ARCAGE) project in 2002, with the participation of 15 centres from 11 European countries. Information on risk factors such as smoking, alcohol consumption, diet, and biological samples were collected using the same protocol from a total of 2,304 cases of upper aero-digestive tract cancer and 2,227 controls.

22.15 **Network meta-analysis**

Network meta-analysis of randomized clinical trials allows comparisons of interventions that may not have been directly compared in head-to-head trials. If, for example, a trial compares treatment A to treatment B and a different trial studying the same patient population compares treatment B to treatment C, network analysis allows one to compare treatments A and C (see 'Further reading').

22.16 **Reporting meta-analysis**

There are guidelines (PRISMA) for reporting results of meta-analysis (see 'Further reading').

22.17 **Statistical software for meta-analysis**

There are dedicated software packages available such as RevMan or Comprehensive Meta-Analysis (CMA), but also some statistical programmes such as Stata, SAS, Excel, and R have additional software available specific to meta-analysis (see 'Further reading').

Further reading and resources

Methodology

Begg CB, Mazumdar M (1994). Operating characteristics of a rank correlation test for publication bias. *Biometrics*, **50**, 1088–101.

Borenstein M, Hedges LV, Higgins JPT, Rothstein H (2009). Introduction to meta-analysis. In: Higgins JPT, Green S (eds) *Cochrane Handbook for Systematic Reviews of Interventions Version 5.1.0* [updated March 2011]. Wiley, Chichester, UK. The Cochrane Collaboration, 2011. Available at: http://handbook. cochrane.org [Accessed July 2018].

Duval S, Tweedie R (2000). Trim and fill. *Biometrics*, **56**, 455–63.

Egger M, Smith GD, Schneider M, Minder C (1997). Bias in meta-analysis detected by a simple, graphical test. *BMJ*, **315**, 629–34.

Higgins JPT, Thompson SG (2002). Quantifying heterogeneity in a meta-analysis. *Stat Med*, **21**, 1539–58.

Higgins JPT, Thompson SG, Deeks JJ, Altman DG (2003) Measuring inconsistency in meta-analyses. *BMJ*, **327**, 557–60.

Li T, Puhan MA, Vedula SS, Singh S, Dickersin K, and The Ad Hoc Network Meta-analysis Methods Meeting Working Group (2011). Network meta-analysis-highly attractive but more methodological research is needed. *BMC Med*, **9**, 79.

Lyons LC. Meta-analysis: methods of accumulating results across research domains. http://www. lyonsmorris.com/lyons/MetaAnalysis.htm [Accessed July 2018].

Orsini N, Li R, Wolk A, Khudyakov P, Donna Spiegelman D (2012). Meta-analysis for linear and nonlinear dose-response relations: examples, an evaluation of approximations, and software. *Am J Epidemiol*, **175**(1), 66–73.

Riley RD, Price MJ, Jackson D, *et al.* (2015). White Multivariate meta-analysis using individual participant data. *Res Synth Methods*, **6**(2), 157–74.

Sedgewick P (2015). Meta-analyses: what is heterogeneity? *BMJ*, **350**, h1435.

Sterne JAC, Egger M, Smith GD (2001) Systematic reviews in health care—investigating and dealing with publication and other biases in meta-analysis. *BMJ*, **323**, 101–5.

Sutton AJ, Abrams KR, Jones DR, Sheldon TA, Song F (2000). *Methods for Meta-Analysis in Medical Research*. Wiley, Chichester, UK.

Trikalinos TA, Olkin I (2012). Meta-analysis of effect sizes reported at multiple time points: a multivariate approach. *Clinical Trials*, **9**(5), 610–20.

Reporting

Hutton B, Salanti G, Caldwell DM, *et al.* (2015). The PRISMA extension statement for reporting of systematic reviews incorporating network meta-analyses of health care interventions: checklist and explanations. *Ann Intern Med*, **162**(11), 777–84.

Stroup DF, Berlin JA, Morton SC, *et al.* (2000). Meta-analysis of observational studies in epidemiology: a proposal for reporting. *JAMA*, **283**(15), 2008–12.

Sutton AJ, Abrams KR, Jones DR, Sheldon TA, Song F (2000). Reporting the Results of Meta-analysis, Chapter 10. In: *Methods for Meta-analysis in Medical Research*. John Wiley & Sons, Chichester, UK.

The Preferred Reporting Items for Systematic Reviews and Meta-Analyses (PRISMA) statement http://prisma-statement.org/ [Accessed August 2018].

Software

Comprehensive Meta-Analysis (CMA) http://www.meta-analysis.com [Accessed September 2018].

Lyons LC, Morris WA. The Meta Analysis Calculator http://www.lyonsmorris.com/ma1/index.cfm [Accessed July 2018].

Meta-analysis Easy to Answer (META) http://davidakenny.net/meta.htm [Accessed July 2018].

Meta-analysis in Stata https://www.stata.com/support/faqs/statistics/meta-analysis/ [Accessed September 2018].

Meta-Essentials: Workbooks for meta-analysis http://www.erim.eur.nl/research-support/meta-essentials/ [Accessed July 2018].

MIX 2.0 http://www.meta-analysis-made-easy.com/ [Accessed September 2018].

OpenMeta[Analyst] http://www.cebm.brown.edu/openmeta/ [Accessed July 2018].

Review Manager 5 (RevMan 5) http://community.cochrane.org/tools/review-production-tools/revman-5 [Accessed April 2018].

Statistics Software for Meta-Analysis http://userpage.fu-berlin.de/~health/meta_e.htm [Accessed July 2018].

The metafor Package: A Meta-Analysis Package for R. http://www.metafor-project.org [Accessed July 2018].

Wilson DB. Meta-analysis macros for SAS, SPSS, and Stata http://mason.gmu.edu/~dwilsonb/ma.html [Accessed July 2018].

Part H

Other practical issues

Chapter 23

Ethical issues in epidemiology

23.1 Introduction

The procedures involved in undertaking most epidemiological investigations do not produce either hazard or discomfort to the individual studied. The most commonly collected information arise either from material already available in databases, material such as hard copies of records that can have key data items extracted, or data that is gathered direct from the subject. Occasionally a limited physical examination is undertaken. Much less often, there is a requirement to take samples of biological fluid such as blood and urine, or to undergo simple investigations such as electrocardiography or plain radiography, but even such investigations are typically associated with trivial risk to health.

Ethical issues do arise in epidemiological studies for several reasons. First, the main focus of most studies is often normal populations and the need to obtain a high response rate from individuals who, unlike a laboratory animal, can refuse to participate without explanation. The study population does not normally 'belong' to the investigator, and the latter frequently requires data that could be considered both confidential and sensitive. The ethical issues relate to preservation of anonymity, a subject's right to refuse to participate, and the avoidance of psychological stress caused by participation There is the possibility that a study may reveal previously unrecognized health problems, which presents issues of whether intervention, not part of the study design, is required.

This chapter considers the major ethical problems that may arise in epidemiological research and discusses approaches to minimize their impact.

23.2 Ethical approval

In most countries, investigators need to seek approval from either their institutional or other local or national authority that their proposed study is ethically sound. The epidemiologist will need to complete the same procedures as a clinical investigator who might, for example, wish to perform a clinical trial with a new drug or to undertake a study involving an invasive procedure such as an endoscopy. Ethical approval is required before access to patient or population groups is permitted and is rapidly becoming a requirement before grant funding will be awarded.

23.3 Scientific validity and ethical research

Increasingly, ethical committees (sometimes referred to as 'human subjects review boards') include a methodologist (who may be a statistician) to consider the validity of the proposed study design. The rationale for considering the latter is the premise that a research study that is incapable of answering the question it poses is unethical because it wastes resources. Further, even in epidemiological enquiries with simple procedures such as a questionnaire, it is unethical for a population to be recruited to a study that is unable to provide an answer. A well-designed study will avoid this problem. In practice the most frequently occurring 'sins' are:

 i) insufficient sample size
 ii) selection bias
iii) information bias, for example, using an invalid method of enquiry.

In addition, it could reasonably be considered unethical to undertake a study on too large a study population if the question can be answered with fewer subjects, for all the reasons stated earlier.

It is a frequent misconception when an epidemiologist either communicates or appears in person before an ethical panel, that there is no need to justify the scientific question and the methods. Ethics committees do have the freedom to respond that 'as this study does not have any likelihood of answering the question it poses in a robust manner, the subjects participating in the study are taking part in an exercise of little merit'. If the study has been peer reviewed by a research funding body prior to ethical submission, then the latter would normally accept the rationale for the study and methods as being satisfactory.

23.4 **Ethical constraints in maximizing response rate**

One of the greatest sources of conflict is the scientific need to minimize non-response/non-participation, conflicting with the ethical requisite not to coerce subjects unnecessarily. There is certainly much that can be achieved to maximize response rates without problem. Often an invitation to participate is not responded to: no answer is not the same as 'saying no'. It is not unreasonable to send one or even two follow-up mailings by post, email, text message, or otherwise to those who have not replied to a first mailing, provided that the accompanying letter is not critical of the previous non-response. Ethics committees may insist that you provide potential participants with an option to indicate they do not want to take part and not receive further communications, usually by means such as returning the questionnaire blank (see Example 23.i). This is useful to distinguish them from those non-responding from apathy or forgetfulness, who might be approached again without anxiety.

Example 23.i Suggested wordings for identifying 'positive' non-responders

'If you prefer not to participate in the study please click below and you will not be contacted again.'
   'If you prefer not to complete the questionnaire please tick here and post it back in the envelope provided, and you will not be contacted again.'

23.4.1 **Non-response vs. drop out**

The appropriate level of contact required is often greater for subjects who have already participated in providing 'baseline information' than to secure their initial participation. Failure to provide follow-up information on those recruited is a significant concern.

A decision should be made, preferably at the outset, as to the strategy to be adopted in the face of an unacceptable level of non-response, either to a postal/electronic/mobile phone contact or attendance for interview/examination at a survey centre. There are several possible approaches:

- repeat contact by the same method;
- telephone contact;
- home visit.

The latter two are probably much more acceptable for following up those who are existing participants. To ensure compliance with ethical standards then permission should be sought from subjects as part of their initial consent (Example 23.ii).

Example 23.ii Type of wording that gives subject consent to be contacted by different methods for follow-up

'I understand that the study team may wish to contact me by mail, telephone, or send me an invitation for a visit to a study centre or at home as part of the follow-up to my participation. I am however free to drop out from such further follow-up in the study at any time by contacting the study team and in such circumstances will thus not be contacted further.'

23.4.2 Opting out or opting in

Studies that require face-to-face contact with the subject normally require that an appointment time is agreed. Alternative approaches include:

i) sending a specific appointment time and asking the subject to telephone or mail back only if they wish to opt out or change the time, and

ii) inviting the subject to telephone or mail back only if they wish to opt in.

The former is more efficient and raises response rates, although it has been criticized for giving the implication, particularly to the less well educated, that attendance is necessary regardless of problems with transport, work, and other constraints. A carefully worded letter should avoid most of these pitfalls.

23.5 Confidentiality and data protection

This is a fairly complex and increasingly important issue that impinges on epidemiological studies. Epidemiologists need to be aware of the changing legal environment at both national and international (especially European Union) level. There are three areas of interest:

i)   legal requirements regarding data registers and storage;

ii) confidentiality of data provided to the study direct by the subject;

iii) access to data held on the study population by other sources and, in particular, their medical records.

23.5.1 Legal requirements

It should be noted that the granting of ethical approval for a study does not imply the study complies with the legal requirements in a specific country or jurisdiction. It is the researcher, and indeed their institution, that has a responsibility to comply with the law. Most societies have a legal framework regarding the acquisition and storage of data from the population. There are, however, several misconceptions about the legal position. In the United Kingdom, under the Data Protection Act (1998) which is still extant at the time of writing (2017), the requirement is for the investigator to register with the appropriate agency that data are being held. The act provides a set of 'principles', which must be adhered to—but they do not provide details of what is and what is not acceptable. Interpretation of the act differs and could only be judged on a case-by-case basis. Instead, researchers are best advised to consult and follow guidelines issued by relevant bodies such as the Medical Research Council. Normally, clinical researchers must ensure that they have consent to hold or use personal information, and in most clinical research this is practicable. When consent is impracticable (and this would have to be justified), it is suggested that confidential information can be disclosed without consent if:

a) it is justified by the importance of the study;

b) there is no intention to contact individuals;

c) there are no practicable alternatives of equal effectiveness; and/or

d) the infringement of confidentiality is kept to a minimum.

Although this discussion is, in some respects, specific to the United Kingdom, a more general point is that, when conducting studies, researchers should be aware of the legal framework and of any recommendations of professional bodies in the country concerned.

In May 2016, it became mandatory for EU member states to enact with national laws data protection legislation that leads to the '*protection of natural persons with regard to the processing of personal data by competent authorities for the purposes of the prevention, investigation, detection or prosecution of criminal offences or the execution of criminal penalties, and on the free movement of such data*'. For researchers in the United Kingdom it is the authors' understanding that existing UK law is compliant with EU directives.

There are also legal requirements in most Organisation for Economic Co-operation and Development (OECD) countries on the security needed in storing data, with protection against hacking. An often-ignored requirement is the length of time it is necessary to store data for, after the study has been completed. When the study was for regulatory purposes, for example, a clinical trial or drug safety surveillance, such requirements may be laid down by the regulatory body. Indeed, the safe and appropriate storage of data may be subject to inspection visits by the appropriate authority.

23.5.2 **Confidentiality of data collected for the study**

There are clear legal and ethical responsibilities on researchers for maintaining confidentiality. The study population should be confident that data provided by them will be kept confidential. There are several simple measures that can enhance this confidence.

Box 23.1 shows a suitable layout for the front sheet for a self-completed questionnaire. It incorporates a study number rather than the subject's name, and, should the form be lost or misplaced, no identification is possible without access to the register of names and study numbers. The simple act of having no data on the front page, although relatively wasteful of space, also engenders a feeling of confidence. A suitable covering letter for such a questionnaire should also address the issue of confidentiality, as in the example shown in Box 23.2. If a form is being completed online, then the subject must be assured that the website is securely protected and indeed the same process whereby identifiable information is not transmitted in the same form can be helpful.

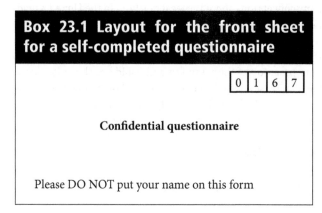

Box 23.1 Layout for the front sheet for a self-completed questionnaire

| 0 | 1 | 6 | 7 |

Confidential questionnaire

Please DO NOT put your name on this form

> ## Box 23.2 Extract from a letter covering the issue of confidentiality
>
> ' ... This information will only be used for the purposes of the research mentioned earlier. The data gathered will be used for looking at groups of individuals and the results presented such that the information from a single individual cannot be identified separately. Access to the information you provide will be limited to members of the research team ... '

The letter emphasizes that the research is interested in looking at groups rather than single individuals, and that it will not be possible to identify individuals from the way that the results will be presented. Subjects are concerned that data given for research may be used for other purposes and given to other bodies and individuals. The letter should reassure the subject that only those involved in the particular project will have access to the original data.

Ethical committees frequently express concern about the inclusion in questionnaires of data concerning sensitive topics like sexual practices and use of addictive substances. The strategies outlined earlier in this chapter should provide sufficient reassurance, but it is not unusual to have questionnaires returned with the study number obliterated! A useful additional tactic is to put the study number on the envelope or elsewhere on the questionnaire to permit identification of the responder.

23.5.3 Access to confidential data from a third party

In epidemiological studies, it is frequently necessary to obtain data from an individual's medical records, perhaps to verify diagnostic or treatment information given in answer to a questionnaire or to uncover new disease episodes in a prospective study. It is the responsibility of the third party to protect the individual's privacy. If a clinician, either in hospital or in general practice, is satisfied by the approvals and permissions that the research team have obtained, then access either to the records themselves, or to specific items of information, may be permitted. This would normally require permission of the patient, although some health service settings may obtain blanket permission from patients attending their service. Thus, patients may be advised that 'the information from your consultation may be used for research purposes and made available to *bone fide* researchers, who have ethical approval to undertake the research. If you do not wish your personal information to be used in this way ... '. More typically, when such blanket consent has not been obtained in the past; the 'custodian' (i.e. the individual who has prior agreed access to the individual subject data) needs to contact the subject and seek their further consent for passing information to an appropriate third-party researcher.

The environment surrounding these issues is continually changing and high-profile instances where personal data is inadvertently released to inappropriate recipients, often results in public outcry and further limitations on release of data. Researchers need to keep abreast of the changing environment and be sensitive to public and political concerns to maintain trust.

The ethical issue is less when the researcher does not hold or need to hold any identifying information (see Example 23.iii), but would require a considerable contribution from the clinician involved.

Example 23.iii

Dear colleague,

We are conducting a follow-up study on patients who had xxx surgery in 2012 and are interested in their current health and status. We would be grateful if you could identify those patients who had that procedure in 2012 and complete a short form about their current status. We do not require any identifying information. Details of the study [...]

It is also easier when the subject has already participated in a study and the clinical record will provide the necessary additional information. Thus, the preferable strategy is to request the permission of the subject in advance, and this is often essential if the subject's recruitment to the study was previously unknown to the physician holding his or her medical records. In such circumstances, a written consent such as that shown in Box 23.3 is appropriate. Note that the consent form provides the name of specific doctors who can be approached. It is the author's experience that this usually results in permission being granted. In addition, the obtaining of such permission before requesting access encourages the third-party physician to participate.

Box 23.3 Extract from a letter seeking consent to obtain medical information

It may be valuable for us to obtain information about your past medical history from your medical records. We would be grateful if you could give us permission to contact your doctor to provide us with such information that is relevant. Please could you complete the tear off slip below and send it back in the envelope provided.

Yours sincerely,

Dr John Smith for the Study Team

Mrs B Jones

21 Pine Road

Newtown   Please circle

I agree to you contacting the doctor(s) below to obtain information   YES
relevant to your research.   NO

General practitioner

    Name   ---

    Address   ---

Hospital doctor

    Name   ---

    Address   ---

        Signed -------------------------   Date --------------------

Some morbidity data on individuals are obtainable from routine data-collection sources although separate ethical approval is normally required, but not necessarily requiring individual patient consent for anonymized data. This is discussed in more detail in Chapter 9 on the use of routine data. Thus, in the many countries with a centralized healthcare system, it is possible to link a patient's primary care record to their subsequent health records in hospital, for example. This linkage may be done 'pseudanonymously' (without the researcher needing to identify specific individuals) but still may require permission.

23.6 Detection of previously unrecognized disease

Many epidemiological studies have as one of their primary aims the ascertainment of morbidity, whether previously recognized by the subject or not. The action to be taken depends on the nature of the problem, its natural history, and the availability of any effective intervention.

23.6.1 Ascertainment of presymptomatic disorders not requiring intervention

There are many instances where such presymptomatic recognition has no practical consequences in so far as no intervention at that stage would alter the prognosis. It might be argued that rather than create anxiety, it is perhaps reasonable not to inform the subject. The best approach is to set out in the consent form the possible results of the survey procedure for an individual and that any relevant information about the condition could be conveyed to the subject's general practitioner. A typical letter is shown in Box 23.4. Such a step is useful in giving the practitioner a baseline for future developments. It should also be made clear what action, if any, is felt appropriate and what information has been conveyed to the subject.

23.6.2 Ascertainment of disorders requiring intervention

Some previously unrecognized disorders, for example, hypertension, do require intervention, and any population-screening survey would need to incorporate in its protocol the action to be taken after case detection even if the intervention is to be handed over to others. An extract from a

---

Box 23.4 Example of a letter to a general practitioner with the results of a study

Dear Dr Brown,

Re: Albert Pink, age 72, 12 Retirement Cottages

Your patient, Mr Pink, agreed to participate in a research study into the occurrence of hip osteoarthritis in retired council gardeners. His X-ray shows evidence of osteoarthritis, particularly concerning the left hip. Mr Pink answered negatively to the presence of hip pain. I am not aware that there is either any treatment or alteration to lifestyle that would be of benefit in such cases. Participants in the study were advised that they would not receive individual results and only those with hip pain, not already under treatment, were advised to visit their general practitioner.

If you require any further information …

suitable letter to be used in such circumstances is shown in Box 23.5. The letter should also explain (as in Box 23.4) how the subject was recruited and the purpose of the study.

The letter gives the relevant result and provides a contact should further information be required. In this example for hypertension, it is reasonable not to give further guidance to the physician about specifics of future action; indeed, it might be resented. By contrast, if the study involves a specialized technique with results requiring interpretation by experts, there may be concern that few general practitioners would feel sufficiently competent to interpret the findings and to plan the appropriate interventions. In such instances, the researcher should provide more guidance in the letter and preferably offer the services of a professional colleague from whom specific advice could be sought, or to whom the patient could be referred.

23.6.3 Ascertainment of unrelated disorders

It is not infrequent that, during the course of a survey, other health problems become apparent that are not part of the study and hence are unanticipated, but are perceived by the researcher, perhaps a junior doctor or nurse, as requiring some intervention. Examples of such include a leukaemia discovered on separating white blood cells for immunogenetic analysis, and diabetes that came to light during an interview with a research nurse for other data. The ethical position is clear. First, managing or even advising about management is not part of the research and should be avoided. Secondly, the subject needs to be advised that there may be a problem and that they should seek medical attention. Simultaneously, the subject's general practitioner should be contacted, either by telephone or letter depending on the circumstances, and given such information as is available. Any such episode should be notified to the project leader and any action taken documented. Obviously, medical omniscience is not expected, but the possession of knowledge that is not followed by appropriate action is culpably negligent.

A related issue is the uncovering of substantial mental distress and psychological disorders. Subjects may indicate they are suicidal or have suicidal thoughts. In other instances, subjects may indicate they are victims of abuse, which might be physical or sexual. These present substantial concerns for the researchers. The first response should be to advise contact with healthcare or other services (and to document that this has been done). How far beyond this is reasonable is debatable. A good source of advice is the parent professional body of the researcher, where relevant.

23.7 Distress among participating subjects

Other than the unanticipated ascertainment of disorders, most questionnaire and interview-based studies will have few other major ethical issues to consider. However, in some instances,

> **Box 23.5 Extract from a letter for a positive result from screening**
>
> ' ... We found his blood pressure to be 210/120 mmHg, which was sustained despite a 10-minute rest. We advised Mr Scarlet that he should seek medical attention for this and to make an appointment to see you within the next week. If you require any further information you can telephone me on ... '

completing a questionnaire or participating in an interview may cause distress to the subject. An example from the authors' recent experience involved conducting a study among war veterans. The study involved a self-complete postal questionnaire which asked both about their current health and about their experiences during deployment. Recalling particularly traumatic events could potentially cause distress. In such circumstances a counsellor was available to the study participants. Alternatively, if conducting home interviews, the interviewer may need to be qualified, or receive special training to deal with circumstances in which the subject is distressed by the nature of questions.

23.8 **Consent**

Consent is necessary for all research investigations on humans. Frequently, in epidemiological studies, the first contact with a subject is the receipt of a request to complete a survey of some form. In that instance written consent is not obtained and participation by completion of the survey assumes *implied* consent (i.e. the subject participated only because he or she was willing to do so). There is no clear distinction between surveys that can rely totally on implied consent and those that require formal written consent. There are certain circumstances where obtaining written consent is probably mandatory. These include:

 i) obtaining information from a third party such as medical or occupational records;
 ii) where an investigation undertaken as part of the survey may uncover previously unrecognized disease that requires further intervention;
 iii) where the survey procedure involves any risk.

By contrast, it may be assumed that a postal or electronic questionnaire will be answered and returned only if the subject consents to do so. Similarly, the subject would attend for a screening examination only if that was his or her wish. The problem comes if such participation is not based on accurate or complete information. It is normally the wording of the letter accompanying the questionnaire or screening invitation that provides the necessary information. If the first contact is by telephone or a home visit, without prior warning, then such information would need to be given either verbally or, preferably, in written form. Ethical committees will look very carefully at the participant information document to ensure that the all the relevant points are covered (Table 23.1). The key points are that the information sheet provides:

 i) a clear statement that the study is for research, and that participation is voluntary;
 ii) the exact nature of the study is given, including its purpose and the procedures to be used;
 iii) a clear statement indicating that non-participation will not jeopardize the medical care they are receiving;
 iv) indicating why they were chosen (e.g. at random);
 v) even if the subject agrees to participate they can, thereafter, withdraw at any time.

An example of letters that should be ethically satisfactory is shown in Box 23.6. The letter comes from the patient's own doctor seeking permission to refer her to the research team and explains why she has been chosen and that she does not have to take part. It does not imply that the study is part of the subject's continuing care and does explicitly give the option of not participating. The research basis is explained, and the subject should not feel it is a necessary part of her management. It is also candid about the tasks involved, which are not trivial.

For many large population-based studies there are multiple parts to participation, for example, completing a questionnaire, agreeing to be examined, giving a blood sample, and to have access to medical records. It is appropriate to seek specific signed consent for each of these individual components and a generic example of such a form is given in Box 23.7.

Table 23.1 Key components of a participant information document

Key components
What is the purpose of the study?
Who is organizing and funding the research?
Do I have to take part?
What will happen to me if I take part?
What will I have to do?
What are the possible disadvantages and risks of taking part?
What are the possible benefits of taking part?
What if there is a problem?
Will my taking part in the study be kept confidential?
What will happen if I don't want to carry on with the study?
What will happen to the results of the research study?
Who has reviewed the study?
How to contact us if you have any questions

Box 23.6 Example of a suitable letter of invitation

Dear Mrs Green,

I am writing to you following your recent discharge from hospital following an episode. I would like your permission to send your details to a research colleague I am working with who would contact you about a research project we are undertaking on whether diet alters the chances of a recurrence. The research aims to look in detail at the diets of 150 patients, such as yourself, and investigate whether there are certain features in the diet that might affect the chances of having another episode.

Your participation in the study would require you to record everything you eat over a period of 24 hours. We would obviously give you full instructions and advise you about the choice of a suitable day. I do hope you will agree to take part in the research, which we hope will help in understanding why some patients develop further episodes.

If you would be interested in participating in this study, please complete the form below and our research dietician, Mrs Blue, will contact you by telephone to follow-up with a home visit when she will explain all the details and answer any questions you have.

If you would prefer not to take part in this research, that is no problem—I will continue to see you in the clinic as arranged.

Yours sincerely

Dr White

Name ---

Address ---

I agree/do not agree (delete where not applicable) to a visit from the research dietician in connection with the study on diet and ulcers

Signature --

Date ---

Box 23.7 Example of participant consent form

Consent

I understand that my participation is voluntary and that I am free to withdraw at any time without giving any reason, without my medical care or legal rights being affected.

Initials..........

I understand that relevant sections of my medical notes and data collected during the study, may be looked at by individuals from the university conducting the study, from regulatory authorities or from the National Health Service, where it is relevant to my taking part in this research. I give permission for these individuals to have access to my records.

Initials..........

I understand that the study will link data from my medical records and questionnaires to national databases containing health information. I give permission for this linking to take place.

Initials..........

I understand that the study questionnaire collects information about my health which might not have been collected previously by the clinic staff, and that my consultant may be interested in seeing my responses to various questions. I give permission for the clinic staff to have access to my questionnaire responses.

Initials..........

I agree to take part in the [study name] study.

Initials..........

....
Name of patient Date Signature

....
Name of person taking consent Date Signature

Further information and contact details:

....

Chapter 24

The costs of an epidemiological study

24.1 **Introduction**

Study design is frequently undertaken without consideration of the cost implications of different available options. Indeed, in many standard texts and taught courses, the student is encouraged to seek the most valid approach to answering a question independently of any cost consequences. Similarly, in refereeing articles submitted to a journal or criticizing published studies it is tempting to suggest that alternative and, frequently, considerably more expensive strategies should have been used. Although in theory the study design influences the costs, in practice the resources available will often constrain the methodological choices. This is important across the range of study sizes from a student undertaking a research project (usually required to be low cost), to an academic consortium making an application to a grant awarding body (where the latter will want the 'return' from the study to be consistent with the costs of undertaking it). What is considered a reasonable cost will also depend on how strong the rationale is for conducting the study.

Example 24.i

Anecdotal evidence from clinical colleagues suggested that some patients with asthma had identified that aspects of their diet might be associated with episodes of the disease. With such limited rationale, prior to undertaking a study on the role of diet in the aetiology of asthma, then the next step may be for a low-cost qualitative study of patients with asthma to collect information on perception of factors precipitating an episode. Alternatively, if the rationale was based on a previous cross-sectional study and there was supportive information, say from ecological studies or animal work, then it may be appropriate to propose a quantitative approach; for example, a case-crossover study looking at 'exposures' before an exacerbation of asthma and a corresponding period without the exacerbation.

Epidemiology should be both the science of the theoretical and the art of the practical—the skill of the epidemiologist lies not in planning the perfect study, but rather in planning the most valid study given the practical limitations of cost and time. Two points, however, are clear. Firstly, no study, however cheap, can be of value if the study design is incapable of producing an answer to the question posed (e.g. a valid estimate of a particular effect). Secondly, and conversely, it is possible that the potential benefit to emerge from a study may not justify the considerable costs of undertaking a methodologically sound study. This is particularly true for relatively rare diseases and could lead to a reassessment of the rationale for undertaking the study.

24.2 **Costing an epidemiological study**

All epidemiological studies incur costs and it is essential to be able to estimate these accurately in advance, both for requesting funding from grant-giving bodies and to ensure that sufficient resources are available for the planned tasks. It is a common mistake to underestimate the costs of conducting a study and then one can be in the uncomfortable situation of realizing that the intended study cannot be completed, or at least that not all aspects of a study can be undertaken with the resources requested. Funding bodies generally do not look favourably on requests for additional resources, particularly if the costs could have been foreseen at the time of application.

Population surveys will vary considerably in their cost, but as there are many common elements it is perhaps useful to take an example to provide a model for how costs can be calculated. The first step is to construct a flowchart of the methodological approach to be used (Fig. 24.1). In this example the plan is to conduct a population study and then use the respondents as a sampling frame to conduct a case–control study. A questionnaire is posted to all persons selected for the study sample. These persons may or may not actually receive the questionnaire and among those who receive it, they will either respond or not. Persons not receiving the questionnaire could have died or moved away, and the mail 'returned to sender'. Those persons who did not respond (and for whom there was no notification of them not having received the questionnaire) were sent another copy of the questionnaire. Among all responders, persons who satisfied specific disease criteria were selected as 'cases' while a sample of responders, who did not meet specific disease criteria, provided an equal number of 'controls'. In preparing a budget for the costs of doing this study, then firstly one should draw up some cost categories (even if some of them will eventually be evaluated as having no costs). These could include:

- Staff salaries and any associated costs of employment. These may relate to:
  - Study recruitment
  - Database design
  - Data cleaning/checking
  - Data analysis

- Estate costs (i.e. will there be any costs for using/hiring offices or clinics in which to conduct the study)
- Consumables (e.g. paper, printing, postage, telephone costs, office stationery costs)
- Equipment (e.g. printer)
- Laboratory services (e.g. processing of biological samples and analysis)
- Contracted special service (e.g. checking study sample for recent deaths)
- Costs for access to data sets
- Volunteer reimbursement (e.g. travel expenses or in recompense for their time)
- Publication (e.g. publishing in open access journals)

There are several ways to cost a study. For example, one can calculate the marginal cost of the study (i.e. the increased costs of conducting the study compared to not conducting the study). Alternatively, one can calculate the full economic costs of conducting a study—this is an estimate of the true cost of conducting such a study in its real-life application.

Example 24.ii

University investigators conducting a large population cohort study were required to cost it on the basis of full economic costs. Therefore, they had to identify the amount of time each academic would spend working on the study and to cost this time. They also had to estimate the amount of accommodation space required and included an 'estates cost' based on the costs if they had to rent such rooms for the conduct of the study.

It is also a common mistake to underestimate the costs involved by not leaving any margin for things not keeping entirely to plan. For example, a particular set of tasks may be calculated to take 800 person-hours and therefore costs are based on this amount of time, forgetting that persons are entitled to holidays and may also have time off sick. It is common practice therefore

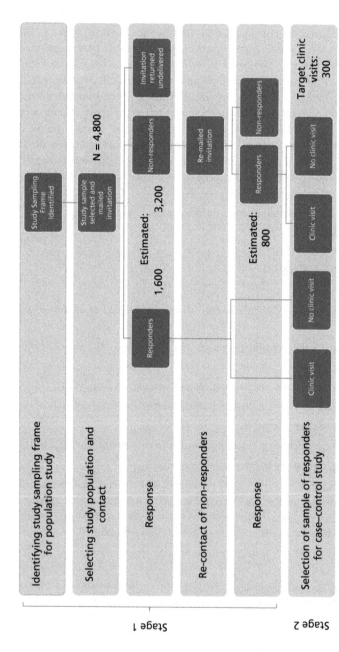

Figure 24.1 Flowchart of a population survey and follow-on case–control study.

to consider that in a year there will be 40 actual working weeks and thus if one had a 40-hour working week, this would provide a total of 1,600 working hours for every year a person was employed. Therefore, to achieve a task taking 800 hours a person would need to be employed for 6 months. Even with all these aspects factored in, there can be other delays out of the investigator's control such as getting access to other data sets, where the timescales in which they are considered and then data sets prepared may not fit in with the study plans!

In terms of staff salaries, one needs to list what tasks are required to be done and estimate how long they will take to complete. Different grades of staff may be needed for different components. For a small study that is part of PhD training, the student may be expected to do all tasks (provided the educational value is assured!). There are staff costs in acquiring the data and separate costs for the handling and analysis of the data obtained. For the former there is often the need for a study coordinator which will include drafting and finalizing the study protocol; applying for permission to conduct the study (including approval from a relevant ethics committee); liaising with study sites (if a multicentre study); recruiting other staff and managing them; and liaising with organizations undertaking the sampling. Project assistants are likely to be required to prepare mailings to be sent out, to receive completed questionnaires and undelivered mail that is returned, enter completed questionnaire data, and prepare follow-up mailings to non-responders. They are also likely to be required to answer telephone calls, emails, and letters from persons invited to take part, some persons will want to contact the study to mention that a person has moved away/is too ill/has died and cannot take part. Others will want to write more about their health—if they felt there was not an opportunity to do so in the questionnaire. It is the authors' experience that more people now object to being invited to take part and will write to query from where the study team have obtained their data and whether the study has all the necessary permissions. All such communication needs to be carefully considered and many will necessitate a reply.

Many of the tasks for the study staff will cover stage 1 and 2, although it will be necessary to estimate the individual times for each member of staff. Additional time will be needed to cost for clinical staff. It is often more efficient to have project assistants undertake all the work involved in actually getting persons to the clinic. Clinic visits will often require nurses or other trained health professionals, depending on the measurements required, and their time will need to be costed both in preparing for the visit, the actual visits themselves, and then completing documentation after the visit. 'No shows' need to be accounted for and their rescheduling in terms of the number time slots to make available. Having nurses available for the more popular clinic time slots (such as in the middle of the day) also needs to be accounted for, as it is unlikely that all available time slots will be filled.

Example 24.iii

It was decided for the aforementioned study that a study coordinator would be required for the full duration of the study in order to undertake tasks associated with protocol development, permissions required to conduct the study, monitor study conduct, and manage staff employed on the study. In addition, an assessment of the person-hours required to do each of the main administrative tasks in the study outlined in Figure 24.1 was estimated, and is shown in Table 24.1.

It was estimated that it took 3 minutes per questionnaire to prepare a questionnaire for mailing and it also took 3 minutes/questionnaire to record a return. After asking staff to type in some questionnaires filled in by other members of staff, it was found that questionnaires took on average 10 minutes to complete (although there was variability depending on the specific responses of the individual). Each clinic visit lasts one hour but a total of two hours were allowed per visit to provide nurses with 30 minutes to prepare for the visit and 30 minutes to complete all the documentation after the visit finished. It was estimated that time should be set aside for training in study operating procedures, in regular team meetings, and for staff professional development. Staff would also be required to attend compulsory training modules when working on research studies and handling data, therefore 15% of time was added for these activities.

Table 24.1 Required staff hours

Project task	Project assistants	Data entry clerks	Clinical research nurses
Preparing initial mailings	240		
Prepare reminder mailings	160		
Record return of questionnaires	120		
Data entry		400	
Issue invitations to cases and a sample of controls	115		
Clinic visits			600
Study team meetings, training, and continuing professional development (15% of time)	95		90
Total study support time (hours)	730	400	690

In order to determine what staffing arrangements would be required, it is necessary to know not only *what* tasks need to be done and *how much* time they will take, but also *when* they are needed to be delivered. Two studies could have similar sets of tasks to be completed but in one study they are conducted sequentially, while in the other they are required to be conducted in parallel. The former study would need fewer persons employed for a longer time compared to the latter. Timelines of a study are often represented in a Gantt chart (named after Henry Gantt) which is a type of bar chart laying out the timelines of a study.

Example 24.iv

A Gantt chart was drawn up incorporating all the tasks involved in the study (Fig. 24.2). The entire study is planned to last 13 months. From this it may be seen that the 730 hours of work for project assistants need to be delivered between 9 May and 13 July, a total of 48 work days. This can be equated to approximately 37 working days (taking account of holidays, time off, and so on) and therefore around 300 working hours. In order to deliver the work required within the timescale, the study will need 730/300 (i.e. approximately 2.5 full-time equivalent persons within this time period).

Using the staffing hours required and the Gantt chart will therefore allow the study investigators to determine what staff they need when in the timeline of a study. Estimating the cost of consumables can sometimes be challenging for a major population survey, particularly if it is being conducted for the first time. How many telephone calls will be required and how much will they cost? How much photocopying will be required? What will be the cost of postage—both outward and return? It is crucial that the correct 'unit costs' are used since these need to be multiplied by many thousands to get the total costs (such as paper, postage, and so on). For mailings it is essential to put together a package, exactly as it will be in the study, in the relevant envelope and then establish the cost of postage outwards and return. In some countries this will be determined by weight, while in others the size of envelope will also contribute to cost.

Example 24.v

The study in Figure 24.1, which involves 4,800 in the study sample, assumes that one-third of persons will respond to the initial mailing (and thus 3,200 will not have responded and potentially require a further mailing).

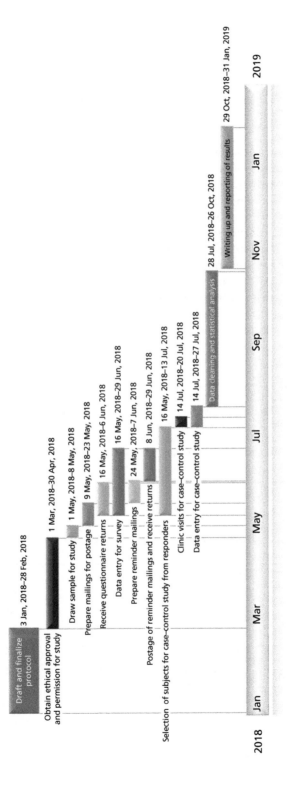

Figure 24.2 Gantt chart of study tasks timeline.

It is further assumed that a quarter of the non-responders will reply to the reminder mailing. Persons will be asked whether they can be contacted again and from these persons 300 cases and 300 controls will be invited (and assuming one-half agree to a clinic visit) this will provide 150 cases and controls. In terms of costing the mailings, these are as shown in Table 24.2.

Therefore, the estimated total cost of the mailings is £25,870. It is wise, however, to build in a small amount of additional 'reserve' funds. If more (or fewer) people return the initial questionnaire than predicted, then the increased (or decreased) costs will be offset by fewer (or more) reminder mailings. However, if there are more returns to the reminder mailings or case–control invitations than predicted, there will be increased costs without opportunity for corresponding savings.

Equipment costs are usually relatively straightforward (although it may be necessary to obtain several quotes for expensive items). In terms of laboratory or special services, cost estimates need to be obtained from the study provider. Although in the past this was often done by 'agreement', it is now the case that most (if not all) services provided by others will require a legal contract, stipulating what has to be delivered, in what timescale, and at what cost.

It is now becoming more common to have patients (or members of the lay public) involved in epidemiological studies. Their roles can include contributing to the research questions (i.e. including research questions which have a priority for patients), bring a patient perspective to practical issues in study conduct (see Example 24.vi), review letters and information leaflets being sent out to patients to make sure they are understandable, and also to help disseminate results through patient organizations. Such involvement needs to be costed, as it is unreasonable to expect patients to provide this for free while the investigators are paid for their role in the study! (See 'Further reading'.)

Example 24.vi

An epidemiological study examining the aetiology of 'disease flares' of rheumatoid arthritis (RA) involved recruiting patients with RA who then reported by mail, email, or telephone when they were experiencing a disease flare. At this time, they would then have a 30-minute telephone interview to collect information on environmental and individual factors related to the period prior to the flare onset. When planning this study, the patient representative, who herself had RA, pointed out that at the time of a disease flare it would be very difficult for patients to hold a telephone for 30 minutes. Therefore, the design was changed to an in-person interview.

Table 24.2 Costing the mailings

Activity	Costing item	Unit cost (£)	Number of units	Cost (£)
Survey questionnaire	20-page questionnaire printing	1.50	8,000	12,000
Survey mailings	Envelopes	0.04	16,000[1]	640
	Postage out	1.20	8,000	9,600
	Postage return	1.20	2,400	2,880
Case–control invitations	Envelope, letter, and information leaflet	0.10	300	30
	Postage out	0.80	600	480
	Postage return	0.80	300	240
Total				25,870

Note: Postage envelope and return envelope for 4,800 initial and 3,200 reminder mailings.

The costs so far relate to actually conducting the study. Once the data has been collected and entered, it then needs to be prepared for analysis and then analysed and reported. Work involved in preparing for analysis will be checking for 'outlying' data, which then may involve accessing the original questionnaires. Then an analysis plan will need to be drawn up, usually between the senior investigator and the study statistician. The statistician will then need to conduct the analysis and produce reports, which will be discussed at investigator meetings. The analysis always takes longer to conduct than originally envisaged—there may be unusual features of the data that were not envisaged (the distribution of certain variables, the level of missing data, high correlation between some variables). Once the analysis is complete, it is common for the statistician to write the statistical methods section of any manuscripts or reports and may also draft all the tables. Of course, if a manuscript is submitted to a journal for publication, reviewers may raise points which require further analyses to be undertaken. Even for a relatively straightforward population-based epidemiological study examining the prevalence of a condition, one is likely to need a statistician for at least six months. One recent cost item which needs to be considered is publishing the results of the study. Open access journals will charge authors whose papers are accepted for publication and the cost can be several thousand pounds. Even if results are published in journals with a traditional publishing model, some funders can insist that manuscripts published from studies which they have funded are made open access. It is therefore important that, if necessary, this is included in the funding costs for the study.

Finally, the cost of archiving and storing the data is almost always forgotten. Most agencies require data to be stored for at least 10 years and perhaps as long as 20 years after the study has completed. Therefore, the cost of storing either the original collected data (on questionnaires) or electronically storing scanned copies of data needs to be estimated and included in the study costs.

For some of the aspects of the planned study, it may be pertinent to consider whether the task could be 'outsourced'. For example, in many countries there are contract research organizations which can undertake large surveys on behalf of researchers. The advantage of using them is that they may be able to undertake the activities faster and at lower cost (although not always). It will reduce the time and work associated with recruiting persons specifically perhaps for a project (and they may only be offered short-term contracts). However, to balance all of this, there is a loss of control over the process. Sometimes things do not go to plan and unless there is very good communication, this may only be evident at the end when it is too late to do anything. Alternatively, companies can undertake to carry out certain tasks, but it transpires that they are unable to do so. This can affect the timeline of the study (and therefore the costs) and may impact on whether the study can be completed. An alternative approach is to design the study so that as much as possible is under the control of the investigators, and to minimize how much the study is dependent on factors out of the researcher's control (Example 24.vii).

Example 24.vii

A case–control study of eczema considered recruiting through general practices. This required the participation of general practitioners who would ask patients consulting for eczema if they would be willing to take part in a research study. However, a feasibility study found that because of limited time in the consultation, general practitioners often forgot to do this and thus patient recruitment was poor. Instead an alternative approach was tried, surveying all adults registered with the general practice and asking respondents (a) if they had been diagnosed with eczema; (b) if they had consulted their general practitioner within the past 3 months for eczema; and (c) whether they were willing for researchers to access their medical records. Although a more costly approach, it proved a much more effective way to identify medically confirmed cases of eczema for the study.

Of course, aspects of design will be influenced by the likely funds available. Even if external funds are applied for, there will be different limits according to the funder approached. Different funders will fund on a different basis (e.g. government funding vs. local charity). Therefore, it is difficult to give one 'formula' for costing a study.

24.3 **Wasting resources**

24.3.1 **Managing timelines**

Irrespective of how much funding a study has, delays in the study once started almost always have a major impact on costs. If the study takes longer to conduct, study staff need to be employed for a longer time and staff costs are usually a major component of study costs. Therefore, it is imperative that such delays are anticipated and minimized. Strategies to do so include prioritizing tasks:

· Which timeline is beyond the research team's direct control (e.g. receiving ethics approval and local research governance approval for the conduct of the study)?

· Which delay has an impact on several other tasks (e.g. make appointments of study staff, such as a study coordinator)?

It may also be prudent in some instances to proceed with a task even though it is not in the final form. If obtaining ethical approval is a key step and can be subject to delays, it might be prudent to proceed with an application even although the list of questionnaire items has not been finalized. There may still be some discussion about items and the project is awaiting data from some ongoing work. At least if the project is able to proceed with an approved questionnaire and if at a later date it is decided to exchange one instrument for another, then a decision can be made, thus balancing the benefits of this against the drawback of a delay by submitting an amendment to the approved protocol.

24.3.2 **Questionnaires**

It is a common mistake, once questionnaire content is finalized, to bulk print study questionnaires. However, even if a questionnaire has been tested in a pilot study, it is the authors' experience that it is worth printing 'in house' and sending out one batch of questionnaires and to examine those returned, before proceeding to print out the remaining questionnaires. This is particularly true for large studies requiring thousands, tens, or hundreds of thousands of questionnaires. Common problems include:

· Typographical errors

  o These are often pointed out by respondents

· Problems with response boxes

  o There is a response box missing or a missing response option. Respondents will often write in a response which they were unable to give with the response options provided

· Items missed out (this is particularly so for individual questions within a questionnaire)

  o This often only becomes evident when the data is analysed and there is seen to be less questions than expected for a scale

· Skip instructions misdirecting respondents to the next question to answer (e.g. 'If no, please proceed to Question 36')

  o Typically these occur when there have been last minute changes to a questionnaire order and it has been overlooked to change some of the skip instructions

Example 24.viii

A questionnaire for use in a large population-based study was tested on a group of individuals, who provided feedback on how understandable the items were and estimates of how long it took to complete. Once they had made some minor changes, some further work with the same individuals confirmed that all items were easily understood and the 15 minutes it took to complete was acceptable.

When the survey was complete, the analyst noted that one question (which should have been completed by everyone) was missing in more than half the respondents. When the investigators checked the questionnaire, the problematic question appeared at the bottom of the page, after body diagrams where respondents indicated the site of symptoms. It seemed likely that many respondents had not noticed the following question and had turned over to the next page without completing it.

Tabulating the responses from the initial questionnaires received would have identified this issue at an early stage.

Finally, study questionnaires should be as short as is compatible with meeting the study objectives. There is a temptation to add additional items on the basis that 'it would be nice to know'. This should be strongly resisted and only items necessary for meeting the study objectives should be included. The cost implications are in a longer questionnaire which uses more paper (and might be more costly in postage), but also the increased time for data entry and analysis. Almost all studies include questions which are not subsequently used—a fact to be remembered when designing a questionnaire—only include items which will be used in the analysis.

Further reading

Involving patients in research

INVOLVE: to support active public involvement in the National Health Service of the United Kingdom, public health and social care research. A source of good practice that is more widely relevant. Available at: http://www.invo.org.uk/

Index

Note: tables, figures, and boxes are indicated by *t*, *f*, and *b* following the page number, for example 4*f* would indicate a figure on page 4.

access to data 95
  clinical records 38
  population registers 30–1
adolescents, data collection 103
advance notification 128, 129*b*
aetiological heterogeneity 216–17
aetiology 63
age-period-cohort models 26, 27
age-specific rates 22, 161*t*–2
  comparisons over time 24–6*f*
age-standardization, DSAR 162–3*f*
agreement of results 115*b*
  categorical measures 117–19
  continuous measures 119–20*t*
  see also repeatability of results
analysis 7*t*, 8
anonymization of data 95
association 5, 211
  Bradford Hill criteria for causation 212–16
  measures of
    attributable fractions 66
    further reading 68
    odds ratios 64–5
    precision 66
    prevalence ratio 63
    rate ratios 64
    risk or rate differences 65–6
    risk ratio 64
  non-causative, possible reasons
    for 211–12
  strength of 213
attributable fractions 66
attributable risk (rate) 66

bias 8, 202, 229
  assessment 119
  direction of 202–3
  information bias 208–9
  in interviews 103
  left censorship 40–1
  major sources 204
  in meta-analyses 237–8
  non-directional misclassification 203
  observer bias 116
  selection bias 204–8
Big Data 91
biobanks 93–4, 97
biological plausibility of studies 214
biomarkers 93–4
birth data 91
Bland–Altman plots 120
Bradford Hill criteria for causation 212–16

cancer registers 92
case ascertainment 39
case–cohort studies 53, 61
  data analysis 187, 190
  further reading 62
case–control studies 48–50, 58*t*, 60
  control groups 81–2
  data analysis 169–78, 190
  flow chart 262*f*
  further reading 61
  minimizing confounding 194–5
  nested 51–2, 59
  odds ratios 64–5
  power calculations 84*t*
  recruitment of cases 71–7
  recruitment of controls 77–81
  study size 82–4, 83*t*
case–crossover studies 52*f*–3, 58*t*, 60
  data analysis 186–7*t*, 190
  further reading 61
case verification 39, 75–7, 76*t*
catchment population approach 29–30, 31
  case ascertainment 39
  case verification 39
  incidence measurement 34, 38–9
  prevalence measurement 41
categorical measures, repeatability analysis 117–19
categorization of exposures 176
causation 4*t*, 5, 211
  aetiological heterogeneity 216–17
  Bradford Hill criteria 212–16
  further reading 218
  reverse causality 212
census data 28, 29, 31, 91
Centre for Evidence-Based Medicine (CEBM) 222
chi-squared (I^2) test
  for heterogeneity 240
  for trend 174–5*t*
citation bias 237
citation management 225, 231
clinical epidemiology 6
Clinical Practice Research Datalinks (CPRD) 91, 92–3
clinical records, access issues 38, 253–5
clinical trials 6
clinic visits, costs 263
closed questions 104–5*b*, 106*t*
cluster (multistage) sampling 33
Cochran's Q test 240
coding data 147–8, 150
  for logistic regression 172
  recoding 153
coding schedules 149*b*, 150

coherence of evidence 215–16
cohort effects 25f–6f
cohort studies 50–2, 58t, 59, 60–1
  data analysis 178–86, 190
  exposure categorization 86
  exposure status ascertainment 87
  feasibility studies 136–8
  follow-up of subjects 130, 132
    ascertaining disease status 132t–4
    duration 88–9
    questionnaires 134b
  further reading 61
  losses to follow-up 135
  multiple exposure data 86
  pilot studies 139
  power calculations 89t
  rate ratios 64
  risk or rate differences 65–6
  risk ratio 64
  selection of subjects 84–9
  study size 87–9, 88t
communicable disease registers 97
comparisons 19–20t
  over time 23–4t
    age-specific rates 24–6f
  standardization 20
    direct 20–2
    indirect 22–3t
competing risks 16
complaints 126–7
confidence intervals 66, 156–8, 169
  for incidence rate 157t
  for incidence rate ratio 179–80
  for odds ratio 170–2
    matched-pairs analysis 177–8
  for prevalence 159–60
  for risk ratio 180t–1
confidentiality
  access to data from a third party 253–5
  of data collected for the study 252–3
  and data linkage 94–5, 153
  legal requirements 251–2
  reassurance of subjects 253b
confounding 8, 19–20, 192–4, 200t
  in case–crossover studies 53
  and conduct of study 195
  investigation of
    baseline comparisons of potential
      confounders 195–6t
    multivariate techniques 199, 201
    standardization 197, 199, 200t
    stratification 196–7t
  matching controls 81–2
  minimization in study design 194–5
  unknown confounders 194–5, 201
consent 38, 250–1, 257
  for access to medical records 253–4b
consent form example 259b
consistency see repeatability of results
consistency checks 152t
consumables, cost estimation 264, 266t
continuous data types 67t
continuous measures, repeatability analysis 119–20
control groups

matching 81–2
  one or two 81
controls
  proportion of 84t
  recruitment 77
    further reading 89
    non-population-based strategies 79–81
    population-based strategies 78–9
cooperation rates, definition of 122
correlation (ecologic) studies 55–7, 56f, 58
  further reading 62
costs 9, 260
  estimation of 260–8
  reimbursement of 126
  sources of wastage 268–9
Cox regression 185–6b, 201
cross-sectional studies 47–8f
  data analysis 169, 190
  left censorship 40–1
  single versus duplicate 40
cumulative incidence 15
cumulative risk see incidence proportion
custodianship of data 95

data access 95
data analysis
  case–cohort studies 187
  case–control studies 169–78
  case–crossover studies 186–7t
  cohort studies 178–86
  confounding 195–201
  costs 267
  Cox regression 185–6b
  cross-sectional studies 169
  crude, age-specific, and standardized rates 161–2
  ecologic studies 189
  effect measurement, interval assessment, and
    significance testing 169
  further reading and resources 167, 190–1
  incidence rate 156–8
  incidence rate ratios 179–80
  life-table methods 181t–2t
  linear trend estimation 174–6
  logistic regression 172–3b, 199
  logrank test 183t–4t
  Mendelian randomization studies 187, 189
  migrant studies 187
  odds ratios 169–74
  population attributable risk 178–9
  prevalence 159–60
  randomized controlled trials 189–90
  rate ratios 178
  risk ratios 180–1
  standardization 165t–6t
    direct 162–3
    indirect 164
  statistical software 165, 166t, 168
  survival curves 182–6
databases
  incidence measurement 37
  recruitment of cases 73–4
  sources of evidence 224–5b
data coding 147–8
data collection 145

approaching subjects 101
  direct and indirect approaches 102*t*–3
  direct electronic entry 150
  hard copy collected by trained interviewers 147
  hard copy direct from subjects 146
  indirect computer entry 150
  missing data 150–2
  role of 101
  typical options 146*t*
data custodians 95
data entry 234
data errors 150, 152–3
data extraction 226, 234
  further reading 231
data extraction form 228*b*
data handling 8, 95
data homogenization 235
data linkage 94–5, 133, 153
  further reading 97
data protection 127, 251–2
data recoding 153
data sharing 153–4
data sources 90–1
  accessing routine data 95
  advantages and disadvantages of secondary
      data 96–7
  biobanks 93–4
  birth and death notifications 91
  census data 91
  combining primary and secondary data 95–6
  disease registers 92
  further reading 97
  healthcare utilization registers 92–3
  normal population surveys 93
data storage 153–4
  costs 267
date of onset of disease 43
death data 91
definition of disease 3, 4*t*
definition of epidemiology 3
delays, management of 268
diagnosis of disease
  case verification 75–7, 76*b*
  disease definition 3, 4*t*
diaries 125
dichotomous exposures 67*t*
direct age-standardized rate (DSAR) 162–3*f*
direct standardization 20–2, 26, 165*t*–6*t*
disagreement
  measurement of 119–20*t*
  see also agreement of results; repeatability
      of results
discomfort avoidance 126
disease causation 4*t*, 5
  see also causation
disease controls 79–80
disease definition 3, 4*t*
disease management 4*t*, 6
disease occurrence 4*t*, 5, 13
  choice of measure 17, 18*t*
  incidence 13–16
  making comparisons 19–20*t*
    over time 23–6
    standardization 20–3

measurement approaches
  incidence 14–16
  prevalence 16–17
prevalence 16–17
disease occurrence studies
  incidence measurement 34–7, 35*f*
    catchment population approach 38–9
    choice of strategy 36*f*
    clinical team compliance 37–8
    diagnosed cases 37
    indirect measures 43–4
    population surveys 40–1
    rare diseases 38
  population selection 28
    access 30–1
    availability 29–30
    data accuracy 31
    representativeness 29
    study size 31–2*t*
  prevalence measurement 41
    catchment population methods 41
    population surveys 42–3
    prospective measurement 42
  sampling from a population 32–3
disease outcome 4*t*, 5–6
disease prevention 4*t*, 6
disease registers 92, 97
disease status ascertainment 132*t*–4
distress 256–7
dose response relationships 214
double data entry 150
drop out, management strategies 250–1
drug registers 93
duplicate population surveys, incidence
      measurement 34, 35*f*, 36*f*–7, 40

ecologic fallacy 57
ecologic studies 55–7, 56*f*, 58
  data analysis 189, 191
  further reading 62
effect measurement 169
  meta-analyses 240–1
electoral registers, recruitment from 78
electronic data capture 150
epidemiological research *see* research
epidemiology 3
  definition 3
  speciality areas 4*t*
episode incidence 14–16, 18*t*
EQUATOR (Enhancing the QUAlity and
      Transparency Of health Research)
      network 155
equipment costs 266
error estimation 66
ethical approval 249
ethical committees 249–50
ethical issues 9, 249
  confidentiality 251–5
  consent 257–9*b*
  detection of previously unrecognised
      disease 255–6
  distress among participating subjects 256–7
  maximising response rate 250–1
  validity of study design 249–50

evidence
definition of 221
levels of 222
reviews of 221, 222
searching for 224–5b
systematic reviews 222
advantages 223
Evidence-Informed Policy Network (EVIPNet) 221
excess risk (rate) 66
exposure opportunity 53
exposures
categorization 67t–8, 86, 176
choice of study design 58t–61
linear trend estimation 174–6
multiple levels of 173–4t
quantifying associations with disease
attributable fractions 66
further reading 68
odds ratios 64–5, 169–74
precision of measures 66
prevalence ratio 63
rate ratios 64
risk or rate differences 65–6
risk ratio 64
recall bias 49
study types 47–58
exposure status
ascertainment of 87
cohort studies 84
external validity 204

face-to-face interviews 104
false positives and false negatives 109t
family controls 80
family relationships, data collection 103
feasibility studies 136–8, 136f
further reading 141
first-ever incidence 14–15, 18t
fixed effect models 241
follow-up, cohort studies 130, 132
ascertaining disease status 132t–4
duration of 88–9
feasibility studies 136–7
losses to 135
questionnaires 134b
forest plots 235–6f, 237f
frequency matching 82
friends controls 80
funnel plots 238–40, 239f

Galbraith plots 236–7, 238f
Gantt charts 264, 265f
generalization of studies 204
general practitioner lists 30
genetic epidemiology 4t
genetic variants, Mendelian randomization
studies 54–5f, 56f, 58t, 217

hard copy data
interviewer-collected 147
preparation for indirect computer entry 147–8, 149b
self-completed questionnaires 146
hazard ratio 181
healthcare utilization registers 92–3

heterogeneity, investigation in meta-analysis 236–40
home visits, inconvenience reduction 126t

identifiers 94
implied consent 257
imputation 151–2
incentives 127
incidence 13–14
choice of measure 17, 18t
measurement approaches 14–16, 18t, 34–7, 35f
catchment population approach 38–9
choice of strategy 36f
clinical team compliance 37–8
diagnosed cases 37
indirect measures 43–4
life-table methods 181t–2t
population surveys 40–1
rare diseases 38
standardized incidence ratio (SIR) 22, 23t
incidence proportion (risk, cumulative
incidence) 13, 14, 15
incidence rate 13, 14
crude, age-specific, and standardized rates 161–2
data analysis 156–8
incidence rate ratios 178
confidence intervals 179–80
inconvenience 125
reduction strategies 126t
indirect standardization 22–3t, 164, 165t–6t
further reading 27
individual patient data (IPD) analysis 233, 243
information bias 208–9
information gathering 7t
information quality 8
information sheets 131b, 257, 258t
'intention to treat' principle 189
internal pilot studies 139
internal validity 204
internet-based interviews 104
interpretation of results 7t, 8
interventions, alteration of disease occurrence 214–15
intervention studies 6
interviews 43, 102–3, 147
face-to-face and telephone 104
invasive procedures 126
invitation letters 129–30b, 258b

J-shaped curves 175–6

Kaplan–Meier curves 182–3f
kappa (κ) statistic 117–19

'Latin square' design 116, 117t
left censorship 40–1
levels of evidence 222
further reading 230
linear trend estimation 174–6
linkage of data 94–5, 133, 153
further reading 97
literature reviews see reviews
logistic regression 172–3b, 199
logrank test 183t–4t
longitudinal studies see cohort studies
losses to follow-up 135

mailing costs 266t
management of disease 4t, 6
Mantel–Haenszel estimate 186–7t, 188t, 196, 198t–9t
marginal costs 261
marginal structural models 218
matched pairs analysis 176–8
matching 50, 81–2
  minimizing confounding 194
  problems with individual matching 82
maximizing participation 128t
  communication strategy 129
    information sheets 131b
    invitation letters 130b
  delivery strategy 128
  incentives 127
  origin of contact 129
  questionnaire design 127–8
media, selection bias 207
medical records, access issues 38, 253–5
MEDLINE searches 225b
Mendelian randomization studies 54–5f, 56f, 58t, 217
  data analysis 187, 189, 191
  further reading 62, 218
meta-analysis 233–4
  calculating the overall effect 240–1
  data entry and homogenization 234–5
  data extraction 234
  description of included studies 235
  description of individual studies' results 235
  forest plots 235–6f, 237f
  further reading 244–5
  investigating homogeneity 236
    funnel plots 238–40, 239f
  network 244
  possible biases 237–8
  prospective 243
  sensitivity analysis 242–3
  statistical software 244
  subgroup analysis 241–2
  using individual patient data 243
meta-regression 242f
migrant studies 53–4, 58
  data analysis 187, 190
  further reading 62
Million Women's Study 93
misclassification 113
missing data 150–2
  on confounders 195
  right censorship 182
mortality rate 14
  standardized mortality ratio (SMR) 22
multiple exposure data, cohort studies 86
multiple publication bias 237
multistage (cluster) sampling 33
multivariate techniques 199, 201

'national' estimates, population selection 29
National Institute for Health and Care Excellence
    (NICE) 221
necessity of exposure 215
negative confounding 192
neighbour controls 79
nested case–control studies 51–2, 59
  further reading 61

network meta-analysis 244
noise 114
non-participation, reasons for 123–4
  antipathy to research 126–7
  avoidance of discomfort 126
  financial cost 126
  inconvenience 125
    reduction strategies 126t
  lack of interest or perceived personal
    relevance 124–5
non-response, management strategies 250–1
non-response bias 205–6
  assessment approaches 206–7
nutritional epidemiology 4t

observational studies 6
observer bias 116, 208
observer variation 114–16
occupational epidemiology 4t
occurrence of disease see disease occurrence
odds ratios 64–5, 169–70t
  confidence intervals 170–2
  further reading 68
  for matched pairs 176–7t
    confidence intervals 177–8
  with multiple levels of exposure 173–4t
  using logistic regression 172–3b
onset of disease, date of 43
open questions 104–5b, 106t
opting out or opting in 251
order effects 116
ordinal exposures 67t
outcome of disease 4t, 5–6
outsourcing 267
overmatching 82

participant information sheets 257, 258t
participation rates
  decline 121, 127
  definition of terms 121–2
  flow chart 123f
  follow-up in cohort studies 130, 132–4
  further reading 135
  gender and age differences 124
  losses to follow-up 135
  maximization 127–30, 128t
    ethical issues 250–1
  measurement approaches 121–3
  reasons for non-participation 123–7
  reporting of 123, 124f
patient contributions 266
'people panels' 31
period prevalence 16–17, 18t
'per protocol' analysis 189
pharmaco-epidemiology 4t
PICO acronym 223
pilot studies 136f, 138–40
  further reading 141
  process issues 140t
  resource issues 140t
  scientific issues 139t
point prevalence 16, 18t
Poisson distribution 156–8, 157t
Poisson regression 201

pooled analysis *see* individual patient data analysis
pooling information 6
population attributable fraction 66, 178–9
  further reading 68
population epidemiology 5
population registers 30
  access 30–1
population selection 7*t*–8, 28
  access 30–1
  availability 29–30
  data accuracy 31
  representativeness 29
  study size 31–2*t*
population surveys 30, 31, 93
  approaches 42–3
  costs 261
  flow chart 262*f*
  incidence measurement 34, 35*f*, 36*f*–7
  prevalence measurement 42–3
  sample size 32*t*
  single versus duplicate 40
population weightings 20–1
postal surveys 43
power calculations
  case–control studies 84*t*
  cohort studies 89*t*
precoded questionnaires 148*b*
presymptomatic disorders, detection of 255
prevalence 13, 16
  choice of measure 17, 18*t*
  data analysis 159–60
  measurement approaches 16–17, 41
    catchment population methods 41
    population surveys 42–3
    prospective measurement 42
    standardized prevalence ratio (SPR) 22
prevalence days 42
prevalence ratio 63
prevention of disease 4*t*, 6
primary data 90
primary data-based studies, use of secondary
    data 95–6
PRISMA Flow Diagrams 226, 227*f*
project assistants 263
propensity modelling 217–18
prospective cohort studies 50, 51*f*, 58*t*, 59, 60, 60–1
  recruitment 85–6
prospective meta-analysis 243–4
prospective notification
  clinical team compliance 37–8
  incidence measurement 34, 35*f*, 36*f*
  prevalence measurement 42
protopathic bias 208
pseudonymization of data 94
publication bias 238
  funnel plots 238–40, 239*f*
  investigating homogeneity, Cochran's Q test 240
publishing costs 267
p values 169

Q test 240
quality assessment 228–9
  further reading 231

quantiles 67*t*
questionnaires 43, 101, 148*b*
  coding schedules 149*b*
  common problems with 268–9
  costs 266*t*
  delivery strategy 128
    advance notification letters 129*b*
  design 105–7
    examples of poor design 107*t*
    further reading 107
  face-to-face and telephone interviews 104
  front sheet layout 252*b*
  inconvenience reduction 126*t*
  interview or subject-completed 102–3
  length of 269
  maximizing participation 127–8
    information sheets 131*b*
    invitation letters 130*b*
  open and closed questions 104–5*b*, 106*t*
  participation rates 121, 122
  precoded 148*b*
  self-completed 146
  use in cohort studies 134*b*
  validation of responses 110*f*, 112

random effect models 241
randomized controlled trials 57*f*–8, 58*t*, 59
  alternatives to 217–18
  data analysis 189–90, 191
  further reading 62
  pilot studies 139, 141
random sampling 32–3
range checks 152*t*
rare diseases
  case–control studies 49
  choice of study design 58*t*
  incidence measurement 38
  recruitment of cases 74
rate differences 65–6
rate ratios 64, 178
recall bias 49, 208–9, 210
receiver operating characteristic (ROC)
    curves 109, 110*f*
recoding data 153
recruitment of cases
  advance notification letters 128–9*b*
  advertising for cases 74–5
  for case–control studies 71–7
  case verification 75–7, 76*b*
  example letter 75*b*
  example patient registration form 76*b*
  exclusion criteria 77
  feasibility studies 136–8
  incident or prevalent cases 71–2
  invitation letters 129–30*b*
  phasing of letters 125*b*
  population-based or hospital-based series 73
  recruitment from colleagues 74
  strategies for case selection 72*f*
  using databases 73–4
recruitment of controls 77
  further reading 89
  non-population-based strategies 79–81

population-based strategies 78–9
registers *see* data sources133
relative risk (risk ratio) 64
   Mantel–Haenszel estimate 186–7*t*, 188*t*
   odds ratios 169–70*t*
     confidence intervals 170–2
reliability of results 115*b*
   see also repeatability of results
repeatability of results 115*b*, 214
   measurement 116
     categorical measures 117–19
     continuous measures 119–20*t*
   observer bias 116
   reducing subject variation 114
reporting study results 155–6*t*
representativeness, target populations 29, 33
reproducibility of results 115*b*
   see also repeatability of results
research
   antipathy to 126–7
   logistical issues 9
   major problem areas 7*t*
   methodology 7–8
   pooling results 6
   scope 3–6
research questions 223
respondents, definition of 122
response rates
   definition of 122
   maximising, ethical issues 250–1
retention, cohort studies 130
retrospective cohort studies 50–1*f*, 58*t*, 59, 85
retrospective reviews, incidence measurement 34, 35*f*,
     36*f*, 37
reverse causality 212
reviews 222
   see also systematic reviews
right censorship 182
risk 5
   see also incidence proportion
risk differences 65–6
risk factors 216–17
risk ratio 64, 180
   confidence intervals 180*t*–1

sample size 8, 31–2*t*
   calculation of 33, 89
   case–control studies 82–4, 83*t*
     influence of increasing the number of
       controls 84*t*
   cohort studies 87–9, 88*t*
sample surveys, assessment of response bias 207
sampling 32–3
   see also population selection
sampling frame 32
sampling units 32
screening 6, 73
   detection of previously unrecognised disease 255–6
   for exposure status 87
   questionnaires 43
   sensitivity and specificity 108–10
secondary data 90–1
   advantages and disadvantages 96–7

use in primary data-based studies 95–6
   see also data sources
selection bias 204–8
   non-response bias 205–7
self-completed questionnaires 146
self-reported diagnosis 77
sensitivity analysis 242–3
sensitivity of tests 108–10
sexual issues, data collection 103
SHARE website 74–5, 89
significance testing 169
simple random sampling 32–3
single population surveys, incidence measurement 34,
     35*f*, 36*f*, 37, 40
social media
   recruitment of cases 74–5
   recruitment of controls 79
specificity of effects 215
specificity of tests 108–10
staff costs, estimation of 261, 263–4*t*
standard error (SE) 66
standardization 20, 165*t*–6*t*
   direct 20–2, 162–3
   further reading 26–7
   indirect 22–3*t*, 164
   investigation of confounding 197, 199, 200*t*
standardized incidence ratio (SIR) 22, 23*t*, 165
standardized mortality ratio (SMR) 22
standardized prevalence ratio (SPR) 22
standard populations 20–1
statistical software 165, 166*t*, 167, 168, 191
   for meta-analysis 244, 245
   multivariate techniques 199, 201
storage of data 153–4
stratification
   investigation of confounding 196–7*t*
     Mantel–Haenszel estimate 198*t*–9*t*
stratified exposure levels 67*t*
stratified random sampling 33
STROBE (Strengthening the Reporting of
     Observational Studies in Epidemiology)
     statement 155
study coordinators 263
study design 7
   choice of 58*t*–61
   ethical issues 249–50
   minimizing confounding 194–5
study identifiers 153
study samples 32
study size 31–2*t*, 66
study types
   case–cohort studies 53, 61
   case–control studies 48–50, 58*t*, 60
   case–crossover studies 52*f*–3, 58*t*, 60
   cohort studies 50–2, 58*t*, 59, 60–1
   cross-sectional studies 47–8*f*
   ecologic studies 55–7, 56*f*, 58
   further reading 61–2
   Mendelian randomization studies 54–5*f*, 56*f*,
     58*t*, 217
   migrant studies 53–4, 58
   randomized controlled trials 57*f*–8, 58*t*, 59
subgroup analysis 241–2

subject bias 208–9
subject selection, cohort studies 84–9
subject variation 114
subspeciality areas 4t
sufficiency of exposure 215
surgical registries 97
surveillance bias 207
survey centre visits, inconvenience reduction 126t
survival curves 182–3f
    comparison
        Cox regression 185–6b
        logrank test 183t–4t
systematic reviews 222
    advantages 223
    assessing quality and risk of bias 228–9
    conduction of 223b–30
    data extraction and management 226–8b
    further reading 230–2
    planning and resourcing 224
    post-publication issues 229–30
    publication 229
    registration of 224
    requests for further information 229b
    searching for evidence 224–5b
    selecting studies for inclusion 226, 227f

target populations 28, 29–30
    access 30–1
    availability 29–30
    data accuracy 31
    representativeness 29
    sample size 31–2t
    sampling 32–3

telephone interviews 43, 102, 104
    participation rates 121
telephone recruitment 79
temporal relationships 213
'test'-based method, confidence intervals for an odds
    ratio 170–1
time, comparisons over 23–4t
    age-specific rates 24–6f
timeline management 268
time-period effects 24
trend, χ2 test 174–5t
twin studies 82

UK Biobank study 93–4
unrecognized disorders, detection of 255–6

validation approaches 111–12, 112t
validity of a study 204
validity of information 108, 109t
    misclassification 113
    non-dichotomous variables 111f
    sensitivity and specificity 108–10
validity of study design, ethical issues 249–50
variation 114
    reducing observer variation 114–16
    reducing subject variation 114

wasting resources 268–9
Woolf's method, confidence intervals for an odds
    ratio 171–2
World Health Organization (WHO), World Standard
    Population 21t, 26
written consent 257

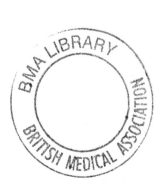